Weinberg's

COLOR ATLAS OF

PEDIATRIC DERMATOLOGY

NOTICE

Medicine is an ever-changing science. As new research and clinical experience broaden our knowledge, changes in treatment and drug therapy are required. The authors and the publisher of this work have checked with sources believed to be reliable in their efforts to provide information that is complete and generally in accord with the standards accepted at the time of publication. However, in view of the possibility of human error or changes in medical sciences, neither the authors nor the publisher nor any other party who has been involved in the preparation or publication of this work warrants that the information contained herein is in every respect accurate or complete, and they disclaim all responsibility for any errors or omissions or for the results obtained from use of the information contained in this work. Readers are encouraged to confirm the information contained herein with other sources. For example and in particular, readers are advised to check the product information sheet included in the package of each drug they plan to administer to be certain that the information contained in this work is accurate and that changes have not been made in the recommended dose or in the contraindications for administration. This recommendation is of particular importance in connection with new or infrequently used drugs.

Weinberg's

COLOR ATLAS OF
PEDIATRIC
DERMATOLOGY

FIFTH EDITION

NEIL S. PROSE, MD, FAAP
Professor of Dermatology and Pediatrics
Duke University Medical Center
Durham, North Carolina

LEONARD KRISTAL, MD, FAAP
Clinical Assistant Professor of Dermatology and Pediatrics
Stony Brook University
Stony Brook, New York

New York   Chicago   San Francisco   Athens   London   Madrid   Mexico City
Milan   New Delhi   Singapore   Sydney   Toronto

Weinberg's Color Atlas of Pediatric Dermatology, Fifth Edition

Copyright © 2017 by McGraw-Hill Education. All rights reserved. Printed in China. Except as permitted under the United States Copyright Act of 1976, no part of this publication may be reproduced or distributed in any form or by any means, or stored in a data base or retrieval system, without the prior written permission of the publisher.

Previous editions published as *Color Atlas of Pediatric Dermatology* copyright © 2008, 1998, 1990, 1975 by The McGraw-Hill Companies, Inc.

1 2 3 4 5 6 7 8 9   DSS   21 20 19 18 17 16

ISBN 978-0-07-179225-7
MHID 0-07-179225-2

This book was set in Minion by Cenveo® Publisher Services.
The editors were Karen G. Edmonson and Robert Pancotti.
The production supervisor was Catherine H. Saggese.
Project management was provided by Kritika Kaushik, Cenveo Publisher Services.
The text designer was Eve Siegel; the cover designer was Anthony Landi.
RR Donnelley was the printer and binder.

Library of Congress Cataloging-in-Publication Data

Names: Prose, Neil S., author. | Kristal, Leonard, author. | Preceded
    by (work): Weinberg, Samuel, 1926-2007 Color atlas of pediatric dermatology.
Title: Weinberg's color atlas of pediatric dermatology / Neil S. Prose, Leonard Kristal.
Other titles: Color atlas of pediatric dermatology
Description: Fifth edition. | New York : McGraw-Hill Education, [2017] |
    Preceded by Color atlas of pediatric dermatology / Samuel Weinberg, Neil S. Prose,
    Leonard Kristal. 4th ed. c2008. | Includes bibliographical references and index.
Identifiers: LCCN 2016014420| ISBN 9780071792257 (hardcover) | ISBN 0071792252 (hardcover)
Subjects: | MESH: Skin Diseases | Child | Infant | Atlases
Classification: LCC RJ511 | NLM WS 17 | DDC 618.92/5—dc23 LC record available at
    https://lccn.loc.gov/2016014420

McGraw-Hill Education books are available at special quantity discounts to use as premiums and sales promotions or for use in corporate training programs. To contact a representative, please visit the Contact Us pages at www.mhprofessional.com.

This book is dedicated to the memory of Dr. Samuel Weinberg.

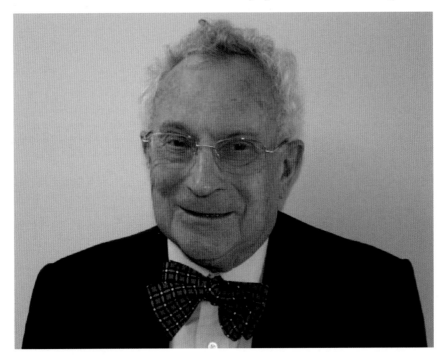

Dr. Samuel Weinberg

Dr. Weinberg graduated from the Chicago Medical School in 1948. After completing an internship and residency in pediatrics, he went into the private practice of pediatrics. Through his personal experience, Dr. Weinberg came to understand the importance of skin disease in children and how little was known about its diagnosis and treatment. After several years of pediatric practice, he began training in dermatology at the Skin & Cancer Hospital, a part of the New York University Postgraduate Medical School.

When his dermatology training was completed, Dr. Weinberg began a private pediatric dermatology practice in Long Island, New York. At Bellevue Hospital in 1962, he founded one of the first clinics in the United States devoted to the care of childhood skin disease. He served there for many years as the Chief of Pediatric Dermatology and remained active as a Clinical Professor at the New York University School of Medicine until the time of his death.

In the 1970s, Dr. Weinberg helped to found the Society for Pediatric Dermatology. His dedication to pediatric dermatology led him to coauthor the first edition of the *Color Atlas of Pediatric Dermatology* in 1975. In 2007, shortly after completing work on the fourth edition of our book, Dr. Weinberg passed away. He will always be remembered as a great teacher, a wonderful mentor, an inspiration to the hundreds of residents he helped to train, and a physician with unparalleled diagnostic acumen and devotion to his young patients. Dr. Weinberg was a great friend to those of us who were privileged to know him.

Neil S. Prose
Leonard Kristal

We would like to thank all of the contributors to this Atlas during the past 40 years.

Arturo Aballi
A. Bernard Ackerman
J. O'D. Alexander
Howard Balbi
William G. Ballinger
Charles S. Baraf
Robert Baron
Alexander G. Bearn
Jerrold M. Becker
Bernard W. Berger
Kassahun Bilcha
Eugene L. Bodian
Alanna Bree
Roman Bronfenbrener
Martin H. Brownstein
William Burke
Hector Caceres-Rios
Philip Charney
Platon J. Collipp
Maurice J. Costello
Vincent Derbes
Ncoza Dlova
Anthony N. Domonkos
Carola Duran-McKinster
Lawrence Eichenfield
Leon Eisenbud
Nancy B. Esterly
Robert P. Feinstein
Ilona J. Frieden

Alexander A. Fisher
Robert W. Goltz
Bernardo Gontijo
Ralph W. Grover
Paul Honig
Jonathan Horwitz
Sidney Hurwitz
Kathleen L. Hussey
Josef E. Jelinek
S. Wayne Klein
Irwin H. Krasna
Jose Kriner
Teresita A. Laude
Lawrence Leiblich
Chester M. Lessenden, Jr.
Moise Levy
Luther B. Lowe
Anthony Mancini
Andrew Margileth
Patricia M. Mauro
Diana McShane
John McSorley
Denise Metry
Dean S. Morrell
Anisa Mosam
Elise Olsen
Seth J. Orlow
Lamar S. Osment
Greg Puglisi

John R. T. Reeves
Perry Robins
Victor Torres Rodriguez
Leah Ronald
Avron Ross
James P. Rotchford
Ramon Ruiz-Maldonado
Ana Saenz-Cantele
Wiley M. Sams
Arthur Sawitsky
Lawrence A. Schachner
Keith M. Schneider
Edward Shapiro
Meyer H. Slatkin
Roy Stephens
Conrad Stritzler
Ronald Stritzler
Virginia Sybert
Joel A. Teisch
Louis Tobin
Donald Waldorf
William A. Welton
Zelma Wessely
David A. Whiting
Mary Williams
Constance Y. Wong
Albert Yan
Alex W. Young, Jr.
Erwin Zimmerman

Department of Dermatology, College of Physicians and Surgeons, Columbia University

New York University School of Medicine (Skin and Cancer Unit) permitted use of photographs
for the following figures: 2-12, 3-40, 4-7, 4-14, 4-30, 6-44, 7-2, 8-10, 8-32, 8-42, 8-43, 8-46, 9-6,
9-11, 11-3, 12-46, 12-47, 12-84, 12-88, 13-4, 13-14, 13-20, 14-8, 14-28, 14-29, 14-42, 14-77,
15-11, 15-52, 15-56, 15-57, 16-6, 17-26, 23-36, 24-9, 26-2, 28-6, 29-5, 29-45, 30-17, 30-18.

The following figures have been used with permission:

Figure 14-61: Listernick RH, Charrow J. The neurofibromatoses. In: Wolff K, Goldsmith LA, Katz SI
et al (eds). *Fitzpatrick's Dermatology in General Medicine.* 8th ed. New York: McGraw-Hill; 2012.
Figures 15-59 and 15-60: Frieden IJ, Esterly NB. Selected genodermatoses in infants and children.
Clin Dermatol. 1985 Jan-Mar;3(1):14-32. © Elsevier. **Figures 18-1 and 18-8:** Prose NS. HIV infection in children. *J Am Acad Dermatol.* 1990 Jun;22:1223-31. © Elsevier. **Figure 18-3:**Prose NS,
Mendez H, Menikoff H, Miller HJ. *Pediatr Dermatol.* 1987 Aug;4(2):67-74. © John Wiley and Sons.
Figures 18-4 and 18-7: Prose NS. Human immunodeficiency virus infection in childhood: The
disease and its cutaneous manifestations. *Adv Dermatol.* 1990;5:113-30. © Elsevier. **Figures 29-36
and 29-37:** Whiting DA. Hair shaft defects. In: Olsen EA (ed). *Disorders of Hair Growth: Diagnosis
and Treatment.* 2nd ed. New York: McGraw-Hill; 2003:138-39.

CONTENTS

Section 13 Nutritional, Metabolic, and Endocrine Diseases Page 145

Section 14 Genodermatoses Page 153

Section 15 Ichthyoses and Disorders of Keratinization Page 175

Section 19 Cutaneous Manifestations of Systemic Disease Page 223

Section 20 Disorders of the Dermis (Infiltrates, Atrophies, and Nodules) Page 237

Contents

The first edition of the *Color Atlas of Pediatric Dermatology* was published in 1975, during the very infancy of our specialty. The book was the product of three brilliant physicians, Drs. Samuel Weinberg, Morris Leider, and Lewis Shapiro, and each brought a unique talent to its creation.

Dr. Shapiro was a dermatopathologist, dermatologist, and highly regarded teacher at Columbia University. For the early editions, he contributed beautiful photomicrographs to accompany the clinical pictures. His contributions to the book in its earliest stages, and to the dermatopathology literature as a whole, are of great value.

Dr. Leider was an illustrious and longtime member of the Department of Dermatology at New York University. He was a wonderful family friend during my early childhood, and he gave me the first edition of the book as a medical school graduation gift in 1975 (NSP). Dr. Leider was the author of a dermatologic dictionary and prided himself on the literary use of words in the medical context. His unique and flowery writing style can still be found in various nooks and crannies of the book, and a particularly wonderful example is located beneath Fig. 16-36.

Dr. Weinberg was one of the founding members of the Society for Pediatric Dermatology and was for many years the Chief of Pediatric Dermatology at Bellevue Hospital in New York. The *Color Atlas of Pediatric Dermatology* was of enormous importance to him throughout his whole life, and he guided its content in a remarkably knowledgeable and thoughtful fashion. He was a wonderful teacher, mentor, and friend to both of us for many years and we sorely missed his insight and humor during the preparation of this edition.

In Dr. Leider's foreword to the first edition of the atlas, we are given a wonderful insight into the special and, we imagine, laughter-filled relationship of these physicians and into their method of conflict resolution. Dr. Leider wrote, "We will spare the reader the gory details of our violent arguments by saying that all contended matter was settled by a 'majority of one' by Dr. Shapiro when it was purely histologic, by Dr. Leider when it was purely literary, and by Dr. Weinberg when it was purely pediatric. For the rest, a true majority ruled."

We are delighted that the *Color Atlas of Pediatric Dermatology* has been in print for over 40 years and are proud to be part of this long tradition. Once again, we ask the reader to bear in mind that this volume is not a textbook and that it should be used in conjunction with one of the several comprehensive references in pediatric dermatology. It is our hope that this atlas will be of practical use to all health practitioners who are involved in the care of children.

Neil S. Prose
Leonard Kristal

Benign Neonatal Dermatoses

Figure 1-1

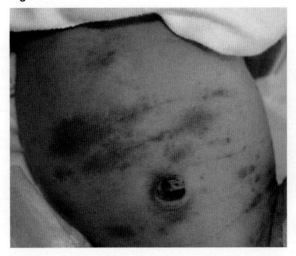

Erythema toxicum neonatorum This very common and completely benign condition usually arises in the first 2 days of life. It is seen in about 30% to 50% of healthy newborns and occurs less frequently in preterm infants. Rarely the onset occurs up to 14 days of age.

Figure 1-2

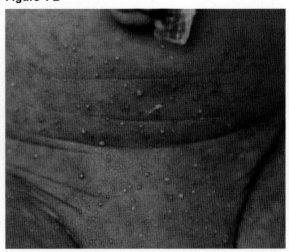

The lesions are erythematous macules, within which papules (Fig. 1-1) and pustules (Fig. 1-2) may develop. The trunk is the most common site, but all other body surfaces, except for the palms and soles, may be involved. In rare cases, these lesions may occur in plaques.

Figure 1-3

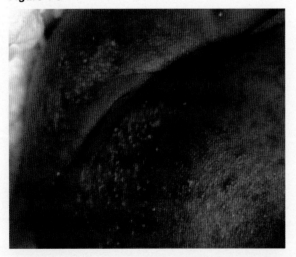

Erythema toxicum neonatorum Occasionally, this unimportant eruption must be differentiated from more serious infectious processes, such as neonatal herpes simplex. Tzanck smear of a pustule of erythema toxicum neonatorum will reveal numerous eosinophils but no multinucleated giant cells or bacteria.

Figure 1-4

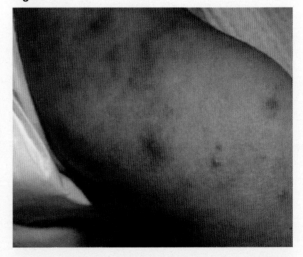

In some newborns, peripheral eosinophilia is also present. The cause of this condition is not known, and it resolves spontaneously within 10 days. No treatment is required.

Figure 1-5

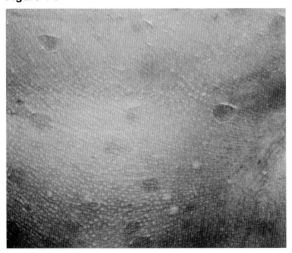

Transient neonatal pustular melanosis This is a benign neonatal dermatosis that is most common among children with more dark-colored skin. The original lesion is a vesiculopustule, which may be present at birth. This small blister quickly ruptures and leaves a typical collarette of superficial scale. Both intact pustules and collarettes are seen in the newborn in Figs. 1-5 and 1-6.

Figure 1-6

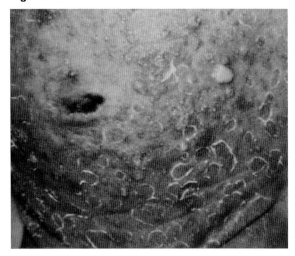

Figures 1-6 and 1-7 show the brownish-pigmented macules that may develop at the site of resolving lesions. These macules may be sparse or numerous and resolve without residua over a period of several weeks to several months.

Figure 1-7

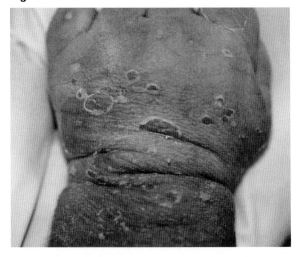

Transient neonatal pustular melanosis In some infants, the pustule and collarette stages seem to occur in utero, and the sole cutaneous manifestations are the typical macules (Fig. 1-8). Lesions of transient neonatal pustular melanosis favor the forehead, neck, chin, and lower back but may be very widespread and may involve the palms and soles.

Figure 1-8

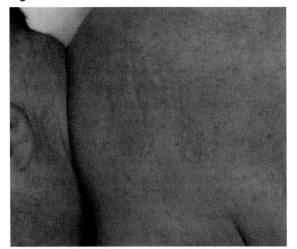

Scraping the base of an unroofed pustule reveals polymorphonuclear leukocytes but no bacteria, pseudohyphae, or multinucleated giant cells. A biopsy of a pustule, which is rarely necessary, shows an intraepidermal collection of polymorphonuclear leukocytes.

Milia, Miliaria, and Pustular and Acneiform Disorders

Figure 2-1

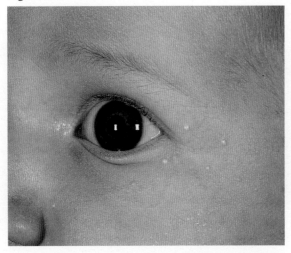

Figure 2-2

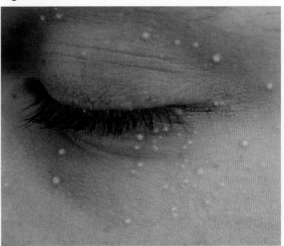

Milia A milium is a white papule, 1 to 2 mm in size, composed of laminated, keratinous material and situated as a solid cyst in a pilosebaceous follicle. Milia are fairly common on the brow, glabella, and nose in newborn infants and in such infants tend to disappear quickly and spontaneously. There may be few or many, and they may develop later in infancy, in childhood, and in adolescence. In older children and adolescents, they tend to persist, may precede acne or be associated with incipient acne

and commonly develop on or around the eyelids. Milia may be ablated, if desirable, by delicate incision and expression of the keratinous content. Lesions that are treated do not recur, but if new lesions appear, they have to be treated in the same way. The operation is trivial and uncomplicated. There are no preventive measures.

Figure 2-3

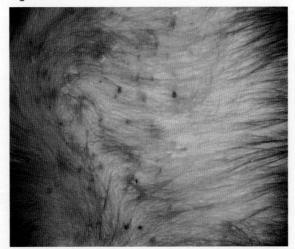

Eosinophilic pustular folliculitis of infancy Children with this rare disorder develop repeated crops of pruritic erythematous papules, yellow or white pustules, which vary in size from 1 to 3 mm. Most lesions are located on the scalp and distal extremities. Tzanck smear may reveal numerous eosinophils, and there may also be a peripheral eosinophilia when flaring. Eosinophilic pustular folliculitis is associated with no systemic symptoms and eventually resolves spontaneously. Therapy with topical steroids is beneficial.

Figure 2-4

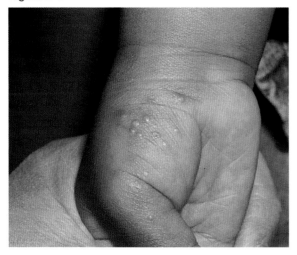

Infantile acropustulosis This cutaneous disorder is characterized by recurrent episodes of intensely pruritic pustules and papulovesicles on the hands and feet. Lesions are most common on the palms and soles but may be seen on the dorsal surfaces as well.

Figure 2-5

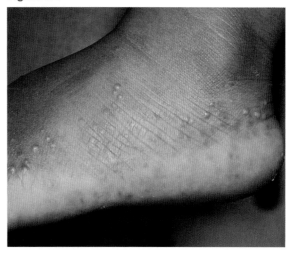

Lesions may also occur on the ankles, forearms, and, rarely, the face, scalp, and upper trunk. The age at onset is typically between 2 and 10 months. Individual episodes last for 7 to 10 days and may recur as often as every 2 weeks at the beginning of the disease. Episodes tend to become less frequent and severe over time.

Figure 2-6

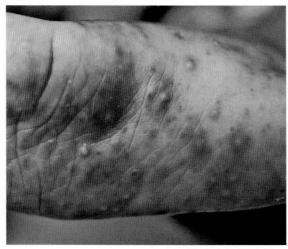

Infantile acropustulosis Stained smears of an individual lesion will reveal numerous neutrophils, although eosinophils may be present early in the course of the disorder. Infantile acropustulosis may also be seen after scabies infestation in infants ("postscabies syndrome").

Figure 2-7

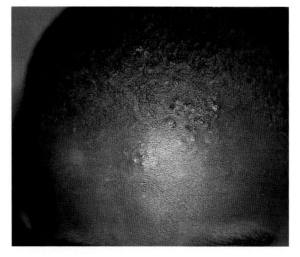

Figure 2-7 shows involvement of the forehead in a patient with infantile acropustulosis. The disease resolves spontaneously by 2 to 3 years of age. The individual lesions in this condition may resolve with scale and postinflammatory hyperpigmentation.

Figure 2-8

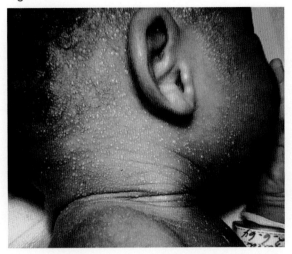

Figure 2-9

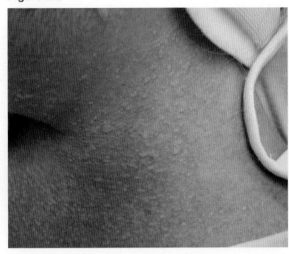

Miliaria crystallina The lesions in this condition are small, clear, thin-roofed vesicles that develop when the sweat duct is obstructed within the stratum corneum. They occur after sunburn or in response to excessive sweating in high environmental heat and humidity. Fever may also be a cause.

The scalp, face, trunk, and intertriginous areas are sites of lesions. Itching is not a symptom. The vesicles resolve rapidly with the elimination of the causative environmental factor.

Figure 2-10

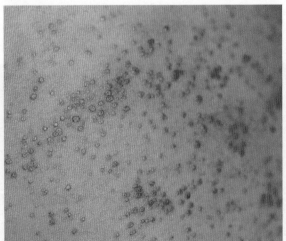

Miliaria rubra (prickly heat) This is the most common form of miliaria. It occurs when there is plugging of the eccrine ducts and release of sweat into the adjacent skin. Miliaria rubra is characterized by discrete erythematous papules and papulovesicles. The forehead, upper trunk, and intertriginous areas are commonly affected. Unlike miliaria crystallina, miliaria rubra is characterized by spasmodic pricking sensations. A decrease in environmental heat and humidity is the only treatment required.

Figure 2-11

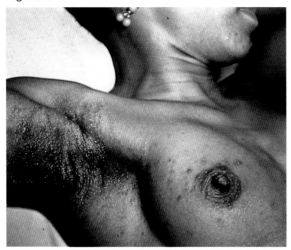

Figure 2-12

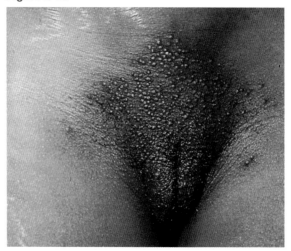

Fox-Fordyce disease (apocrine miliaria) This chronic and intensely pruritic papular eruption is localized to the axillae, areolae, and pubic areas where apocrine glands are found. It occurs almost exclusively in young women, frequently with the onset during adolescence. The follicular papules result from the obstruction of the intraepidermal sweat duct, with the release of apocrine sweat into the surrounding skin.

Figure 2-11 shows the process in an axilla; Fig. 2-12 shows it in the pubic area. The etiology of Fox-Fordyce disease is unknown and the treatment is difficult. Topical retinoids, hormonal therapy, and antimicrobial therapy are sometimes helpful. Pimecrolimus, a topical immunomodulator, has recently been shown to be beneficial.

Figure 2-13

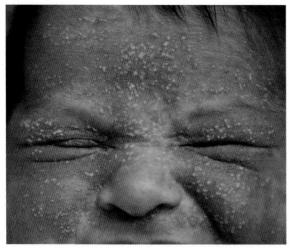

Figure 2-14

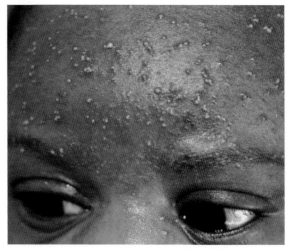

Neonatal cephalic pustulosis This disorder is characterized by the development of numerous very small erythematous papulopustules over the scalp, face, and neck. Lesions usually develop during the second or third week of life. Researchers believe that this eruption is identical to that which was previously termed

as neonatal acne. Recent research suggests that the cause is the lipophilic yeast, *Malassezia. M furfur* or *M sympodialis*, can be isolated from the skin of most patients. Topical ketoconazole is a safe and effective treatment.

Figure 2-15

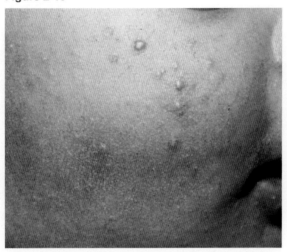

Neonatal and infantile acne Mild comedonal acne is fairly common in the newborn. The typical eruption consists of closed comedones. Open comedones, inflammatory papules and pustules, and small cysts may also occur. Neonatal acne is due to the stimulation of sebaceous glands by androgens from both mother and infant.

Figure 2-16

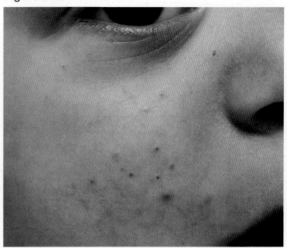

The lesions of neonatal acne usually resolve during the first few months of life. Acne, in varying degrees of severity, may also appear in infants after the neonatal period. This form of infantile acne may persist for 1 or 2 years and may rarely eventuate in scarring.

Figure 2-17

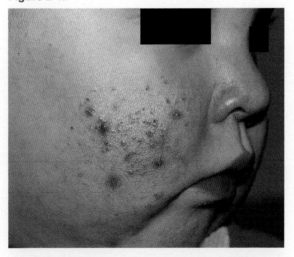

Neonatal and infantile acne Children with an early onset of acne and a strong family history are particularly at risk for a severe course of the disease during puberty. Most cases of neonatal and infantile acne do not require treatment. If necessary, a mild benzoyl peroxide preparation may be used.

Figure 2-18

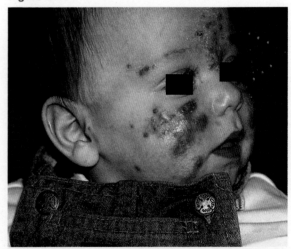

Infantile cystic acne Comedones generally predominate in infantile acne, although more inflammatory papules and pustules may be seen. Rarely, an infant may develop cystic nodules, as seen in Fig. 2-18, that occasionally heal with scarring. Infants with severe acne should be evaluated for sexual precocity or abnormal virilization.

Figure 2-19

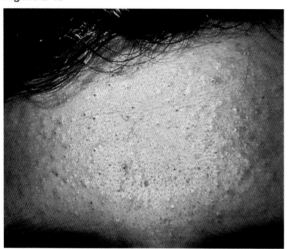

Figure 2-20

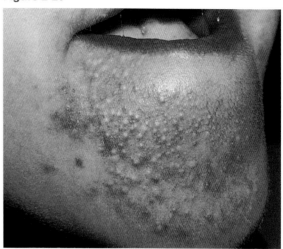

Acne vulgaris The common varieties of acne generally begin to develop in late childhood or early adolescence. Acne during adolescence is caused by the effect of androgenic hormones on the pilosebaceous unit. The increased activity of the sebaceous gland provides a substrate for *Propionibacterium acnes*, whose lipolytic enzymes convert triglycerides in sebum to free fatty acids. Abnormal keratinization in the pilosebaceous follicle also plays a role in the development of acne. The earliest lesions are open or closed comedones. Figures 2-19 and 2-20 show the comedo stage, with open and closed comedones represented.

Figure 2-21

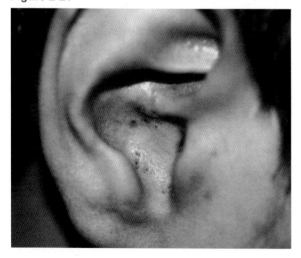

Figure 2-22

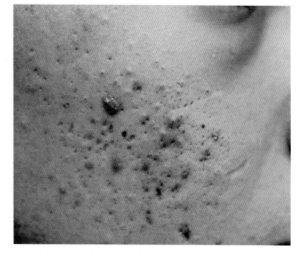

Acne vulgaris Comedones may be found in the ears, most commonly in the conchal area as seen in Fig. 2-21. Comedones in this area can be quite large and can at times resolve with pitted scarring.

Figure 2-22 shows open and closed comedones, a few inflammatory papules and pitted scarring.

Figure 2-23

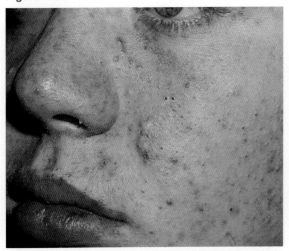

Acne vulgaris Many cases of acne progress from open and closed comedones (blackheads and whiteheads) to inflammatory forms that are marked by papules, pustules, and cysts. Figure 2-23 shows the beginning of progression to inflammatory papules and pustules. Figure 2-24 shows the progression from the comedonal to a more severe inflammatory phase of acne.

Figure 2-24

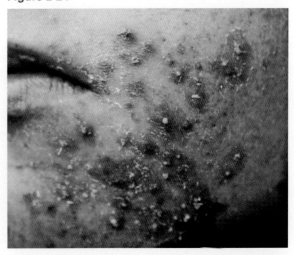

Topical therapies are aimed at decreasing skin colonization by *P acnes* (topical antibiotics) and at normalizing keratinization within the follicle (tretinoin). As acne becomes more inflammatory, systemic antibiotics may be needed to decrease the inflammation and to prevent possible scarring. Avoidance of irritating soaps and scrubbing is advised.

Figure 2-25

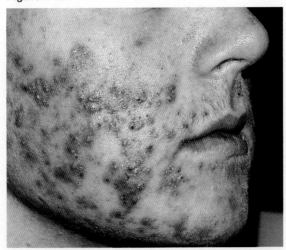

Cystic acne Figure 2-25 shows a combination of inflammatory acne with cysts. Figure 2-26 indicates the further progression with numerous inflammatory cystic nodules. Severe cystic acne is more difficult to control or cure and may cause scarring. Although, topical therapy with combinations of antibiotics and topical retinoids is of value, systemic antibiotics, such as doxycycline and tetracycline may also be required because of their antibacterial and anti-inflammatory properties.

Figure 2-26

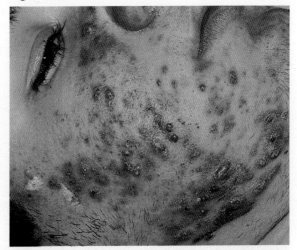

The intralesional injection of corticosteroids may also be helpful. Isotretinoin is indicated for nodulocystic acne that may cause scarring or recalcitrant acne that is not responding to therapy. Side effects of this therapy range from dry lips and skin to elevation of cholesterol and triglycerides. In addition, all female patients must be advised that isotretinoin is a potent teratogen and that pregnancy must be avoided.

Figure 2-27

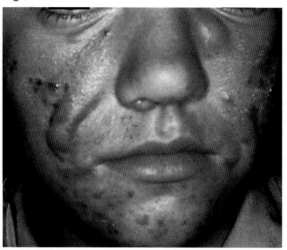

Acne conglobata In conglobate acne, the most severe form of acne, cysts tend to be large, irregular, and intercommunicating and tend to result in severe scarring. Severe cystic acne can sometimes be controlled with topical therapy and systemic antibiotics. The patient who does not respond to these measures may be a candidate for isotretinoin.

Figure 2-28

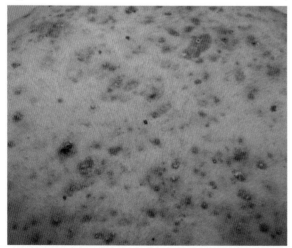

Figure 2-29

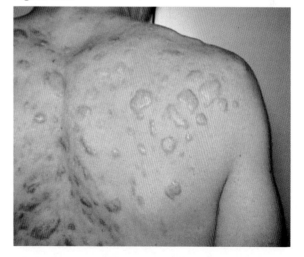

Scarring following acne Atrophic scars, hypertrophic scars, and keloids following resolution of inflammatory lesions of acne are an uncommon but particularly distressing complication. The chest and upper back are the sites of predilection. Figure 2-28 shows atrophic scarring with ongoing inflammatory lesions. Figure 2-29 shows the keloids that may result. Keloids occur less commonly on the face. The tendency toward keloid formation is more common in African American adolescents and is sometimes familial. Successful control of the acne itself, through topical or systemic therapy, may minimize the extent of future scarring. The use of intralesional corticosteroids is the most effective treatment of keloids once they have formed.

Figure 2-30

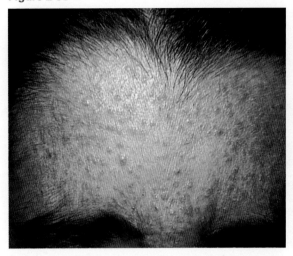

Acne and precocious puberty from a pinealoma In this 4-year-old child, persistent acne, precocious puberty, and frequent headache were the presenting signs and symptoms of a pinealoma. Occasionally, acne in a preadolescent may be an indication of an endocrine abnormality in which either androgen or glucocorticoids are present in excess. For example, a typical eruption of monomorphic follicular papules, usually concentrated on the back and chest, is seen in Cushing disease.

Figure 2-31

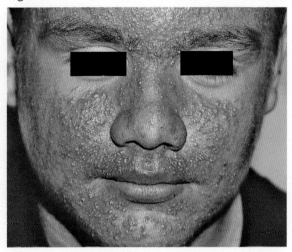

Steroid acne (dexamethasone) This form of acne may be caused by systemic or topical corticosteroids, as is seen in Fig. 2-31 of a patient receiving systemic dexamethasone. The eruption is monomorphous, characterized by the presence of small erythematous papules or pustules primarily seen on the upper trunk, arms, neck, and, less commonly, the face.

Figure 2-32

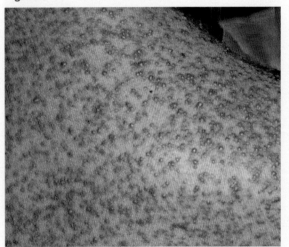

Figure 2-32 shows numerous monomorphous follicular papules in a patient undergoing systemic steroid therapy with dexamethasone.

Figure 2-33

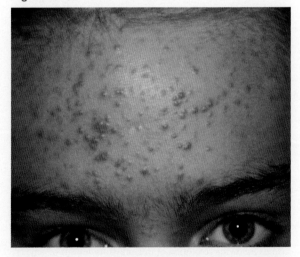

Steroid acne (dexamethasone) Figure 2-33 shows a young girl who has applied a fluorinated topical steroid cream to her face. This has resulted in a monomorphous eruption of inflammatory acneiform papules.

Figure 2-34

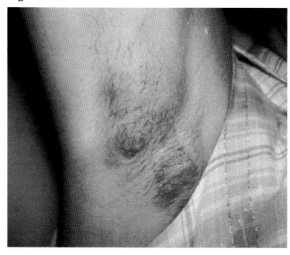

Hidradenitis suppurativa This condition is a chronic, recurrent inflammatory process of unknown etiology that involves the follicular epithelium of apocrine bearing areas. The favored locations are the axillae, groin, and buttocks. The disease begins just before or during puberty and persists, with remissions and exacerbations, for years. It is more common in women and is

Figure 2-35

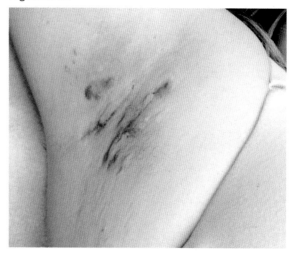

sometimes associated with acne conglobata and dissecting cellulitis of the scalp. Worsening of the disease may be seen during summer months or at the time of menstruation. Hidradenitis suppurativa is aggravated by obesity. The involved areas in the axilla or groin may present with pustules, nodules, abscesses, and sinus tracts.

Figure 2-36

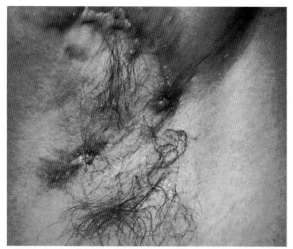

Hidradenitis suppurativa In Fig. 2-36, the condition has partially, and temporarily, abated. Corded hypertrophic and keloidal scarring has developed. The treatment of hidradenitis suppurativa is often difficult. Topical and systemic antibiotics are most commonly used; a combination of oral rifampin and clindamycin has been documented to be effective. Treatment with biologic agents may also provide relief in patients with severe involvement.

Figure 2-37

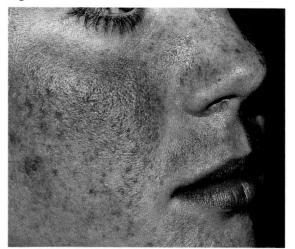

Rosacea This is an inflammatory condition of the midface characterized by the presence of erythema, papules, pustules, telangiectasias, and, in the later stages, hyperplasia of the sebaceous glands of the nose. The absence of comedones helps distinguish this condition from acne vulgaris, although the two conditions may coexist. Although usually seen in middle age, this condition may start in late adolescence.

Figure 2-38

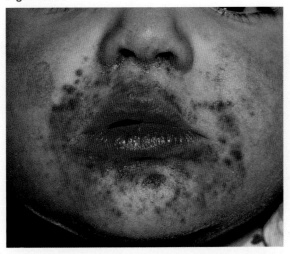

Periorificial dermatitis This condition is a chronic eruption of fine papules and pustules located on the skin around the mouth and nose and sometimes around the eyes. The condition may initially present with perinasal scaling, which then progresses to involve the perioral area.

Figure 2-39

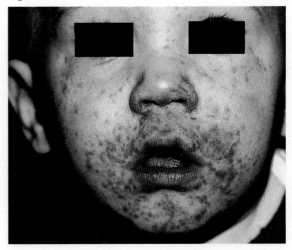

The etiology of this condition is not completely understood. It usually begins in early childhood, with men and women equally affected. It may be more common in children with skin of color.

Figure 2-40

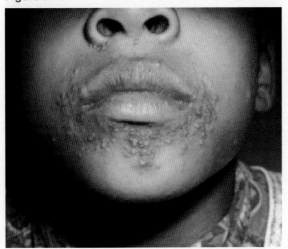

Periorificial granulomatous dermatitis Topical steroids may cause severe worsening of this disorder. In most instances, perioral granulomatous dermatitis responds to oral erythromycin or to the application of topical metronidazole.

Figure 2-41

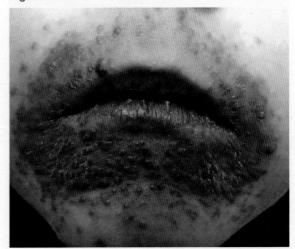

In most cases, this is a clinical diagnosis and biopsy need not be performed. However, the lesions do have a granulomatous infiltrate, and, on the basis of both the appearance and the histology, the condition may be confused with sarcoid.

Figure 2-42

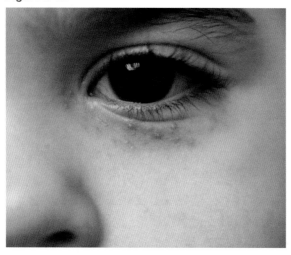

Periorificial dermatitis Occasionally an infant or young child may present with an inflammatory papular or papulopustular eruption in the infraorbital area. This may be the initial presentation of periorificial dermatitis. In a brief period of time, most patients develop a more typical eruption located around the mouth.

Figure 2-43

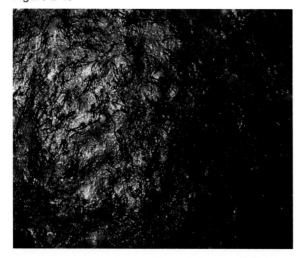

Figure 2-44

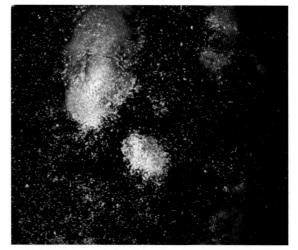

Dissecting cellulitis of the scalp This condition was originally called *folliculitis et perifolliculitis capitis abscedens et suffodiens,* which translates into an inflammation in and around hair follicles of the scalp that flows (pus) and channels under or through (tissue). This chronic condition resembles, and sometimes accompanies, acne conglobata and hidradenitis suppurativa (the follicular occlusion triad). Like them, it is marked by inflammation, purulence, intercommunicating abscesses, cysts, sinuses, and scarring. This disease appears to be somewhat more common among African Americans, and the onset may occur during adolescence. A number of therapies are routinely used. These include topical and systemic antibiotics, incision and drainage of abscesses, and intralesional steroids. More recently, there is some evidence that treatment with biologic agents may be of benefit. There are usually many remissions and exacerbations, and the process often eventuates in a scarring alopecia.

Bacterial Infections

Figure 3-1

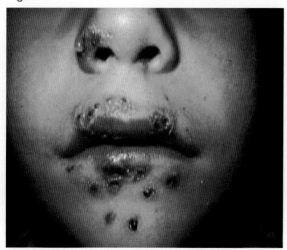

Figure 3-2

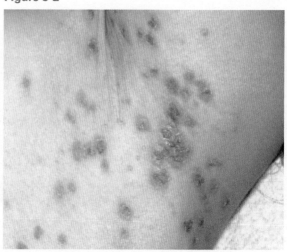

Impetigo Impetigo is a primary superficial infection of the skin. It is more prevalent in humid climates and occurs most commonly in the summer months. Trauma to the skin, such as a small abrasion or insect bite, sometimes provides the site of entry for the infective bacteria. The lesions evolve from discrete small vesicles into pustules. The fluid content of the primary lesions dries into a thick yellowish crust (Fig. 3-1), and removal of the crust may reveal bright-red and shiny erosions (Fig. 3-2).

The most common cause of impetigo is *Staphylococcus aureus*. Because the "honey-crusted" lesions of impetigo may be caused by a combination of *S aureus* and *Streptococcus pyogenes*, systemic antibiotic therapy should be effective against both organisms. The use of topical mupirocin ointment appears to be an effective treatment and may replace the need for systemic therapy in some patients with localized lesions.

Figure 3-3

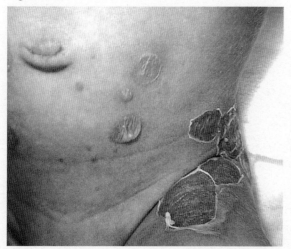

Figure 3-4

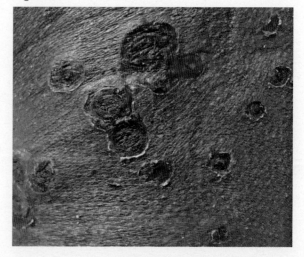

Bullous impetigo This form of impetigo consists of flaccid blisters that quickly rupture and evolve into superficial round or oval erosions with a varnished surface and minimal crust. Blisters are caused by the local effect of staphylococcal toxin. Figure 3-3 shows blisters and superficial erosions.

Figure 3-4 shows the collarettes of scale following rupture of the bullae. Bullous impetigo is associated with a pure culture of *S aureus*. Oral treatment with dicloxacillin or a cephalosporin is an effective mode of therapy. If methicillin-resistant *Staphylococcus aureus* (MRSA) is suspected, oral clindamycin is frequently recommended, and can be used pending results of culture.

Figure 3-5

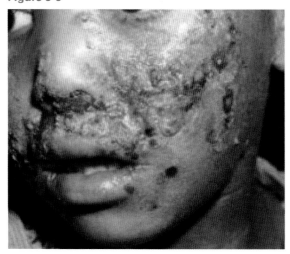

Impetiginization This is the term for impetigo imposed upon preexisting dermatoses, most commonly insect bites and atopic dermatitis. Eruptions that are pruritic are particularly susceptible to secondary infection. The most common organisms are *S pyogenes* and *S aureus*. Figure 3-5 shows a case of impetiginized atopic dermatitis. The development of such "honey-crusted" lesions in a child with eczema suggests the need for systemic antibiotic therapy.

Figure 3-6

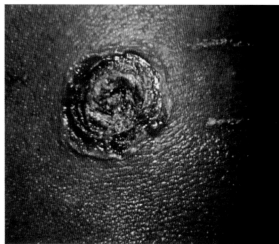

Ecthyma Ecthyma occurs when there is ulceration beneath the surface of a skin infection. If impetigo is infection by streptococci and/or staphylococci superficially in the epidermis, ecthyma is infection by the same organisms through the entire thickness of the epidermis (0.1 mm) to the upper reaches of the dermis (perhaps to a depth of 0.5 mm). Clinically, there is often a firm crust covering a superficial ulcer, surrounded by erythema.

Figure 3-7

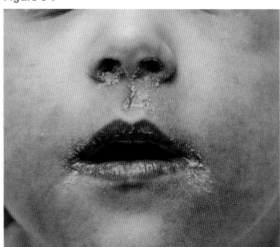

Staphylococcal scalded skin syndrome This eruption occurs most commonly in children under the age of 5 years. It is characterized by a generalized tender, macular erythema, which is most prominent on the skin around the mouth and nose and in intertriginous areas. Within 1 or 2 days, the rash begins to peel. Typically, the large superficial flaccid bullae ("scalded skin") are quickly unroofed, revealing areas of slightly erythematous and shiny skin. These areas crust and then heal. Children with this syndrome are often extremely irritable and febrile, but the

Figure 3-8

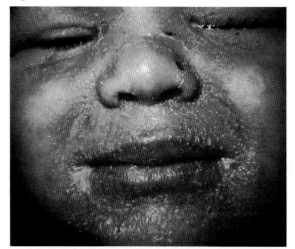

overall prognosis is good. Figures 3-7 and 3-8 illustrate superficial blistering and erythema around the mouth. The scalded skin syndrome is caused by an epidermolytic toxin that may be produced by several strains of *S aureus*. These causative organisms may be present in the nose, throat, conjunctiva, or an infected wound. Staphylococcal scalded skin syndrome resolves without scarring within a period of 2 weeks. Treatment consists of appropriate supportive care and penicillinase-resistant antibiotics.

Figure 3-9

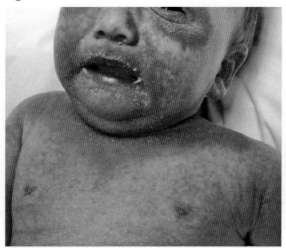

Figure 3-10

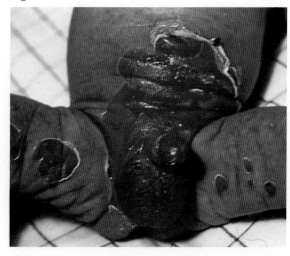

Staphylococcal scalded skin syndrome Figure 3-9 shows a generalized light-colored erythema which is accentuated in skin folds. The staphylococcal toxin exfoliatin may sometimes produce extensive areas of desquamation. Other clues to diagnosis include areas of denuded skin in sites of anatomic stress, and skin tenderness.

Treatment in severe cases consists of intravenous antibiotics that are effective against strains of *S aureus* that are prevalent in the geographic area. Infants with this degree of involvement (Fig. 3-10) must be managed carefully with respect to fluid and electrolyte levels.

Figure 3-11

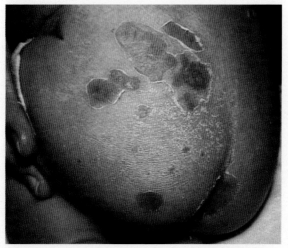

Figure 3-12

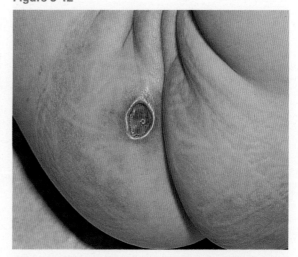

Staphylococcal scalded skin syndrome Scalded skin syndrome must be differentiated from scarlet fever, Kawasaki disease, toxic shock syndrome, and drug-induced toxic epidermal necrolysis.

Chancriform pyoderma Infection with a *Staphylococcus*, or more often with organisms such as *Pseudomonas aeruginosa* or *Proteus* and combinations thereof, can result in chancriform ulcers. These lesions are more difficult to treat. In addition to effective systemic antibiotics, attention must be paid to skin care of the entire diaper area, and topical antibiotics may be required.

Figure 3-13

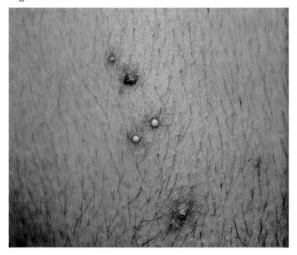

Folliculitis This is a common form of bacterial skin infection in both children and adolescents. Typically, the lesions are erythematous papules or pustules, arising at the openings of hair follicles. Pruritus or mild discomfort may be associated with the infection.

Figure 3-14

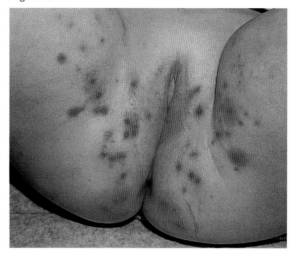

Involvement of the buttocks and perineum is particularly common in infants and young children (Fig. 3-14). Infants may be predisposed to folliculitis in this area secondary to occlusion by diapers.

Figure 3-15

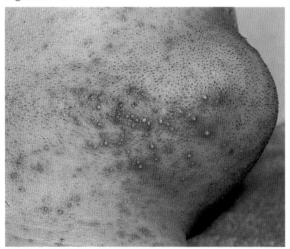

Folliculitis, shown in Fig. 3-15 in the beard area, is most commonly caused by infection with *S aureus* and responds to treatment with oral antibiotics that cover this organism. In areas where methicillin-resistant organisms are common, antibiotic therapy needs to be adjusted accordingly.

Figure 3-16

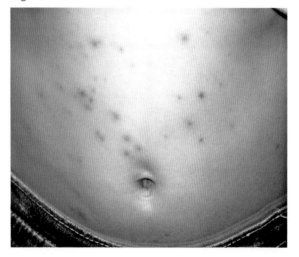

Hot tub folliculitis This condition is seen after immersion in a hot tub in which gram-negative organisms, predominantly *Pseudomonas* species, proliferate as a result of improper maintenance. Patients develop numerous discrete erythematous papules and pustules on the upper trunk, groin, buttocks, and thighs. Lesions may be tender. The eruption is self-limited, although topical gentamicin and/or diluted white vinegar soaks may hasten resolution. Hot tubs must be properly cleaned and maintained.

Figure 3-17

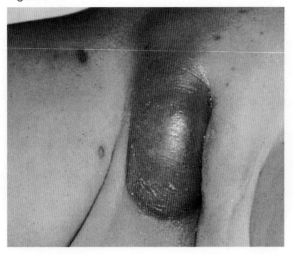

Figure 3-18

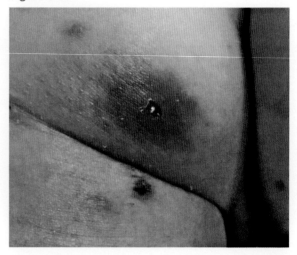

Furuncle A furuncle is a skin abscess or boil. Lesions of this type shown in Fig. 3-17 on the right labia, are usually caused by *S aureus*. It is important to culture these lesions to rule out the possibility of MRSA. The organism invades through either an area of damaged skin, a hair follicle, or a sebaceous gland. As bacteria multiply, a deep cavity containing polymorphonuclear leukocytes and bacteria is formed. Abscesses can form anywhere on the body but are most common on the extremities, neck, buttocks, and axillae.

Many individuals with recurrent furuncles are found to be harboring the causative strain of *S aureus* in the nares. Rarely, recurrent furunculosis is a sign of an underlying immune deficiency. In the earliest stages, intermittent warm compresses and systemic antibiotics may abort or mature lesions quickly. When lesions are pointed, incision and drainage is the treatment of choice. A carbuncle is a multiloculated abscess that forms when two or more neighboring furuncles become confluent.

Figure 3-19

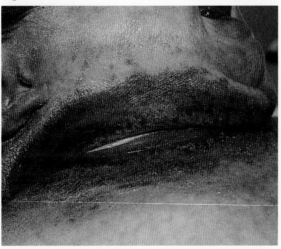

Figure 3-20

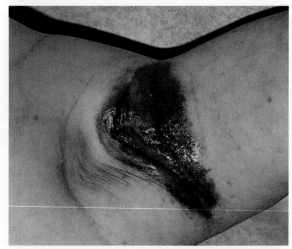

Streptococcal intertrigo Some infants develop a sharply demarcated, intensely erythematous and sometimes macerated intertriginous eruption in the neck folds (Fig. 3-19), axillae (Fig. 3-20), or groin area caused by group A β-hemolytic streptococcus. Identical lesions can be caused by infection with *S aureus*.

This is associated with a distinctive foul odor but with an absence of satellite lesions (differentiating it from *Candida albicans* intertrigo). Treatment with topical and oral antibiotic therapy is advised. Family members may also suffer from streptococcal pharyngitis or other strep infections.

Figure 3-21

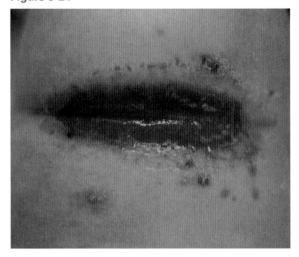

Figure 3-22

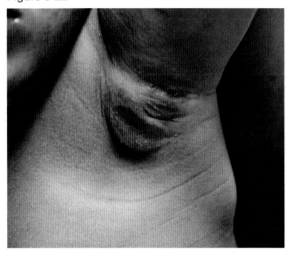

Streptococcal intertrigo Figure 3-21 shows a strep infection of the popliteal fossae. Note the beefy red, weepy erythema with some crusting at the periphery. There are also some pustules at the periphery.

This young child has a strep infection in the axillae. One or multiple flexural areas may be involved. There may be a characteristic odor in the area of involvement.

Figure 3-23

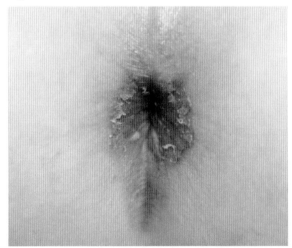

Figure 3-24

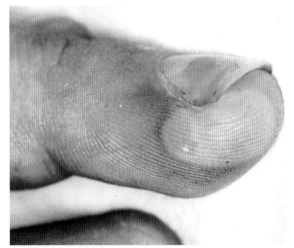

Perianal streptococcal disease Group A β-hemolytic streptococcus is sometimes the cause of perianal inflammation in a child. This localized infection is accompanied by painful defecation or pruritus. Examination of the area reveals a bright-red erythema surrounding the rectum and oozing from the infected area of skin. Diagnosis may be confirmed by perianal swab and culture. *S aureus* has also been reported to cause a similar clinical picture, and so treatment should be guided by culture results.

Blistering distal dactylitis This is a distinctive cutaneous infection that is caused by group A β-hemolytic streptococcus. The clinical appearance, as shown in Fig. 3-24, is a superficial blister over the anterior fat pad of the distal phalanx. One or more fingers may be involved. The blister fluid is culture-positive for the causative bacteria, and treatment consists of incision and drainage along with the appropriate antibiotic by mouth.

Figure 3-25

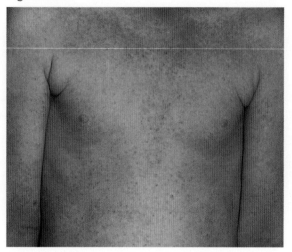

Figure 3-26

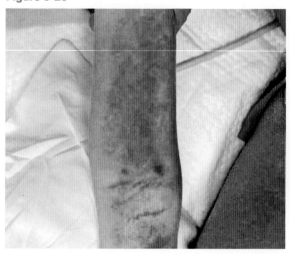

Scarlet fever Scarlet fever is a generalized exanthem of childhood, with the highest incidence between the ages of 5 and 15 years. The cause is infection (usually of the oropharynx) by group A β-hemolytic streptococcus. The rash results from an erythrogenic toxin produced by these bacteria. The disease begins after a short incubation period of 2 to 4 days with a pharyngitis, fever, and malaise. The skin then begins to show a diffuse punctate erythema with a fine "sandpaper" texture.

The face may become flushed but does not become as erythematous as the body. Characteristically, there is pallor around the mouth and the tip of the nose. Erythema is deepest in skin folds, especially the antecubital fossae and the axillary lines, where petechiae in linear arrangement may develop. These typical lesions, known as Pastia lines, are seen in Fig. 3-26. Tender cervical adenopathy is common.

Figure 3-27

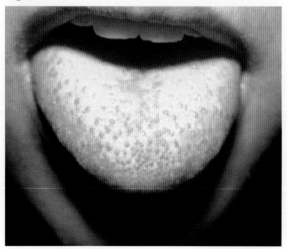

Figure 3-28

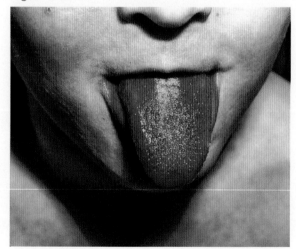

A red pharynx, purulent tonsillitis, and palatal petechiae may be present. During the first 2 days of the illness the tongue develops a thin white coating with erythema and mild swelling of the papillae ("white strawberry tongue"), as seen in Fig. 3-27.

By the fourth to fifth day, the white membrane sloughs off revealing prominent papillae on a shiny red tongue as seen in Fig. 3-28.

Figure 3-29

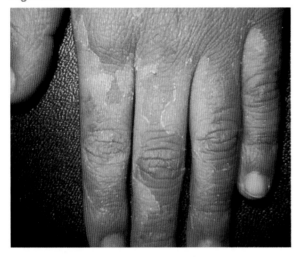

Scarlet fever Desquamation of the hands, feet, elbows, and knees occurs during healing.

Figure 3-30

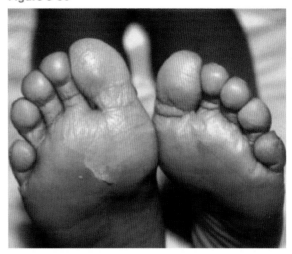

Occasionally, peeling in these locations may be the sole cutaneous manifestation of a mild, resolving streptococcal infection.

Figure 3-31

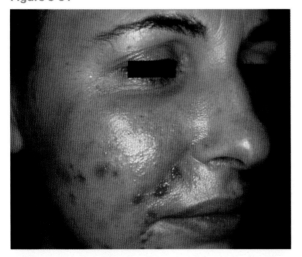

Erysipelas This is a rare form of superficial cellulitis caused by group A β-hemolytic streptococci. Erysipelas frequently occurs on the face and presents as a tense, warm, and tender erythematous plaque with a well-demarcated border. In this patient, there is edema of right cheek and multiple erosions. The patient may be severely ill with fever and local lymphadenopathy. A parenteral antibiotic is often required in the initial, acute phase.

Figure 3-32

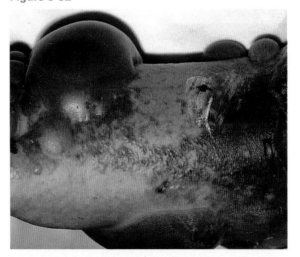

Invasive group A streptococcal disease Group A β-hemolytic streptococcus may, though rarely, cause severe invasive disease with clinical findings such as pneumonia, septicemia, necrotizing fasciitis, and a toxic shock-like illness. A small proportion of patients with varicella also may develop secondary infection with streptococcus, leading to severe invasive disease.

Figure 3-33

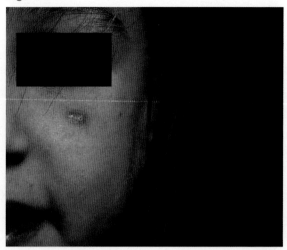

Figure 3-34

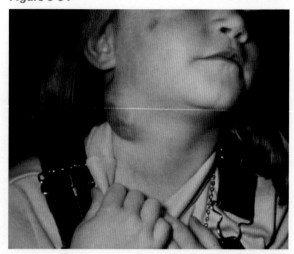

Cat-scratch disease This disease is characterized by the appearance of a papule or pustule at the site of a scratch from a cat. Within several weeks, enlarged regional lymph nodes (Fig. 3-34) develop and become tender and fluctuant. Cat-scratch disease is accompanied by fever and malaise in about one-third of cases.

Localized adenopathy may last from several weeks to months and then resolves spontaneously. Central nervous system involvement is a very rare but sometimes serious complication. The disease is caused by *Bartonella henselae*. Treatment with erythromycin, azithromycin, or doxycycline is usually effective.

Figure 3-35

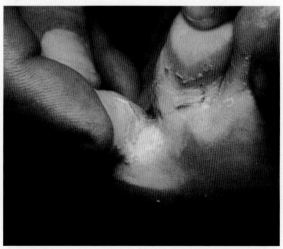

Figure 3-36

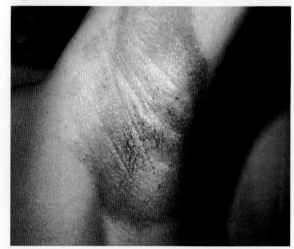

Erythrasma This is a fairly common condition that is occasionally seen during childhood and increases in frequency with age. Lesions occur in the axillae, groin, and toe webs. The causative organism is a diphtheroid, *Corynebacterium minutissimum*. Involvement in the axilla, as seen in Fig. 3-36, appears as a well-demarcated brown-to-red plaque. Maceration and scaling

between the toes (Fig. 3-35) is another clinical presentation. A characteristic of the lesion is that it fluoresces coral-red under the Wood's light (3650 Å) because the causative organism produces porphyrins in the stratum corneum. Erythrasma is exceedingly superficial but can become extensive. A 10-day course of oral erythromycin, 250 mg 4 times a day, is the treatment of choice.

Figure 3-37

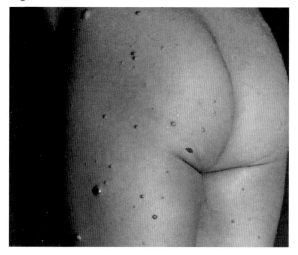

Figure 3-38

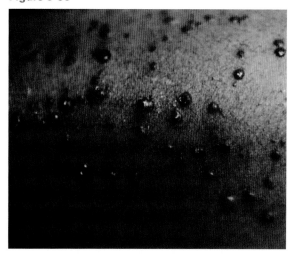

Verruga peruana (Carrion disease) This infection, caused by *B bacilliformis,* is seen in the Peruvian Andes and is transmitted by the *Lutzomyia* sand fly. It also may be seen in travelers from this area. An acute phase of this infection, called Oroya fever, is characterized by fever and commonly hemolytic anemia, thrombocytopenia, and elevated liver transaminases. Patients may also have dyspnea, mental status changes, and seizures. Patients with

the eruptive phase develop crops of small nodules that enlarge and develop a vascular appearance. These lesions then may ulcerate, bleed, and subsequently heal with fibrosis over several months. Different stages of lesions may coexist. A persistent bacteremia is common. The preferred treatment is chloramphenicol, although doxycycline may be effective. Cutaneous lesions may resemble those of bacillary angiomatosis.

Figure 3-39

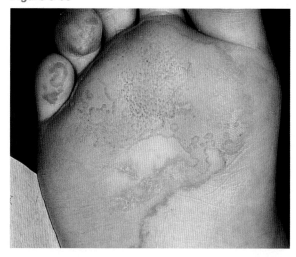

Figure 3-40

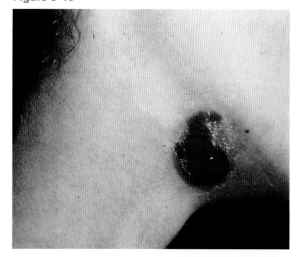

Pitted keratolysis This condition is characterized by numerous shallow, discrete pits on the plantar surface of the feet, usually in the weight-bearing areas. Although the condition is asymptomatic, there is usually hyperhidrosis and the feet may be malodorous. Painful erosions may occur. The condition is caused by *Micrococcus* species. Topical clindamycin or topical erythromycin are the treatments of choice.

Actinomycosis This is a chronic granulomatous disease of worldwide distribution caused by gram-positive obligate parasites that are most closely related to bacteria. Illustrated in Fig. 3-40 is the most common cervicofacial form of the disease. Deep to this superficial neck mass is a focus of actinomycosis. The purulent discharge from the underlying sinus contains yellowish particles, the so-called sulfur granules. These granules are colonies of the causative agent, which is usually *Actinomyces israelii.* Diagnosis is made by culture of the organism on anaerobic media, and the treatment of choice is penicillin.

Figure 3-41

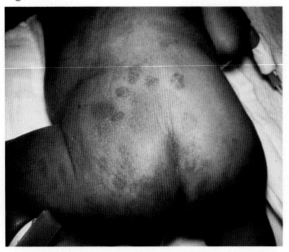

Figure 3-42

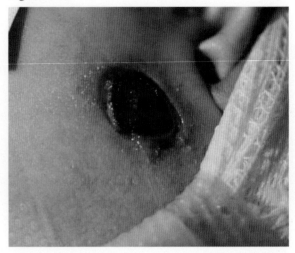

Cutaneous effects of *Pseudomonas* sepsis Sepsis caused by *Ps aeruginosa* occurs most commonly in the child with an underlying illness. It is seen in children with immune deficiency due to cancer chemotherapy, in those with malnutrition, and in those with extensive burns. Some of the less specific cutaneous manifestations, specifically erythematous macules and petechiae, are shown in Fig. 3-41. *Pseudomonas* sepsis may also present with discrete small nodules and bullae.

The classic skin lesion of *Pseudomonas* sepsis is termed *Ecthyma gangrenosum*. This form characteristically progresses quickly from a well-circumscribed area of edema to a centrally located blister and then to a gangrenous ulcer with a gray eschar. Multiple lesions in different stages of evolution may be present, and the lesions may appear on any body surface. Gram stain and culture of tissue scraped from the base of a blister will be positive for *Pseudomonas*.

Figure 3-43

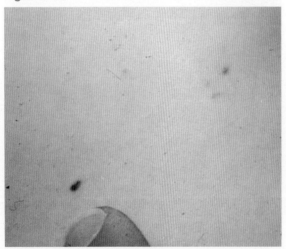

Figure 3-44

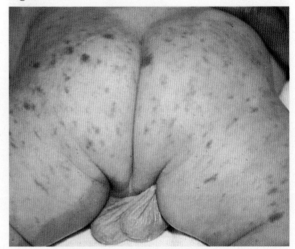

Cutaneous effects of meningococcemia The early treatment of meningococcemia with appropriate parenteral antibiotics can often be lifesaving. Cutaneous manifestations of this disease may provide the single most important diagnostic clue in the acutely ill child. The most common findings on the skin are petechiae and purpura. The small petechial lesion shown in Fig. 3-43 develops early in the course of the disease, and a scraping yields gram-negative diplococci on both Gram stain and culture. Subsequently, the lesions arise in additional crops, enlarge, and coalesce.

The numerous ecchymoses shown in Fig. 3-44 are the result of this rapidly ongoing process. These areas may become necrotic and develop eschars. Other cutaneous manifestations, occurring subsequently, include peripheral gangrene and purpura fulminans, with confluent areas of necrosis of the skin. These are the result of vasospasm, shock, and a consumption coagulopathy. A deficiency in protein C may be another cause of this process.

Figure 3-45

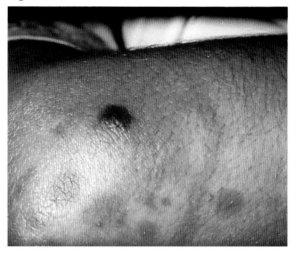

Figure 3-46

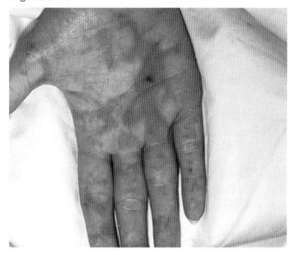

Cutaneous effects of gonococcemia Infection with *Neisseria gonorrhea* may manifest as a purulent conjunctivitis in the newborn or as a genital discharge in the sexually abused child or sexually active adolescent. Disseminated gonococcal infection, as shown in Fig. 3-45, is quite rare. Gonococcemia presents with a migratory polyarthralgia or septic arthritis and fever.

The skin lesions are few, are often located on extremities, and may overlie the involved joints. Initially, there are small erythematous macules that progress to papules. These tender lesions may develop a small vesicle and then a gray, umbilicated center. Rarely, bullae, petechiae, and larger hemorrhagic lesions are also seen. Figures 3-45 and 3-46 show the macules and necrotic papules that are typical of disseminated gonococcal infection.

Spirochetal, Protozoal, Mycobacterial, and Rickettsial Diseases

Figure 4-1

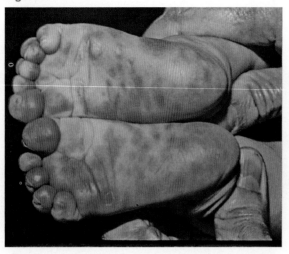

Congenital syphilis In utero infection by the spirochete *Treponema pallidum* can occur after the 16th week of gestation. Intrauterine disease, especially during early pregnancy, may result in spontaneous abortion or in a severely affected infant. Severe disease that is present at birth presents with hepatosplenomegaly, ascites, meningoencephalitis, and severe anemia. Osteochondritis is the most characteristic bone change. The cutaneous findings in severe congenital syphilis include bullae, pustules, macules, and papules.

Figure 4-2

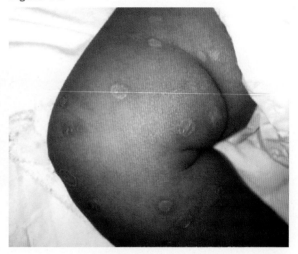

Fissuring and peeling of the skin are also characteristic. The palms, soles, and periorificial skin are sites of predilection. Syphilitic rhinitis, with a copious and bloody nasal discharge, is an associated finding. If infection occurs late in pregnancy, signs and symptoms may be delayed for several weeks. In these cases, diagnosis is usually made on the basis of a positive syphilis serology in mother and infant. If the disease is allowed to progress, rhinitis, cutaneous macules, and mucous patches may be the presenting signs.

Figure 4-3

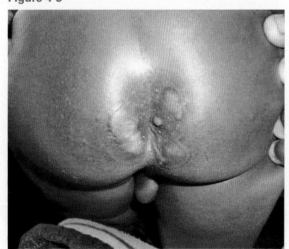

Acquired syphilis Unlike congenital syphilis, acquired syphilis in infants, children, and adolescents follows the classic course of syphilis in adults. Such an infection in a child should be assumed to be the result of sexual abuse. The first event in the development of syphilis is a dark-field positive chancre at the portal of entry of the treponeme. Shortly thereafter, serologic tests for syphilis become positive.

Figure 4-4

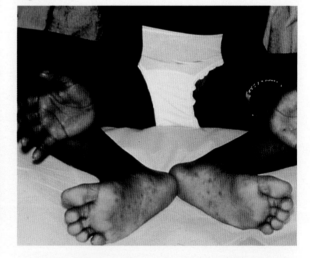

Secondary syphilis usually develops 6 to 8 weeks after the appearance of the chancre. Malaise, low-grade fever, myalgias, and lymphadenopathy are accompanied by a wide variety of cutaneous manifestations. The lesions shown in Fig. 4-3 are condylomata lata around the rectum. Note the moist papules and plaques. Figure 4-4 shows the most common presentation: copper-colored papulosquamous lesions, most commonly on the palms and soles.

Figure 4-5

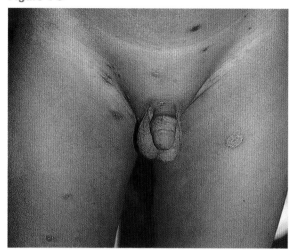

Acquired syphilis Sometimes the eruption resembles pityriasis rosea, as seen in Fig. 4-5. Other cutaneous manifestations of secondary syphilis include papular lesions, pustules, nodules, and plaques.

Figure 4-6

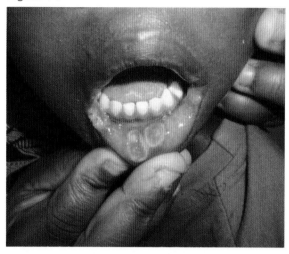

Mucous patches are a common manifestation of acquired syphilis, and appear as white slightly raised plaques on an erythematous base with a serpentine, well-defined border.

Figure 4-7

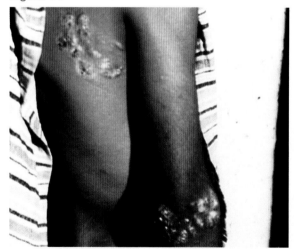

Yaws This is a nonvenereal treponematosis that is caused by *T pertenue*. It is endemic in areas of Central and South America, Africa, and Southeast Asia. The disease is acquired by physical contact, and the majority of cases occur during childhood. An ulceration occurs at the site of the primary inoculation. Secondary lesions are cutaneous nodules or moist or hyperkeratotic plaques; they appear within several weeks and resolve spontaneously. Recurrence of latent disease, with gummata of the skin and bones, may occur many years later.

Figure 4-8

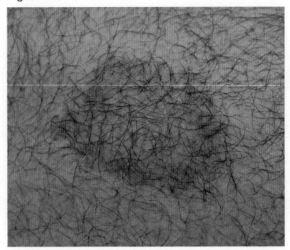

Erythema migrans (Lyme disease) Lyme disease is caused by the spirochete *Borrelia burgdorferi* and is transmitted by the pinhead-sized *Ixodes* ticks. The illness is endemic in large areas of the continental United States. The early cutaneous manifestation, termed *erythema migrans*, is shown in Figs. 4-8 and 4-9. It consists of an expanding annular lesion around the original tick bite.

Figure 4-9

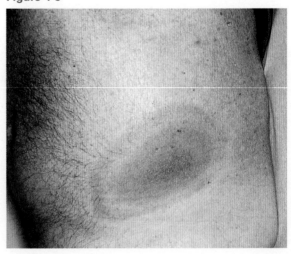

Satellite areas of involvement may also be present. Multiple lesions of erythema migrans may represent early disseminated Lyme disease as seen in Fig. 4-11.

Figure 4-10

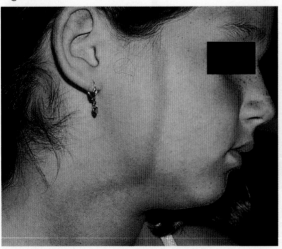

Erythema migrans (Lyme disease) Pruritus or burning may be present at the site of the lesion, and the rash may be accompanied by fever, malaise, and regional lymphadenopathy. The systemic manifestations of Lyme disease include neurologic dysfunction (eg., Bell's palsy), cardiac conduction abnormalities, and arthritis.

Figure 4-11

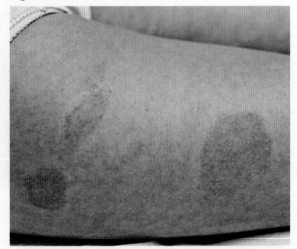

Early antibiotic therapy for the typical skin lesion will often prevent the development of the more serious and long-lasting systemic illness. Serologic testing is of some value in diagnosis but results may be negative early on, especially in the absence of neurologic or joint symptoms.

Figure 4-12

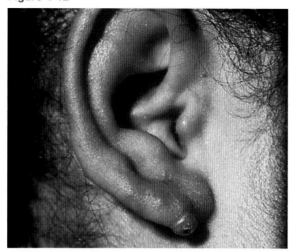

Figure 4-13

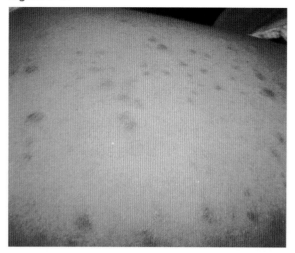

Lepromatous leprosy Leprosy, or Hansen disease, is a chronic multisystem disease that is caused by *Mycobacterium leprae*, an acid-fast bacillus. The highest incidence of the disease is in areas of South America, Africa, and Asia. It is not rare in children. The clinical manifestations of this illness depend on the host response to infection. At one end of the spectrum is lepromatous leprosy (LL), which represents a diminished host response to the leprosy bacillus. Cutaneous lesions in this form of the disease vary. Macular lesions are symmetrically distributed hypopigmented and erythematous patches. When widespread involvement occurs, the lesions may be difficult to differentiate from normal skin. The lesions pictured here are more infiltrative. Nodular lesions of the earlobe, as shown in Fig. 4-12, are particularly common in LL. Annular plaques and papules (Fig. 4-13) may also be present. LL is the form most likely to cause widespread nerve damage and ocular disease.

Figure 4-14

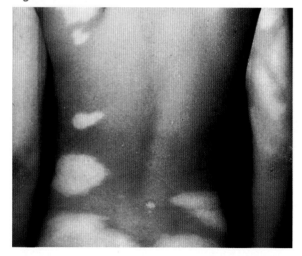

Figure 4-15

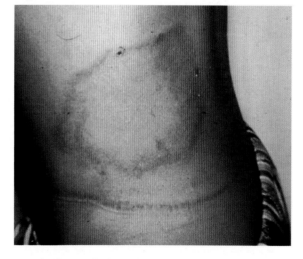

Tuberculoid leprosy Patients with tuberculoid leprosy (classification TT) are those who have the strongest immune response to chronic infection. The cutaneous lesions are typically sharply demarcated plaques with a firm raised border. Varying degrees of erythema, hypopigmentation, and anesthesia may be present. Note the large, sharply demarcated areas of decreased pigmentation in Fig. 4-14, and the raised border of the lesion in Fig. 4-15.

In early disease, the loss of sensation and normal sweating in involved areas may be difficult to detect, and the lesions can easily be confused with vitiligo and pityriasis alba. TT tends to remain a localized disease and spontaneous resolution may occur. Nerve damage tends to be limited to one or two nerves. Combinations of rifampicin, clofazimine, and dapsone are required in many cases.

Figure 4-16

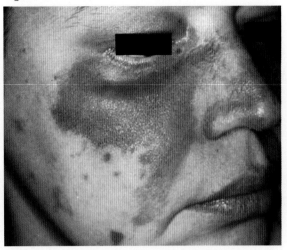

Figure 4-17

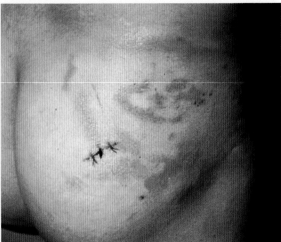

Dimorphous leprosy The terms *borderline* and *dimorphous* leprosy are used to refer to patients whose disease shows features of both the lepromatous and tuberculoid forms. Patients with dimorphous leprosy (classified as BL, BB, or BT) have varied skin lesions, including the plaques and annular lesions shown in Figs. 4-16 and 4-17. They often suffer widespread and rapidly progressive nerve damage. Knowledge of the proper treatment of leprosy must include an understanding of the acute

exacerbations that may accompany therapy. Treatment of non-lepromatous leprosy with antibiotics may induce erythema and edema of the skin lesions, accompanied by rapid damage to the peripheral nerves (type I reaction). Type II reaction, also termed as *erythema nodosum leprosum,* is most common in patients who have LL. It consists of painful dermal nodules accompanied by ocular disease, peripheral neuropathies, and a wide variety of constitutional symptoms.

Figure 4-18

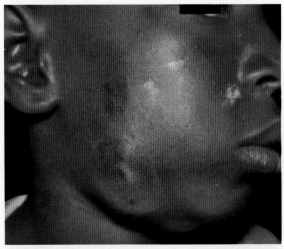

Figure 4-19

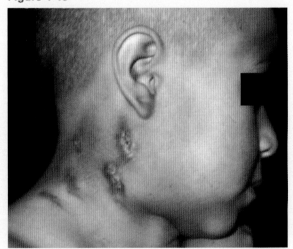

Primary complex of tuberculosis in the skin A child who has an area of injury to the skin may develop a primary complex in that location when exposed to someone with active tuberculosis. After an incubation period of 1 to 3 weeks, a red papule develops and evolves into a nodule or plaque with ulceration (tuberculous chancre). The tuberculous ulcer is accompanied by regional lymphadenopathy. This form of cutaneous tuberculosis is a self-limited disease, and a slow healing with scar formation occurs.

Scrofuloderma The skin lesions of scrofuloderma result from extension of tuberculosis from areas of infection in the bones, joints, muscle, or most commonly lymph nodes. The lesion begins as a nodule and evolves into an ulcer with draining sinuses. Figure 4-19 shows a case of tuberculous cervical lymphadenitis, with the channeling of sinuses to the skin surface. This form of cutaneous infection by *M tuberculosis* is particularly common in children.

Figure 4-20

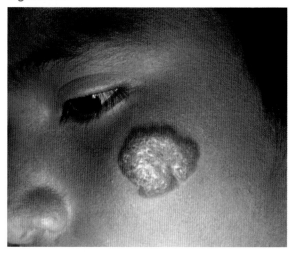

Figure 4-21

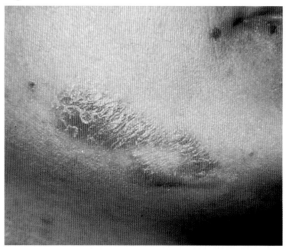

Lupus vulgaris This is a progressive form of cutaneous tuberculosis that results from either primary inoculation or the hematogenous spread of *M tuberculosis*. It is seen in patients who are very sensitive to the organism. Favored locations are the central face, earlobes, and other parts of the head and neck.

The lesions may be papules, nodules, or plaques, and the color is often described as "apple jelly." Older lesions, as shown in Fig. 4-21, are brownish annular plaques; the area of central clearing represents an attempt at healing.

Figure 4-22

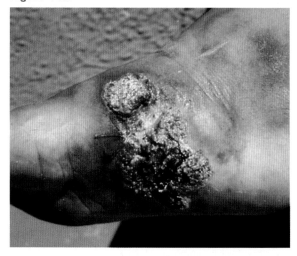

Figure 4-23

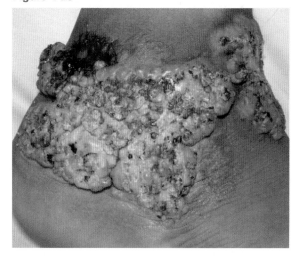

Tuberculosis cutis verrucosa This form of cutaneous tuberculosis caused by *Mycobacterium tuberculosis or Mycobacterium Bovis* results from exogenous reinfection of an already tuberculin-sensitive individual. Although this reinfection can occur from contact with tuberculous tissue, children can develop this after contact with tuberculous sputum. There is most likely a history of prior injury to the foot.

Lesions most commonly occur in children on the lower extremities. When the lesions are located on the hands or feet, they tend to develop a distinctly verrucous surface, beneath which is inflammation. This may start with a small warty growth which slowly progresses peripherally. The resultant large warty plaque may develop central scarring, as is seen in Fig. 4-22. Purulent material may be expressed.

Figure 4-24

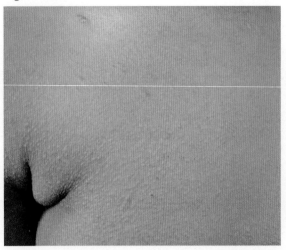

Lichen scrofulosorum This term describes a condition that consists of grouped lichenoid papules on the trunk. It occurs in children who have active tuberculosis in other locations. The individual lesions are flat-topped follicular papules and are either erythematous or flesh-colored. The condition is asymptomatic and follows a benign course to spontaneous resolution. Recurrences are common.

Figure 4-25

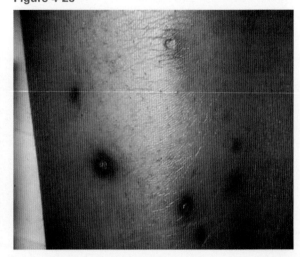

Papulonecrotic tuberculid Clinically this condition is highly stereotypic. It consists of dusky red match head- to pea-sized sterile papules that arise in symmetrical crops on the extensor aspects of the extremities, usually on the elbows and knees. Occasionally the buttocks are also involved. The condition is asymptomatic and heals spontaneously with varioliform scars. Polymerase chain reaction (PCR) amplification has detected tuberculosis DNA in these lesions.

Figure 4-26

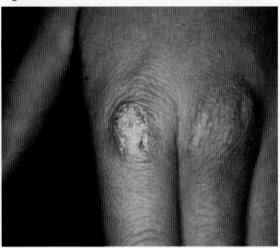

Infection with atypical mycobacteria There are a number of cutaneous infections that are caused by mycobacteria other than *M tuberculosis* or *M leprae*. Illustrated here is infection by *M marinum*. This organism is known to contaminate fish tanks and swimming pools, and the cutaneous infection is sometimes termed *swimming pool granuloma*. In fact, the case shown in Fig. 4-26 was traced to a fish tank and that in Fig. 4-27 to a swimming pool.

Figure 4-27

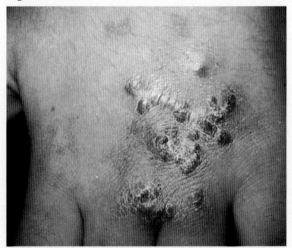

The lesions usually appear at a point of trauma and the hands, feet, elbows, and knees are particularly common locations. After an incubation period of 2 to 6 weeks, the lesions evolve from small papules into single or grouped violaceous nodules. Satellite lesions may be present. Biopsy of a mature lesion reveals a caseating granuloma, and acid-fast organisms within histiocytes can sometimes be identified. Diagnosis can also be made by culture of biopsied material.

Figure 4-28

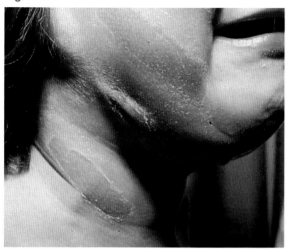

Figure 4-29

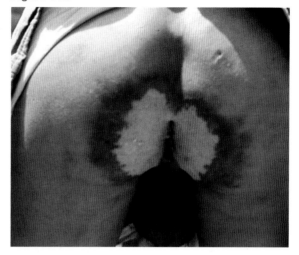

Infection with atypical mycobacteria Figure 4-28 is another instance of a granulomatous process caused by a *Mycobacterium* other than that of tuberculosis. In this case, the organism was *M avium-intracellulare.* The lesion resembles that of tuberculosis cutis colliquativa. The causative organism was cultured from the discharge that issued from sinuses emerging from infected lymph nodes. The patient was positive in reaction to conventional tuberculin and to tuberculins derived from the atypical mycobacteria.

Amebiasis cutis *Entamoeba histolytica,* the cause of intestinal and cutaneous amebiasis, extends to the skin from intestinal infestation. Discharging from the ulcerous process in the lower part of the gut, viable amoebas contaminate and may infect the perianal region. When the infection is seen in an active state, the process is a continually creeping, painful ulceration that has little tendency to heal spontaneously. When the infection is healed, the clinical appearance is a scar, as shown in Fig. 4-29.

Figure 4-30

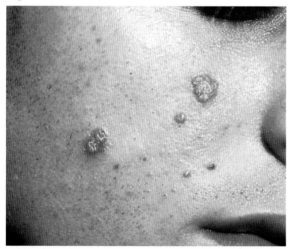

Figure 4-31

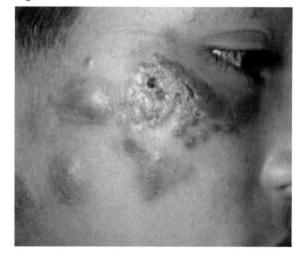

Leishmaniasis The cutaneous form of leishmaniasis is caused by a protozoan *(Leishmania tropica)* that is transmitted by the bite of a sandfly (of the genus *Phlebotomus*) in certain endemic regions (the Middle East, China, Africa, India, the former Soviet Union). The primary process in the skin starts as a macule of erythema, evolves into a papule (Fig. 4-30), and then develops into a granulomatous or ulcerous process (Fig. 4-31). The lesion takes up to 1 year to heal spontaneously in the form of a vacciniform scar.

Systemic or *visceral leishmaniasis* (kala-azar) is caused by the related protozoan *L donovani.* This form is characterized by fever, anemia, leukopenia, emaciation, and severe hepatosplenomegaly. The skin develops a grayish pigmentation, usually on the face. Finally, mucocutaneous leishmaniasis caused by *L braziliensis,* is characterized by destructive mucosal lesions, and is endemic in some areas of Latin America.

Figure 4-32

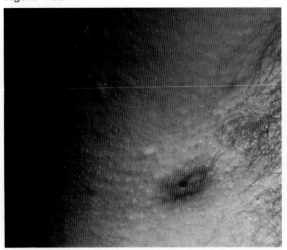

Figure 4-33

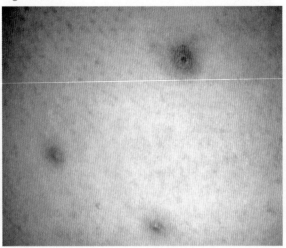

Rickettsialpox This self-limited febrile illness is caused by *Rickettsia akari*. It is transmitted to man by a mite that is an obligatory parasite of the common house mouse. One to two weeks after exposure, a nodule develops at the point of entry of a parasitized mite. The nodule becomes vesicular and then crusted with a black eschar (the pock, seen well developed on the neck in Fig. 4-32). Regional lymphadenopathy is usually present.

Within several days, the patient develops intermittent fever, photophobia, headache, myalgia, and lassitude. Two to three days later, a generalized exanthem, consisting of discrete macules that quickly become papular, appears (Fig. 4-33). Firm vesiculopustules arise atop the papules and these subsequently form crusts. The eruption lasts for 1 to 2 weeks. The disease must be treated on clinical suspicion. Serologic tests for antibodies and biopsy for culture, direct fluorescent antibody, and PCR can all be used to confirm the diagnosis.

Figure 4-34

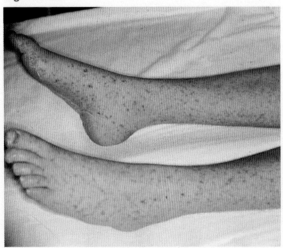

Figure 4-35

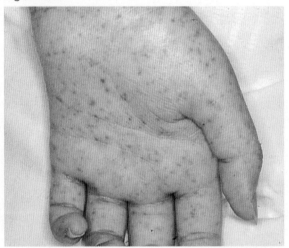

Rocky Mountain spotted fever This disease is caused by *Rickettsia rickettsii* and is transmitted by a number of different ticks. Despite its geographical title, Rocky Mountain spotted fever is present in many locations throughout the United States and the entire Western Hemisphere. After infection by tick bite, there is an incubation period of 2 to 14 days. The abrupt onset of the disease includes severe headache, fever, chills, arthralgia, and myalgia. After 2 to 3 days of these constitutional symptoms, erythematous macules erupt on the wrists, hands, forearms, legs, and ankles, as

seen in Figs. 4-34 and 4-35. Lesions then spread to the palms and soles and the trunk. The macules originally blanch with pressure but soon become purpuric and even necrotic. The disease causes a severe vasculitis and complications include disseminated intravascular coagulation, hemorrhage into the gastrointestinal and urinary tracts, and cardiovascular collapse. The high fatality rate is markedly reduced by prompt antibiotic therapy and the disease must be treated immediately upon clinical suspicion. PCR or immunohistochemical staining of a skin lesions can confirm the diagnosis.

Viral Diseases

Figure 5-1

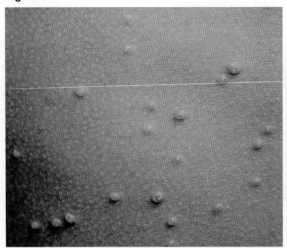

Molluscum contagiosum This condition is a benign viral infection that appears as crops of discrete, slightly umbilicated, flesh-colored, or shiny papules. It is extremely common among children and may be seen in several children within a family. The lesions may become inflamed if traumatized or infected and sometimes become inflamed spontaneously as they resolve.

Figure 5-2

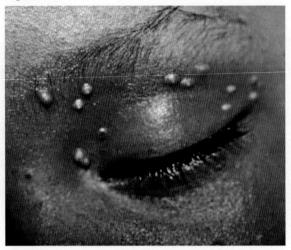

The lesions tend to be grouped, and the average size of a lesion is 2 to 3 mm in diameter and height. The trunk, face, genitalia, and intertriginous areas are the most common sites of infection. Pruritus is an occasional symptom and an eczematous eruption may develop in the area of the molluscum.

Figure 5-3

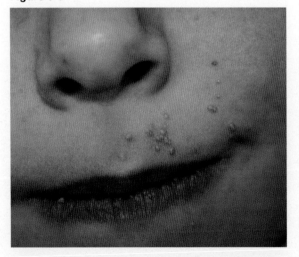

Molluscum contagiosum This viral infection is self-limited, but treatment is often required because of discomfort or out of concern for appearance. Treatment should be individualized to the age and extent of involvement in each patient.

Figure 5-4

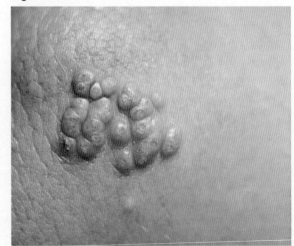

As the infection is self-limited, observation is an acceptable option. In the cooperative patient, destruction of lesions with curettage or light cryotherapy may be attempted for treatment of limited lesions. Some dermatologists treat this disorder with the office application of topical cantharidin. The child with numerous lesions poses a particular therapeutic challenge.

Figure 5-5

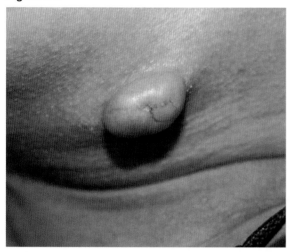

Figure 5-6

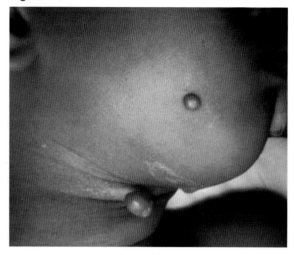

Molluscum contagiosum Occasionally, a lesion of molluscum contagiosum may grow to as large as 3 cm in diameter. Two photos of such "giant mollusca" are shown in Figs. 5-5 and 5-6. The diagnosis is usually suggested by the presence of more typical, smaller lesions on adjacent or distant skin surfaces. Note the presence of a central umbilication in Fig. 5-5. Treatment is by surgical removal when possible.

Figure 5-7

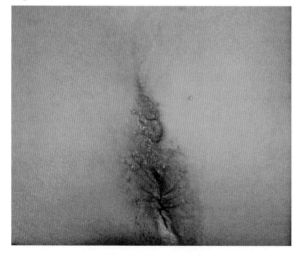

Figure 5-8

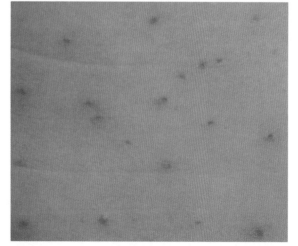

Molluscum contagiosum When molluscum contagiosum appear in the groin or especially the intergluteal cleft area, they may be misdiagnosed as warts. Molluscum in the intergluteal cleft area may appear like "fleshy" skin tags, and upon close examination that can be aided by magnification, a central umbilication can be seen. If the diagnosis is in question, a biopsy would yield the diagnosis.

Some patients with molluscum contagiosum will develop scarring from this viral infection. Large and even small molluscum may scar even without any treatment. Figure 5-8 shows a patient who developed scarring without any treatment given for the molluscum.

Figure 5-9

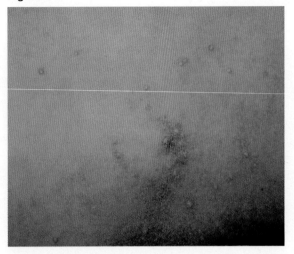

Figure 5-10

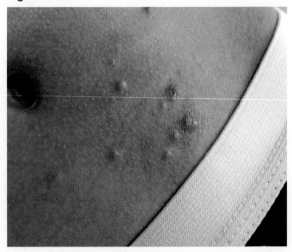

Molluscum contagiosum dermatitis Many children with molluscum contagiosum infection develop an eczematous, pruritic dermatitis surrounding the affected area of involvement. Low potency topical corticosteroids can alleviate the dermatitis. At times, the lesions in the involved area may have to be treated in order to permanently clear the dermatitis.

Figure 5-11

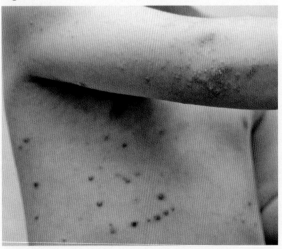

Figure 5-12

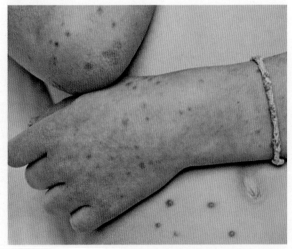

Molluscum contagiosum id reaction Some patients may develop a hypersensitivity eruption as a result of the immune response to the virus. This eruption favors the extremities, particularly the elbows (Fig. 5-11) and knees, with skin colored to erythematous papules and grouped papulovesicles. The buttocks may also be involved. Inflamed molluscum is seen elsewhere. Note the inflamed mollusum on the abdomen in Figs. 5-11 and 5-12. The papules on the elbow and hand in Fig. 5-12 are related to the id reaction and are not inflamed molluscum.

Figure 5-13

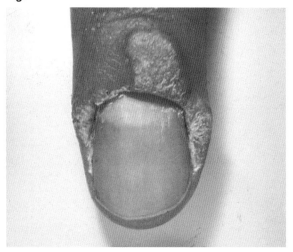

Verruca vulgaris The common wart is a benign growth caused by localized infection with one of the many types of human papillomavirus. These small DNA viruses are part of the papovavirus group. Warts are especially common among children and adolescents and may occur on any mucocutaneous surface. The hands are a particularly frequent location.

Figure 5-14

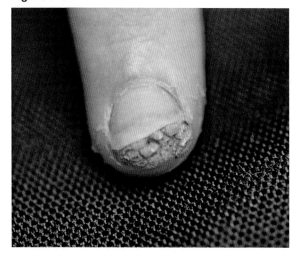

The typical wart is a rough-surfaced nodule that may be either lighter or darker than the surrounding skin. Lesions involving the proximal and lateral nail folds are common and present particular treatment difficulties.

Figure 5-15

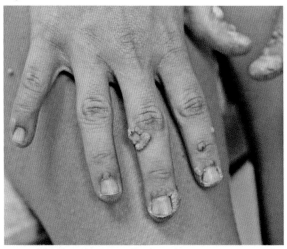

Verruca vulgaris Gentle cryotherapy or topical salicylic acid preparations may be of value in the treatment of warts. However, severe warts such as those shown in Fig. 5-15 may require additional therapies, such as injection with intralesional candida antigen.

Figure 5-16

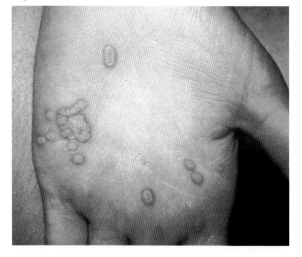

Figure 5-16 illustrates multiple warts located on the palmar surface of the hand. In general, treatment must be individualized to the age and cooperative abilities of the patient and to the size and location of the warts.

Figure 5-17

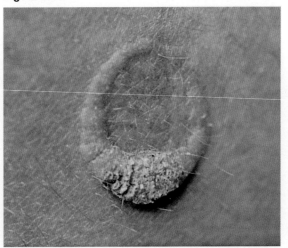

Verruca vulgaris Following the application of cantharidin or liquid nitrogen, blister formation may result. Upon resolution of the blister, a ring wart may develop, as seen in Fig. 5-17.

Figure 5-18

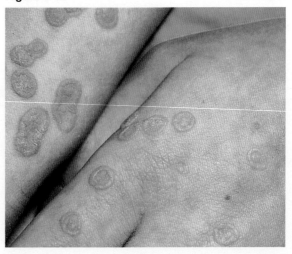

Multiple ring warts are seen in Fig. 5-18.

Figure 5-19

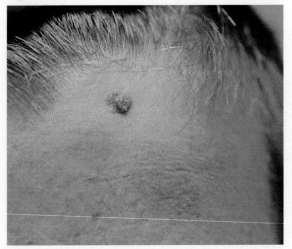

Verruca vulgaris Although the hands are the most common location for warts in children, they may occur on almost any part of the skin surface.

Figure 5-20

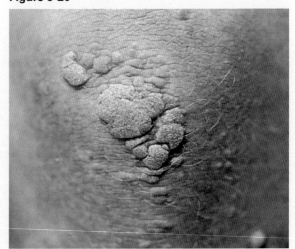

Figure 5-20 illustrates the appearance of multiple clustered warts on the knee.

Figure 5-21

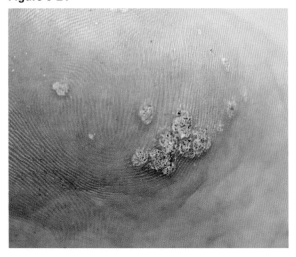

Figure 5-22

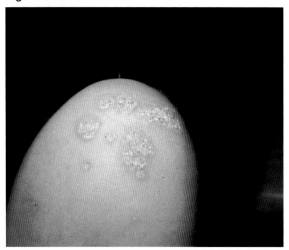

Plantar warts Plantar warts appear as flat areas of firm hyperkeratosis on the soles of the feet. Lesions that occur at points of pressure may be associated with severe pain on walking. Figure 5-21 illustrates solitary and multiple plantar warts. Note the obliteration of skin markings, which does not occur in a callus. The lesions in Fig. 5-22 on the heel are numerous and mosaic. Treatment of plantar warts requires perseverance on the part of both patient and physician.

Attempts at a rapid cure may result in scarring. One practical method involves the daily application of salicylic acid plasters or liquid salicylic acid preparations along with repeated paring of the necrotic surface of the wart. The success of this routine may be hastened by gentle cryotherapy.

Figure 5-23

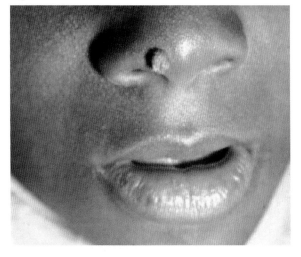

Figure 5-24

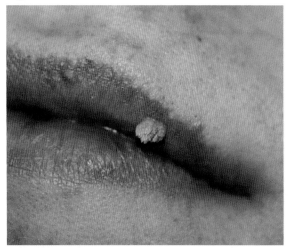

Filiform warts The surfaces of common warts are influenced by their position on the body. In general, they have a rough surface. On hands, the surfaces of warts are doomed from wear and tear, so that troughs and crests are shallow; on soles, they are flat and smooth from the weight of the body, but where they are undisturbed, common warts tend to grow with fimbria or fingerlike projections. They are then called *filiform* or *digitate* warts.

The face and scalp are the most common sites where warts grow in this fashion Filiform warts may also occur on the lips as shown in Fig. 5-24.

Figure 5-25

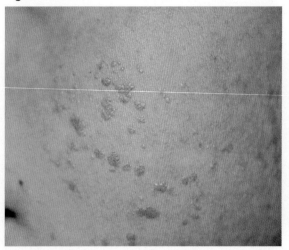

Verruca plana Plane, or flat, warts may be caused by several types of the human papillomavirus. They are common in children. The lesions are slightly raised, flesh-colored papules, and usually 2 to 4 mm in diameter.

Figure 5-26

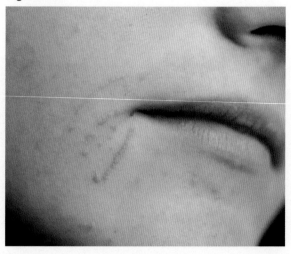

The face and hands are the most frequent locations for these multiple small warts. The lesions may be discrete or confluent, and a linear array of flat warts, as shown in Fig. 5-26, may result from autoinoculation in a scratch.

Figure 5-27

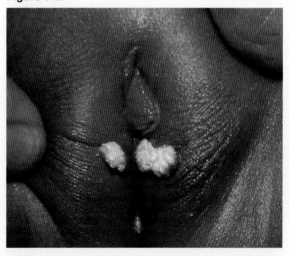

Condyloma acuminatum Warts with this "cauliflower" appearance on the labia (Fig. 5-27), penis, or around the rectum (Fig. 5-28) are termed *condylomata acuminata*. The presence of lesions of this type in a child should prompt the physician to consider the possibility of sexual abuse, although the true incidence of this association is not known. In very young children, perinatal transmission is probably the most common cause.

Figure 5-28

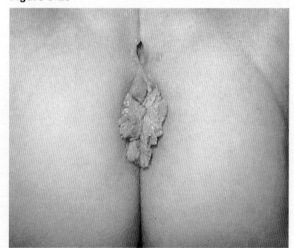

In some cases, as well, condylomata acuminata may be the result of innocent contact with another infected individual. The use of topical products containing podophyllum or imiquimod are effective treatments.

Figure 5-29

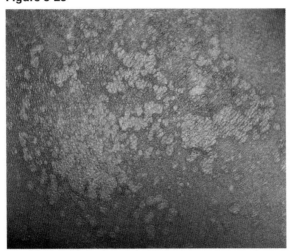

Epidermodysplasia verruciformis This rare familial disease usually has its onset during childhood. Patients develop numerous flat warts, initially involving the face and upper trunk. A number of human papillomavirus types have been implicated. As the lesions tend toward confluence, they may mimic the appearance of tinea versicolor. Most patients with epidermodysplasia verruciformis have depressed cell-mediated immunity, and they are also at risk for squamous cell carcinoma. A similar presentation may be seen in children with HIV infection.

Figure 5-30

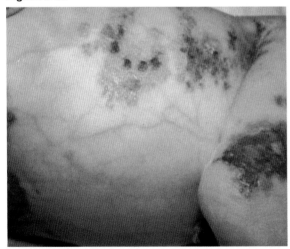

Neonatal herpes simplex Neonatal herpes simplex infection is acquired during passage through an infected birth canal. The cutaneous involvement may be as extensive as shown in Fig. 5-30, or it may be subtle. The scalp is the most common site for the typical clustered vesicles.

Figure 5-31

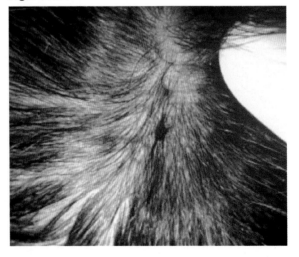

Because of the very high frequency of concurrent disseminated disease, cutaneous herpes simplex in the newborn must be considered a pediatric emergency. Early treatment with an intravenous antiviral agent minimizes complications and offers the infant the best possibility of survival.

Figure 5-32

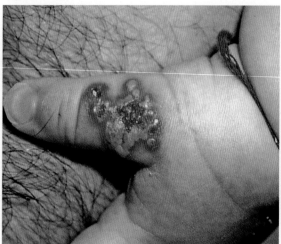

Herpes simplex Herpes simplex infection of the fingers may occur in infants and young children. The first episode may accompany herpetic gingivostomatitis.

Figure 5-33

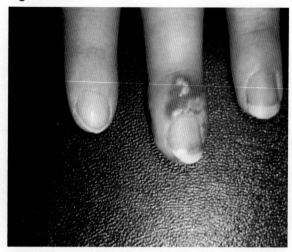

Herpetic whitlow Herpetic whitlow presents with pain or paresthesia and with erythema and vesicle formation. The original infection is sometimes misdiagnosed as a bacterial or candida paronychia, but subsequent recurrences lead the practitioner to the correct diagnosis.

Figure 5-34

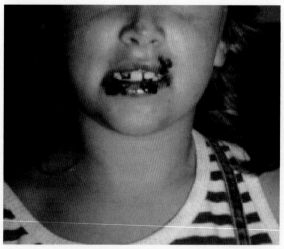

Herpetic gingivostomatis Primary infection with herpes simplex may cause a severe gingivostomatitis that is severely painful and interferes with eating and drinking. Treatment consists of topical analgesics, supportive care, and oral or intravenous acyclovir.

Figure 5-35

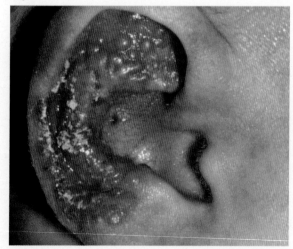

Recurrent herpes simplex Recurrent herpes simplex infections can occur in a wide variety of locations, including, as shown in Fig. 5-35, the ear. The original episode could easily be mistaken for a bacterial infection.

Figure 5-36

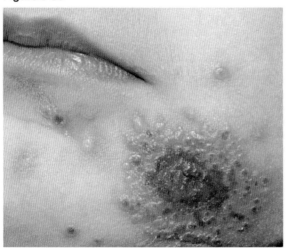

Herpes simplex, recurrent Following an episode of primary herpes simplex, the virus may remain dormant within a nerve ganglion. Represented in Fig. 5-36 and Fig. 5-37 are lesions on the face showing a less common location serving to illustrate that recurrent herpes simplex may occur on any area of the skin.

Figure 5-37

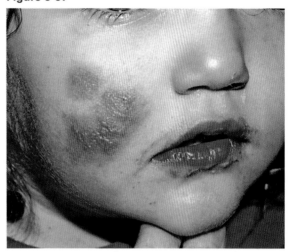

A number of triggering factors including febrile illness, emotional or physical stress, excessive sun exposure, and trauma may cause the virus to replicate and spread to the skin surface.

Figure 5-38

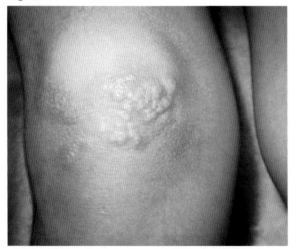

Herpes simplex, recurrent Patients with recurrent disease will often experience prodromal pain or paresthesia in the involved area. Most episodes last from 7 to 10 days. Figure 5-38 shows lesions on the knee. This is a less common location, serving to illustrate that recurrent herpes simplex may occur on any area of the skin.

Figure 5-39

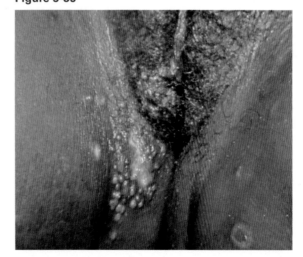

Genital herpes simplex Herpes simplex infection in the genital region is a sexually transmitted disease. It is common in the sexually active adolescent as shown in Fig. 5-39. In the young child, genital herpes simplex should create a high index of suspicion for sexual abuse. This figure illustrates the multiple painful erosions that may occur in primary infection. Regional lymphadenopathy and fever may also be present. Recurrences of genital herpes are very common but are generally much milder in both extent and duration than the primary disease.

Figure 5-40

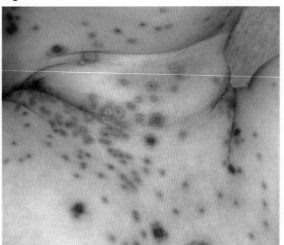

Figure 5-41

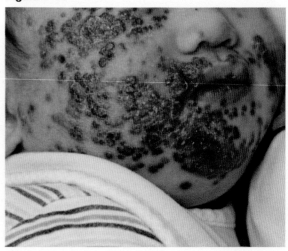

Eczema herpeticum (Kaposi varicelliform eruption) Disseminated cutaneous herpes simplex infection is a serious complication of atopic dermatitis. It may also occasionally occur in individuals with other dermatologic disorders. Patients rapidly develop numerous umbilicated vesicles in the areas of eczematous involvement. Children with eczema herpeticum often become seriously ill with high fever. Bacterial superinfection and sepsis can be a complication, and the disease is occasionally fatal.

The patients pictured here developed involvement of the entire skin surface. The lesions in Fig. 5-40 are typical umbilicated vesicles, and the lesions in Fig. 5-41 are equally extensive and are beginning to crust. Skillful and attentive supportive treatment is required in order to maintain fluid and electrolyte balance and prevent superinfection. Treatment with intravenous acyclovir hastens clinical improvement and is recommended for children with extensive or rapidly increasing involvement.

Figure 5-42

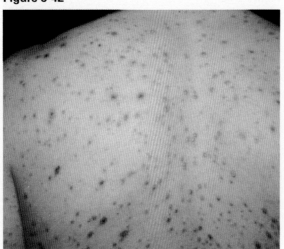

Figure 5-43

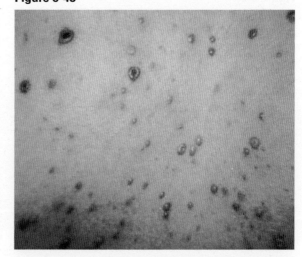

Varicella Chickenpox is caused by a virus of the herpes group. The disease is highly contagious and is spread by droplet or direct contact. The incubation period for chickenpox ranges from 11 to 21 days. Prodromal symptoms consist of low-grade fever, headache, anorexia, and malaise. On the following day, the characteristic rash begins to appear. The lesions evolve from erythematous macules to form small papules. Quickly, a clear vesicle arises on this erythematous base.

The classic lesion of chickenpox has been poetically described as a "dewdrop on a rose petal". Over the next several days, the vesicles rupture and then crust. The rash begins on the chest and back and spreads centrifugally to involve the face, scalp, and the extremities. New lesions of chickenpox arise in crops over a period of several days. Since crops of macules, papules, vesicles, and crusts are successive and overlapping, one sees lesions at all stages of development in given locations. Itching is a symptom and may be severe.

Figure 5-44

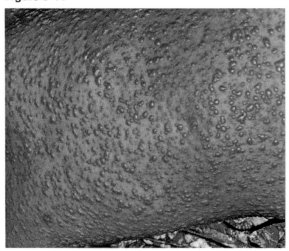

Figure 5-45

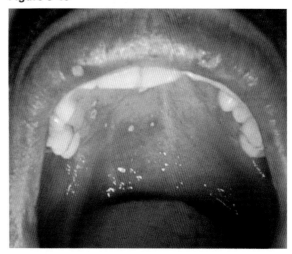

Varicella Figure 5-44 depicts a case of chickenpox of unusual severity. The lesions tend to be large blisters and to become hemorrhagic. Cases of this type are more likely to occur in children with reticuloendothelial malignancies or immunologic defects, or in those under immunosuppressive or prolonged corticosteroid therapy. This patient had scarlet fever 2 weeks prior to the varicella outbreak.

Lesions on the oral mucous membranes, which are common, are pictured in Fig. 5-45. They are most common on the palate and quickly evolve into small, superficial erosions.

Figure 5-46

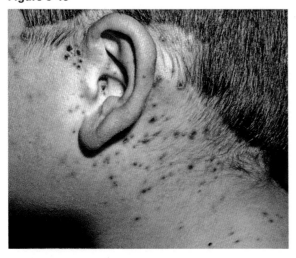

Figure 5-47

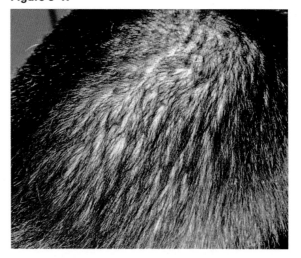

Varicella Other, less frequent, sequelae include thrombocytopenia, purpura fulminans, and postinfectious encephalitis. Finally, a significant number of cases of Reye syndrome occur after chickenpox, and aspirin should therefore not be used as an antipyretic.

Involvement of varicella in in the scalp is shown in Fig. 5-47. Complications of chickenpox may include varicella pneumonia, myocarditis, and hepatitis. Secondary bacterial infection of the skin lesions is by far the most common complication of chickenpox.

Figure 5-48

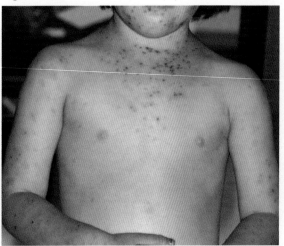

Varicella In rare cases of chicken pox, lesions occur primarily or exclusively in sun-exposed areas. Figure 5-48 shows an example of photo-related varicella, with a concentration of lesions on the sun-exposed areas of the mid-upper chest.

Figure 5-49

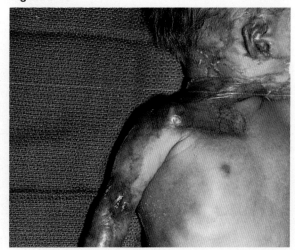

Congenital varicella syndrome On rare occasions, the infants of women who develop chickenpox during the first trimester of pregnancy are born with congenital defects. The congenital varicella syndrome is characterized by asymmetrical arm or leg lengths, ocular abnormalities, microcephaly, and intrauterine growth retardation. Cutaneous scarring in a dermatomal distribution is particularly characteristic of the constellation of birth defects caused by the varicella zoster virus.

Figure 5-50

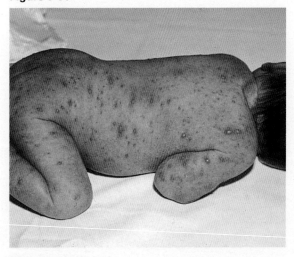

Neonatal varicella Maternal chickenpox during several days before or after the birth of a child may lead to a significant health risk for the infant. The newborn who is exposed to varicella without the benefit of transplacental maternal antibody may go on to develop severe disseminated infection with pulmonary

Figure 5-51

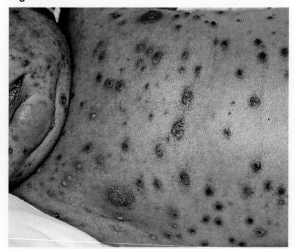

and hepatic involvement. This disease may sometimes be fatal. Pictured here are newborns with numerous typical chickenpox lesions. The hemorrhagic lesions that may be part of neonatal varicella are not present in these cases.

Figure 5-52

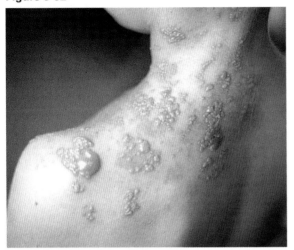

Herpes zoster Herpes zoster, or shingles, is an acute eruption characterized by vesicles and small bullae. Lesions are usually unilateral and confined to a single dermatome. The cause of herpes zoster is the varicella zoster virus. After an initial episode of chickenpox, the virus lies dormant in the dorsal root or cranial nerve ganglia. Reactivation of the virus, usually years later, leads to the typical eruption.

Figure 5-53

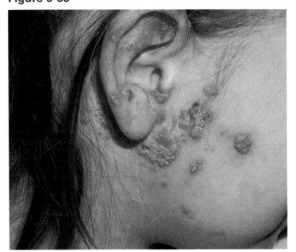

Herpes zoster is a relatively rare disease in children and is seen more frequently in those young people who had chickenpox at a very early age. Localized pain may precede the onset of the rash, but postherpetic neuralgia is unusual in childhood. Children with lesions around the eye or on the tip of the nose may have involvement of the nasociliary nerve and should be observed carefully for ocular involvement. Children with involvement of the ear, shown in Fig. 5-53, may develop severe otalgia and when associated with facial paralysis it is known as Ramsay Hunt syndrome.

Figure 5-54

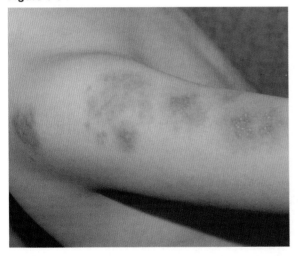

Herpes zoster The child with herpes zoster may, in the normal course of the illness, develop several chickenpox-like lesions outside of the involved dermatome. However, rapid and widespread evolution of such lesions—generalized herpes zoster—is a problem of greater concern. Hematogenous spread of the viral infection in this fashion may be an indication of an underlying immune deficiency.

Figure 5-55

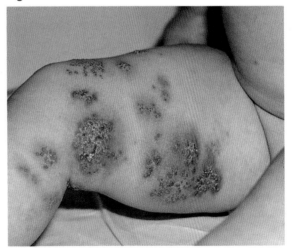

Infants born to mothers who developed primary varicella infection during pregnancy may likewise have been infected during fetal life. These infants may develop herpes zoster without a clinical history of previous varicella. Associated with this may be a temporary paresis of the affected area.

Figure 5-56

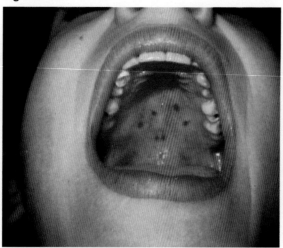

Figure 5-57

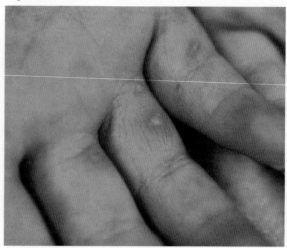

Hand-foot-mouth disease This common and benign viral disease of childhood is usually caused by the A16 strain of coxsackievirus, although other strains of the same virus have been implicated. It most often occurs in late summer and early fall. The prodrome consists of low-grade fever and malaise.

Shortly thereafter, vesicular lesions arise on the soft palate (Fig. 5-56), tongue, buccal mucosa, and uvula. The lips are usually spared. Occasionally, these lesions may be painful and cause some difficulty in eating. The cutaneous lesions develop 1 or 2 days after those in the mouth. They consist of asymptomatic round or oval vesiculopustules that evolve into superficial erosions. The edges of the palms (Fig. 5-57) and soles (Fig. 5-58) are a favored location.

Figure 5-58

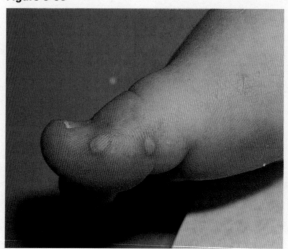

Hand-foot-mouth disease The dorsa of the hands and feet may also be involved. There is sometimes an accompanying macular and papular eruption on the buttocks. The eruption lasts from 7 to 10 days and no therapy is required. Although culture of the virus is possible, the diagnosis of hand-foot-mouth disease is usually made on clinical grounds.

Figure 5-59

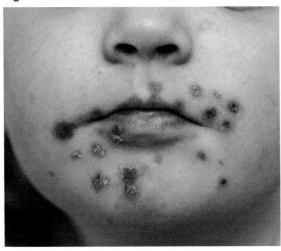

Atypical hand-foot-mouth disease Since 2008, outbreaks of an atypical form of hand-foot-mouth disease, caused by coxsackie virus A6, have been documented in countries throughout the world. The development of skin lesions is often accompanied by fever, chills, malaise, and diarrhea. Perioral lesions, along with involvement inside the mouth, are common, and, as seen in Fig. 5-59, may be confused with impetigo.

Figure 5-60

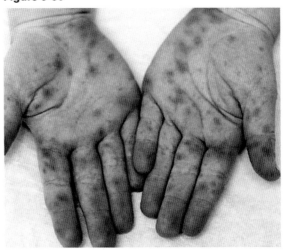

Figure 5-60 illustrates the development of numerous lesions on the palms of the hands. Although hand, foot and mouth are sites of predilection for this atypical form, lesions tend to be more widespread, and, in children with atopic dermatitis, occur in areas of involvement of the eczema itself, such as the antecubital and popliteal fossa ("eczema coxsackieum").

Figure 5-61

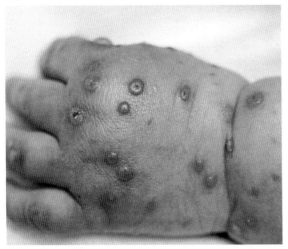

Atypical hand-foot-mouth disease Vesicles and bullae, some with central umbilication, are frequently seen in this variant of hand-foot-mouth disease. The lesions may be tender.

Figure 5-62

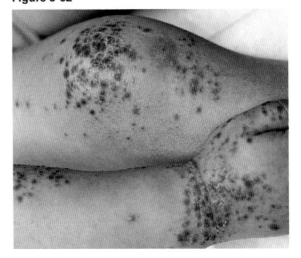

The bullae in atypical hand-foot-mouth disease rapidly evolve into superficial erosions, and, in severe cases, this may involve a large part of the skin surface. In the resolving phase of the disease, it is not uncommon for children to shed fingernails and toenails.

Figure 5-63

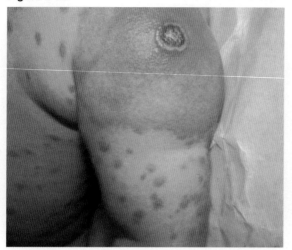

Figure 5-64

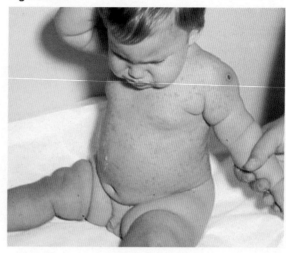

Complications of vaccinia The worldwide eradication of small-pox has eliminated the need for vaccination with the modified cowpox virus. Over the many years when this medical practice was necessary, a number of benign and some more serious dermatologic complications were observed. The sequelae of small-pox vaccination are as follows: 3 to 4 days after inoculation, there develops an area of erythema and edema at the injection site (usually an arm or thigh); this rapidly evolves into edema, vesiculation, ulceration, crusting, and scar formation over a period of about 3 weeks. For most children, fever, malaise, and local discomfort are the major side effects. The complications of a severe local reaction (Fig. 5-63) and of a generalized eruption (Figs. 5-64 and 5-65) are illustrated here.

Figure 5-65

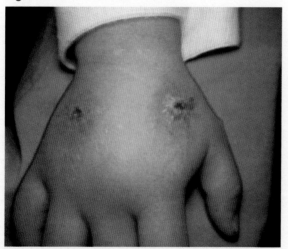

Figure 5-66

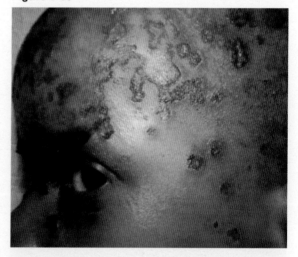

Complications of vaccinia Still another complication of vaccinia vaccination was accidental autoinoculation on an undesirable site while the primary pock was in progress. Auto-inoculation then resulted in a new lesion that began in 1 day (a reaction time) and rapidly repeated the whole process. The seriousness of such accidents was site-specific: on the face, particularly around the eyes, blindness, and elsewhere on exposed skin, cosmetic defects, were serious consequences.

Eczema vaccinatum Disseminated vaccinia was the most dreaded complication of smallpox vaccination. Like eczema herpeticum, eczema vaccinatum occurred in children with underlying eczematous disorders. It was more serious because of the severity of the acute illness, the tendency toward scarring, and a higher incidence of mortality. Figure 5-66 suggests that the scarring from eczema vaccinatum can be disfiguring.

Figure 5-67

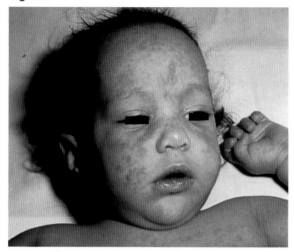

Exanthem subitum (roseola) Roseola is a common childhood illness that is now known to be caused by human herpes virus 6. Most cases occur during the first year of life. The disease is characterized by 3 to 5 days of high fever accompanied by minimal constitutional symptoms. Pharyngitis, periorbital edema, and cervical adenopathy may be present and febrile seizures sometimes occur.

Figure 5-68

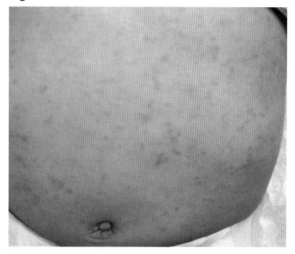

The disappearance of fever is accompanied by the onset of rash. The typical eruption is macular and papular, and it is concentrated on the neck and trunk. The eruption clears in hours or at most a day or two. Note the light pink macules on the infant pictured in Fig. 5-68.

Figure 5-69

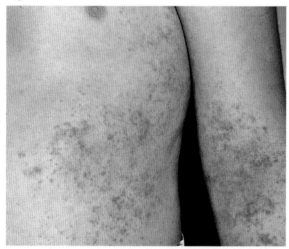

Unilateral laterothoracic exanthem This condition of unknown etiology begins as an eruption in a periflexural area, the axillary fold being the most common. Other flexural areas including the inguinal fold and popliteal areas may be involved initially. The eruption then spreads unilaterally in an asymmetric fashion, at times involving an entire side of the body.

Figure 5-70

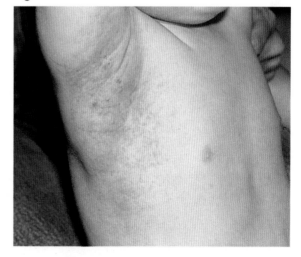

The eruption may then generalize to the rest of the body, typically maintaining predominance on the original side. Clinically, the eruption is scarlatiniform or eczematous in nature. About 50 percent of patients may develop pruritus. Spontaneous resolution usually occurs in 4 to 6 weeks.

Figure 5-71

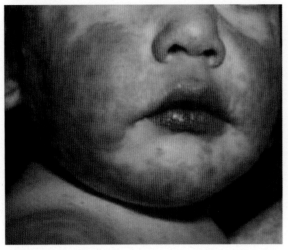

Papular acrodermatitis of childhood (Gianotti-Crosti syndrome) This condition is characterized by the eruption of firm erythematous papules on the extremities, cheeks, and buttocks. The papulonodular lesions may become confluent in some areas, as illustrated in Figs. 5-71 and 5-72.

Figure 5-72

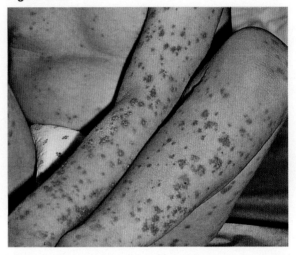

This disease was originally seen in children with anicteric hepatitis B infection in Europe. Since that time, this syndrome has been found to occur primarily in association with Epstein-Barr virus infection, although other causes include coxsackie, parainfluenza, poliovirus, vaccinia, β-hemolytic streptococcus, and bacille Calmette-Guérin (BCG).

Figure 5-73

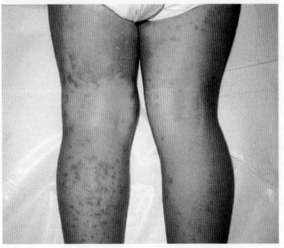

Papular acrodermatitis of childhood (Gianotti-Crosti syndrome) Figures 5-73 and 5-74 both illustrate lesions occurring on the legs, with relative sparing of the popliteal fossae.

Figure 5-74

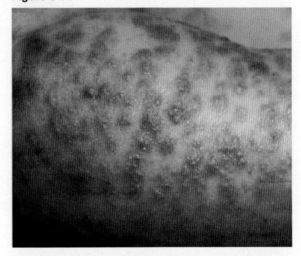

The papules in Gianott-Crosti syndrome are, at first, brightly erythematous and extremely firm to the touch. The disease is self-limiting, lasting 6 to 8 weeks.

Figure 5-75

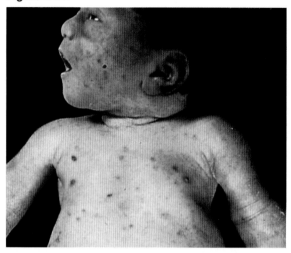

Congenital cytomegalovirus infection Congenital infection with cytomegalovirus, a DNA virus of the herpes group, results in disease of varying severity. While some neonates are completely asymptomatic, severely affected infants display intrauterine growth retardation, microcephaly, and hepatosplenomegaly. The cutaneous manifestations, shown in Fig. 5-75, are petechiae and purpura. The "blueberry muffin" spots are an indication of extramedullary hematopoiesis.

Figure 5-76

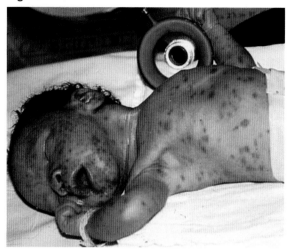

Congenital rubella In utero infection by the rubella virus during the first 20 weeks of gestation may result in severe multisystem involvement and a variety of developmental defects. Illustrated in Fig. 5-76 are the dark-blue-to-purple "blueberry muffin" lesions in the severely affected neonate. They are a sign of extramedullary hematopoiesis. Thrombocytopenic purpura is an additional cutaneous manifestation. Congenital cataracts, deafness, and cardiac malformations form a classic triad in infants with the severe intrauterine infection.

Figure 5-77

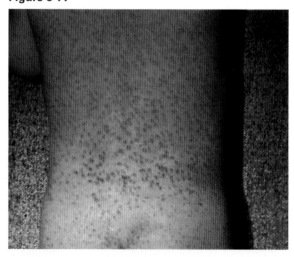

Rubella This viral disease affects both children and young adults. A mild prodrome consists of headache, coryza, and low-grade fever. The rash itself varies enormously in its course and duration. Most typically, it begins on the face and neck and spreads to the trunk and extremities, as pictured in Fig. 5-77, over 1 or 2 days. The lesions are small pink macules and maculopapules, which rapidly coalesce and then fade. The rash is so evanescent that it may begin to disappear on the face before developing on the trunk and extremities.

Figure 5-78

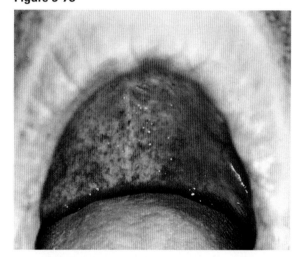

Petechiae on the soft palate, termed *Forchheimer sign,* are present in some patients and are illustrated in Fig. 5-78. Systemic illness is generally mild. Enlargement of suboccipital and posterior auricular lymph nodes is a characteristic physical finding. The most serious aspect of rubella is the severe developmental delay that may result from intrauterine infection during the first trimester. Routine childhood immunization has resulted in fewer epidemics and therefore in a lower incidence of viral exposure to pregnant women.

Figure 5-79

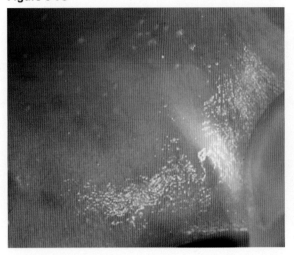

Measles Rubeola, or measles, is a systemic illness caused by an RNA paramyxovirus. The incidence of this previously common childhood disease has decreased markedly since the advent of an effective vaccine, but measles has by no means been eradicated. After an incubation period of 1 to 2 weeks, the infected child develops fever, conjunctivitis, photophobia, and a distinctive brassy or barking cough. Frequently, the fever and constitutional symptoms are severe.

Figure 5-80

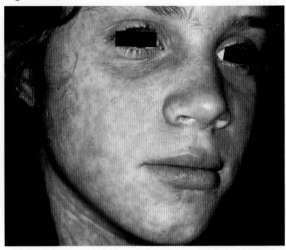

A day or two after the onset of these constitutional signs and symptoms, the enanthem (Koplik spots) appears as bright-red puncta with central blue-white flecks on the buccal mucosa opposite the second molars (Fig. 5-79). The characteristic rash is maculopapular and erythematous. It begins on the forehead and behind the ears and spreads to the face (Fig. 5-80), neck, trunk, and extremities. The rash disappears in the same sequence, sometimes leaving areas of fine desquamation. The duration of the entire illness is usually 5 to 7 days.

Figure 5-81

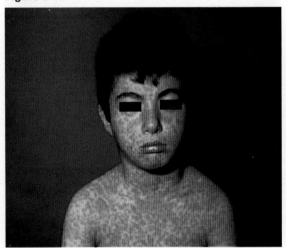

Measles Figure 5-81 shows the "measly" appearance of a child who clearly feels miserable. The disease is brief and self-limited for most children, and the treatment is entirely supportive. The incidence of complications is higher, however, than in other childhood exanthems. Otitis media is the most common. Serious complications include bronchopneumonia and encephalitis, which may cause permanent neurologic damage. Subacute sclerosing panencephalitis is a late sequela of measles.

Figure 5-82

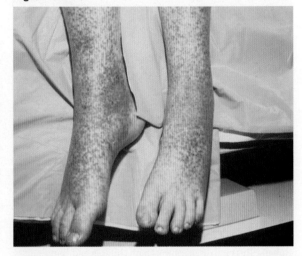

Atypical measles This can occur in individuals who were given the old killed-virus vaccine (no longer available) or were given a live measles vaccine that was inactivated by improper storage. Atypical measles is characterized by high fever and severe respiratory symptoms. The accompanying rash is similar to that of Rocky Mountain spotted fever (Figs. 4-34 and 4-35). The exanthem, which typically begins on the hands and feet, may be macular, vesicular, or purpuric.

Figure 5-83

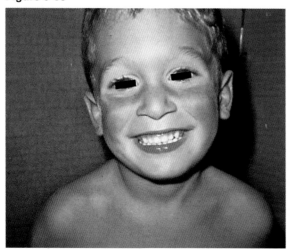

Erythema infectiosum (fifth disease) Erythema infectiosum is a mild childhood disease that is caused by human parvovirus B19. This condition develops after a mean incubation period of 14 days. There are few if any prodromal symptoms. The rash evolves in three clinical stages. The first stage is characterized by the abrupt appearance of a bright-red malar blush.

Figure 5-84

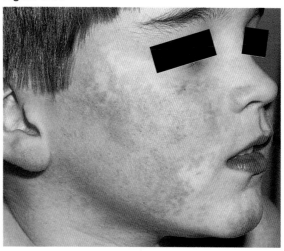

The appearance is so startling that it has been given the suggestive description of "slapped cheeks" (Figs. 5-83 and 5-84). During the second stage, the facial rash begins to fade, and a maculopapular, urticarial, or morbiliform exanthem develops on the extremities and trunk. Pruritus may be present.

Figure 5-85

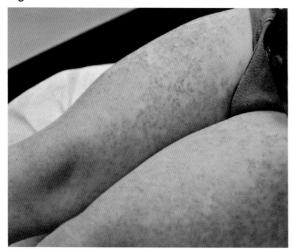

Erythema infectiosum (fifth disease) As portions of this rash fade over a period of several days, a reticular pattern emerges, mainly on the extremities, which gives the arms and legs a marbled appearance (Fig. 5-85 and 5-86). This reticular eruption, which is the third stage of the disease, may last for only 1 week, or it may last continuously or by relapses for as long as 8 weeks. Exercise and variations in temperature may make the rash appear more or less prominent. No treatment is required.

Figure 5-86

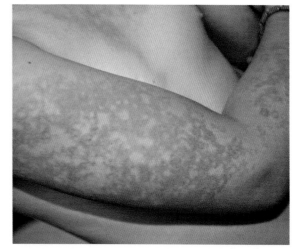

Human parvovirus B19 is also the cause of transient aplastic crisis in children with hemoglobinopathies, and of hydrops fetalis in the children of women exposed to the virus during pregnancy. In addition, adults who are exposed to children with fifth disease may acquire human parvovirus infection, and are likely to develop severe arthralgias as part of their illness. It is of note that children with fifth disease are contagious only before the occurrence of the rash.

Figure 5-87

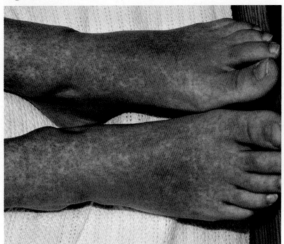

Figure 5-88

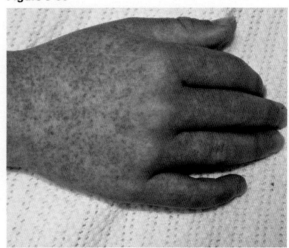

Papular purpuric sock and glove syndrome In its most characteristic form, patients develop a papular and purpuric eruption on the hands and feet, with sharp demarcation at the wrists and ankles. Other areas of involvement may include the face, buttocks, and inguinal creases.

This syndrome was originally described in conjunction with parvovirus B19 infection, but it has also been attributed to measles virus, cytomegalovirus, coxsackie virus B6, human herpesvirus 6, and hepatitis B. Systemic symptoms are rare and the condition usually resolves in 1 to 2 weeks.

Superficial Fungal Infections

Figure 6-1

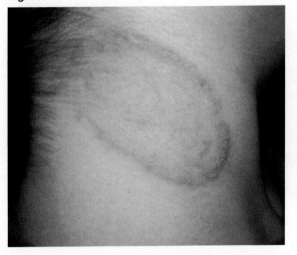

Tinea corporis Superficial fungal infections of the skin are among the most common of all pediatric dermatoses. These are illustrations of more superficial fungal infections of hairless skin. The annular lesions in Figs. 6-1 and 6-2 resulted from infection with *Trichophyton tonsurans*.

Figure 6-2

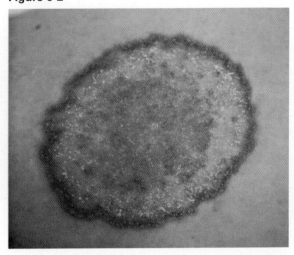

In the cases illustrated, clinical diagnosis of a superficial fungal infection is reasonably certain, and one may guess that the causative fungus is a *Microsporum* or *Trichophyton*. A potassium hydroxide preparation of a scale obtained from the edge of a lesion will identify the hyphae.

Figure 6-3

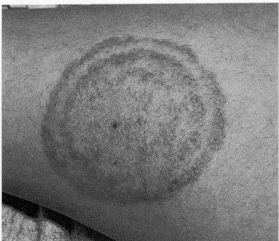

Tinea corporis In some cases, tinea corporis presents with concentric rings (Fig. 6-3). Definitive diagnosis depends on mycologic culture of the scale from a lesion. In cases of candidiasis, tinea imbricata and favus, the causative organism can frequently and confidently be guessed correctly. In general, one may say that *Microsporum canis*, *Microsporum audouinii*, *T tonsurans*, and *T schoenleinii* can infect scalp and hairless skin, and *Trichophyton rubrum* and *Candida albicans* can infect hairless skin and nails.

Figure 6-4

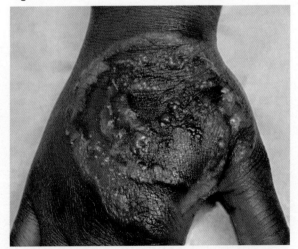

Tinea corporis-vesicular On rare occasions, a marked inflammatory response to the presence of a dermatophyte leads to a vesicular or bullous eruption. The clinical presentation seen in Fig. 6-4 must be differentiated from acute contact dermatitis, bullous impetigo, or an autoimmune blistering disease such as linear IgA dermatosis.

Figure 6-5

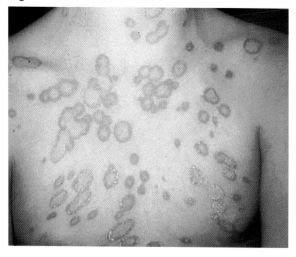

Tinea corporis The numerous scaly rings illustrated in Figs. 6-5 and 6-6 are due to *M canis*. The majority of cases result from exposure to infected cats, many of which have no symptoms of ringworm.

Figure 6-6

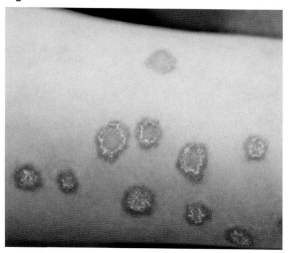

Kittens appear to have a higher frequency of infection than adult cats, and shedding of the fungus occurs more during the winter months. In addition, cats that live both outdoors and indoors appear to be more commonly infected with *M canis* than do indoor cats.

Figure 6-7

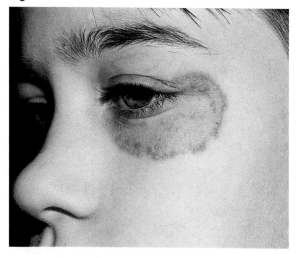

Tinea corporis (faciei) Infection at the sites shown in Fig. 6-7 may also be termed *tinea faciei*. Note the ring shape of the active periphery of the lesions in this patient.

Figure 6-8

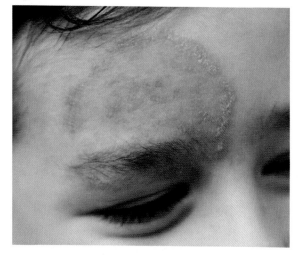

Facial lesions may be due to *T tonsurans*, *T rubrum*, or *T mentagrophytes*. Cutaneous infection with zoophilic species, such as *M canis*, may also occur on the face. As noted in Fig. 6-8, this usually results from close contact with a household pet.

Figure 6-9

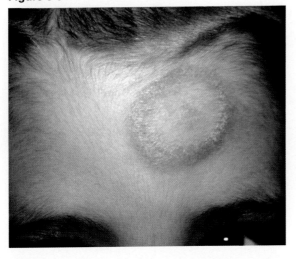

Tinea corporis (faciei) Topically applied antifungal agents, such as the azole and allylamine agents, are effective therapies. There may be temporary hyperpigmentation or hypopigmentation after successful treatment, but even severe lesions such as these resolve without scarring.

Figure 6-10

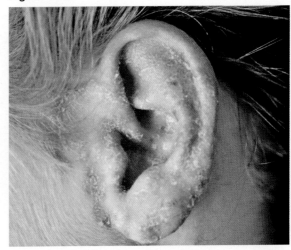

In some patients, the occurrence of fungal infection in locations such as the ear may make it difficult to appreciate the ring morphology of the lesion, and thus lead to misdiagnosis as atopic or contact dermatitis. In that situation, the application of topical steroid creams will make the infection worse.

Figure 6-11

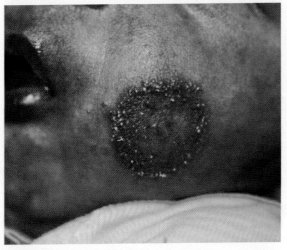

Neonatal tinea Tinea corporis can occur during the first weeks or months of life, and is sometimes misdiagnosed because the primary care provider has not considered that possibility.

Figure 6-12

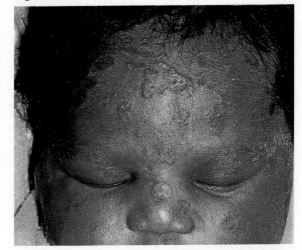

This infant developed typical arcuate lesions on the face. The child's caretaker had a fungal infection of the hand.

Figure 6-13

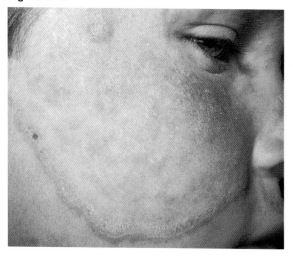

Tinea incognito This Latin term for "tinea unrecognized" refers to lesions of tinea corporis that are made worse by the application of topical corticosteroids. The areas of involvement may become unusually large and develop multiple concentric rings.

Figure 6-14

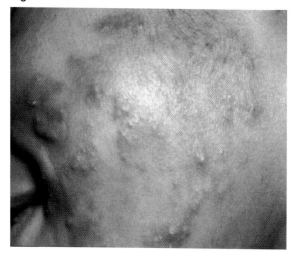

In this case of tinea incognito, the patient applied a topical corticosteroid, previously prescribed for atopic dermatitis, to an undiagnosed ringworm infection on the face. The papules and nodules develop when fungal elements penetrate the hair follicle and cause a deeper infection. This form of infection, termed *Majocchi granuloma*, may also occur on the legs of adolescent girls, where it is spread by shaving.

Figure 6-15

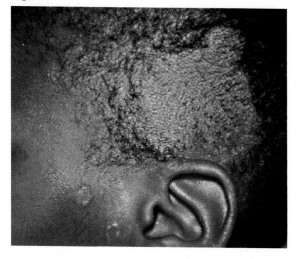

Tinea capitis Fungal infections of the scalp are extremely common in children. The diagnosis of tinea capitis should be entertained in any child in whom patches of incomplete alopecia, crusting, or scaling are found in the scalp. In previous decades, *M canis* and *M audouinii* were the most common pathogenic fungi infecting the scalp. The latter frequently causes a discrete grayish patch of hair loss, as shown in Fig. 6-16.

Figure 6-16

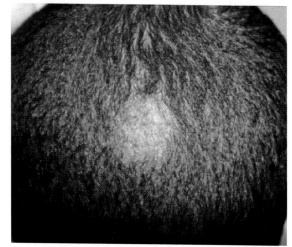

In most parts of the United States and in many other parts of the world, *T tonsurans* is now the predominant organism causing tinea capitis. In the United States, this form of tinea capitis is seen almost exclusively in African-American children. In some children, this dermatophyte causes discrete and dramatic areas of hair loss studded by the stubs of broken hair, so-called black-dot ringworm (Fig. 6-18).

Figure 6-17

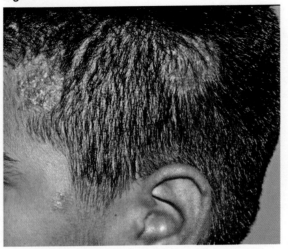

Tinea capitis Because *T tonsurans* does not fluoresce, the Wood's light is no longer of use in most cases. However, diagnosis can be confirmed by the use of either potassium hydroxide preparation or fungal culture. Pictured here is a child with significant scaling and hair loss due to infection with *T tonsurans*. There is also a small circular lesion on the facial skin. Similar lesions may develop on the back and chest and provide a clue to diagnosis.

Figure 6-18

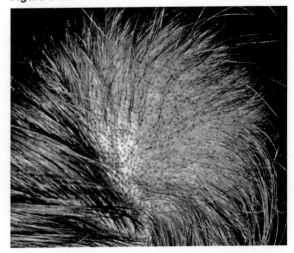

In some cases, there are only small and unimpressive patches of "seborrheic" scale with minimal hair loss or groups of small pustules. Attempts to treat tinea capitis with topical antifungal agents alone are doomed to failure. Oral griseofulvin is the most effective form of therapy. The use of selenium sulfide shampoo may be effective in preventing spread to classmates and siblings.

Figure 6-19

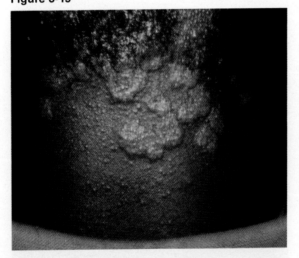

Tinea capitis Figure 6-19 shows an exuberant inflammatory response to *T tonsurans*. The lesions have spread onto the neck, but the primary source of infection is in the hair follicles in the scalp, and systemic therapy is required.

Figure 6-20

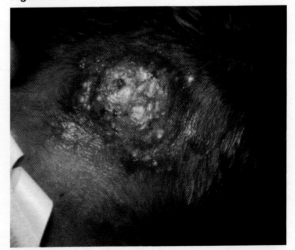

Kerion In some children, an exuberant inflammatory response to the infecting dermatophyte may occur. This boggy and tender mass is termed a *kerion*, a word that in Greek means a honeycomb, honey, or beeswax and is intended to describe the clinical appearance. Children with a kerion may also develop localized lymphadenopathy and fever. Although bacterial superinfection may sometimes occur, misdiagnosis of a kerion as a bacterial infection of the scalp is an all too common pitfall. The proper treatment is oral griseofulvin along with, in some cases, systemic therapy for the bacterial component.

Figure 6-21

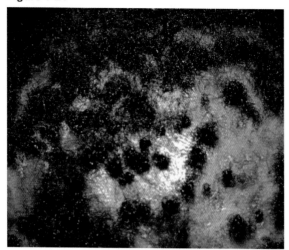

Figure 6-22

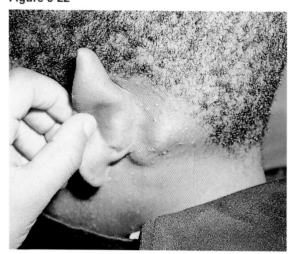

Kerion Children who develop a severe inflammatory response to infection with *T Tonsurans* may develop significant and prolonged hair loss after the condition has been adequately treated. Even in cases that are as severe as this (Fig. 6-21), it is most common for the hair to return to normal.

Id reaction to tinea Lymphadenopathy is a common occurrence in children with tinea capitis. Before treatment or shortly after starting griseofulvin for tinea capitis, some patients also develop a pruritic eruption that is a hypersensitivity reaction. These patients develop numerous fine papules, concentrated on the face, neck, trunk, and upper extremities. There is no need to discontinue the griseofulvin, for the eruption resolves in 1 to 2 weeks. Relief can be obtained with the application of low-potency topical corticosteroids. It is important to differentiate this from a true drug eruption.

Figure 6-23

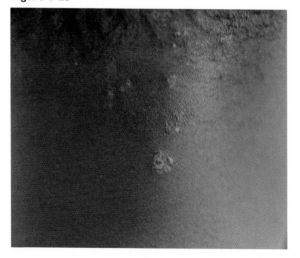

Figure 6-24

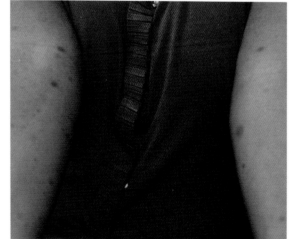

Tinea corporis secondary to scalp infection with *T tonsurans* Children with tinea capitis frequently develop small round scaly lesions on the face, upper arms, and neck, as pictured in Fig. 6-23. These can be treated with a topical antifungal medication, but the underlying scalp infection must be treated with a systemic medication. Frequent recurrences of lesions of this type provide an important clue to infection of the scalp.

It is not unusual for young family members of children with tinea capitis to also develop the same condition. Adult caregivers are likely to develop small round lesions without scalp involvement, and this can also be a clue to the diagnosis in the child. In Fig. 6-24, the patient's mother developed such lesions on the inner aspects of her arms, probably from the contact that occurred while combing her daughter's hair.

Figure 6-25

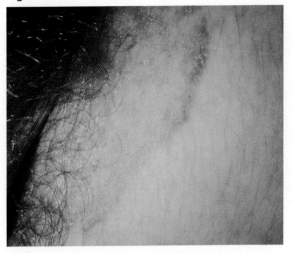

Tinea cruris The groin is a common site of acute and then enduring superficial fungal infection (Figs. 6-25 and 6-26). *Epidermophyton floccosum, T rubrum,* and *C albicans* are the most common infecting fungi. In infants, *C albicans* is the usual pathogen; in older children and adults, all are common.

Figure 6-26

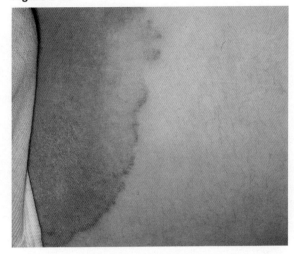

Intertriginous spaces, such as groin, axillae, and digital webs, are particularly susceptible to fungal infection because the pH of these areas is less acidic than elsewhere, temperature is higher, and humidity is greater.

Figure 6-27

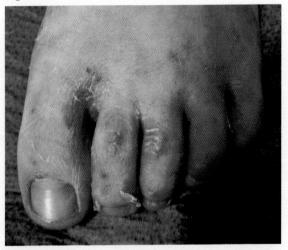

Tinea pedis Superficial fungal infection of the feet is somewhat unique because of the location. Between the toes (most commonly the fourth and fifth), the condition appears as erythema, maceration, and scaling. It is attended by itching or vague discomfort. On the sole and the lateral aspects of the feet, scattered pustules and vesicles with surrounding erythema and edema may occur. More commonly, there is persistent dry scale in a "moccasin" distribution with minimal inflammation.

Figure 6-28

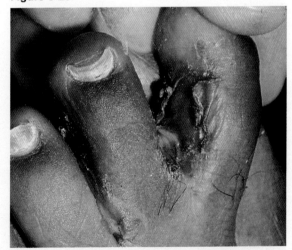

In some cases, as shown in Fig. 6-28, this may become secondarily infected. The fungi that are commonly found are *E floccosum, T mentagrophytes, T rubrum,* and *C albicans.* Fungal infections of the feet, although rare in infants and young children, must be considered when presented with erythema and scaling of the feet. More likely diagnoses with this presentation are atopic dermatitis, juvenile plantar dermatitis, and contact dermatitis.

Figure 6-29

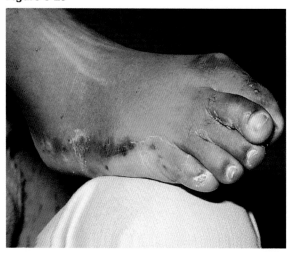

Tinea pedis Figure 6-29 shows a typical "moccasin distribution" with scaling along the side of the feet. Sweating, friction, and debris promote fungal infection. During early adolescence, there is a marked increase in the incidence of tinea pedis.

Figure 6-30

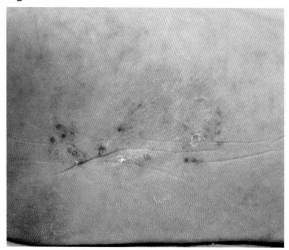

Occasionally, intensely pruritic vesicles along the side of the foot are a key to diagnosis. For most patients, the use of topical antifungal therapy, along with the wearing of sandals and light cotton socks, is an adequate therapy.

Figure 6-31

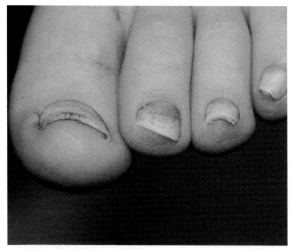

Onychomycosis Tinea unguium (fungal infection of the nails) is somewhat uncommon during childhood. After puberty, its frequency increases with age. Usually, onychomycosis is associated with tinea pedis. Fungal culture of the nails is sometimes difficult but extremely important in confirming the diagnosis. Onychomycosis is the most difficult of the superficial fungal infections to treat because the nail plate is not easily penetrated by topically applied agents. However, lacquer medications containing antifungal agents are sometimes effective.

Figure 6-32

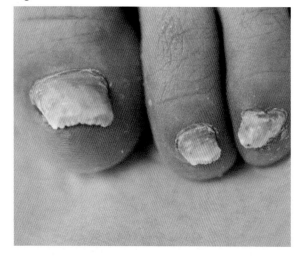

Systemic antifungal agents such as itraconazole and terbinafine are effective in the treatment of onychomycosis, but laboratory monitoring may be necessary during treatment. Figures 6-31 and 6-32 show infection with dermatophytes. Note the thickening and discoloration of nail plates in both photos. Infection by dermatophytes usually proceeds in a distal-to-proximal direction. Infection of nails by *C albicans* is different in that it is more acute (frequently purulent) and tends first to involve the lateral and proximal nail folds.

Figure 6-33

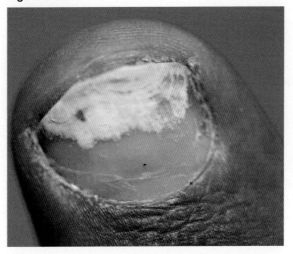

White superficial onychomycosis This relatively rare form of onychomycosis usually affects the toenails. It occurs when fungi directly invade the superficial part of the nail plate and form opaque "white islands" on the plate. As this worsens, the nails become soft and rough. The most common cause is *T mentagrophytes.*

Figure 6-34

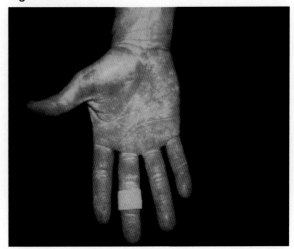

Tinea manuum Superficial fungal infection of the palms usually presents with erythema and whitish scale, predominantly in the palmar creases. It is almost always associated with tinea pedis. Generally tinea manuum involves one hand, but when both hands are involved, it is not symmetrical. The causative organism is usually *T rubrum.* The condition may be treated with either topical imidazole creams or with oral antifungals. On the dorsa of the hands, the infecting fungi are more likely to be those that cause tinea corporis elsewhere.

Figure 6-35

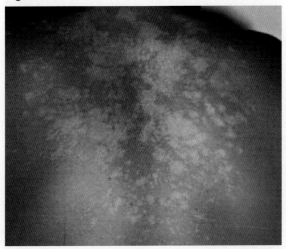

Tinea versicolor This title designates a superficial fungal infection *(tinea)* that changes color *(versicolor).* The causative organism was originally called *M furfur* and is now more commonly called *Pityrosporum orbiculare.* Tinea versicolor typically causes numerous patchy scaling macules on the upper chest and back, proximal arms, and neck.

Figure 6-36

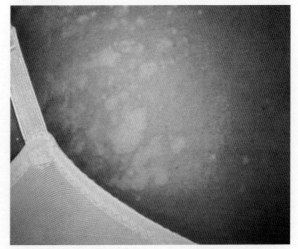

The lesions may be hypopigmented, as shown in Fig. 6-36, or brown-orange, depending on the skin color of the patient and the degree of recent sun exposure. The organism is believed to prevent either the formation of melanin or the transfer of melanosomes into keratinocytes. The formation of azelaic acid is another suggested mechanism for the resultant hypopigmentation.

Figure 6-37

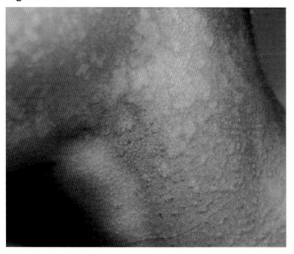

Tinea versicolor Although it is most common on the back and chest, involvement of the neck and face are often seen, especially in hot and humid environments.

Figure 6-38

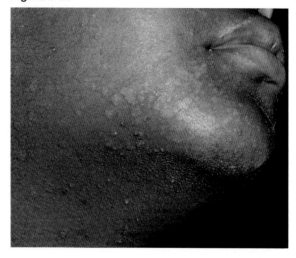

Tinea versicolor is usually asymptomatic but may itch slightly. The organism cannot be cultured, but diagnosis is aided by the orange or brown glow of lesional skin under a Wood's light and by the "spaghetti and meatballs" appearance of clustered hyphae and spores on potassium hydroxide preparation.

Figure 6-39

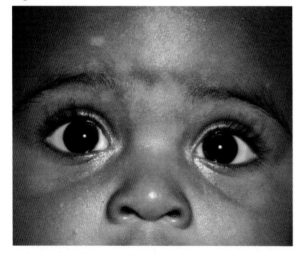

Tinea versicolor Although tinea versicolor usually makes its appearance after puberty, it can develop in childhood and facial lesions are even occasionally seen in breast-fed infants.

Figure 6-40

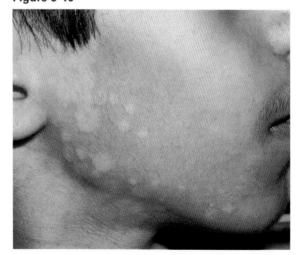

There are several approaches to the treatment of tinea versicolor. Small areas of involvement can be eradicated by the use of an imidazole cream. In patients with more extensive disease, the best approach is the use of a selenium sulfide or sodium thiosulfate lotion. Patients should be warned that treatment of tinea versicolor does not diminish the very high rate of recurrence and that the return to normal skin color may be delayed for weeks to months after the completion of therapy.

Figure 6-41

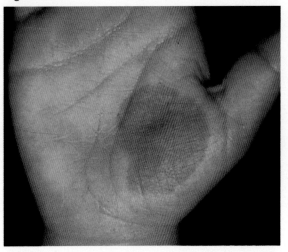

Tinea nigra This is an infection of the stratum corneum, commonly on a palm, that is caused by the dematiaceous fungus *Exophiala (Cladosporium werneckii)*. It occurs most commonly in tropical regions. The clinical appearance is a tan-to-black discoloration with sharp borders that enlarge slowly.

Figure 6-42

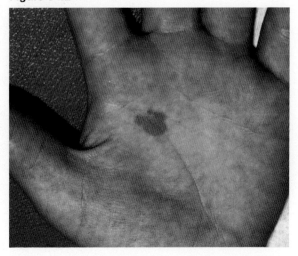

Tinea nigra can be mistaken for a melanocytic nevus, melanoma, or simple artifact. The correct diagnosis can be confirmed by potassium hydroxide examination or fungal culture. Treatment consists of a keratolytic lotion or topical imidazole cream.

Figure 6-43

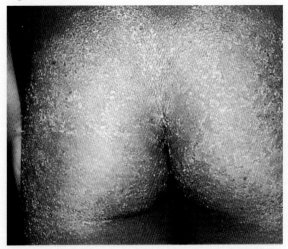

Tinea imbricata Tinea imbricata is a superficial fungal infection of the glabrous skin that is seen in a number of tropical countries. The causative organism is *T concentricum*. Brown papules evolve into annular plaques. As the infection continues, many concentric ring lesions develop, which resemble the patterning of a tortoise shell. Oral antifungals are effective therapy but relapses occur.

Figure 6-44

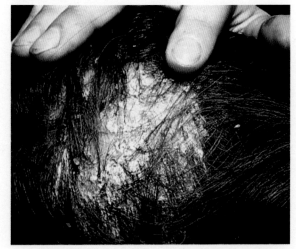

Favus This chronic form of tinea capitis is caused by *T schoenleinii*. It occurs in parts of Europe, Africa, and South America as well as in some rural areas of the United States and Canada. Pictured here are the typical scaly patches seen in favus. The yellowish cup-like crusts, called scutula, are a distinctive part of this disease. The coalescent crusts form a plaque that emits a characteristic mousy odor. This form of fungal infection of the scalp may persist into adult life.

Figure 6-45

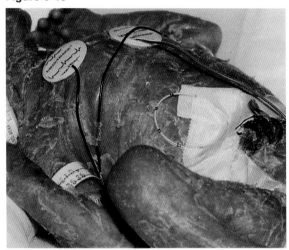

Congenital cutaneous candidiasis The presence of a generalized candidal dermatitis at birth is the result of intrauterine infection.

Figure 6-46

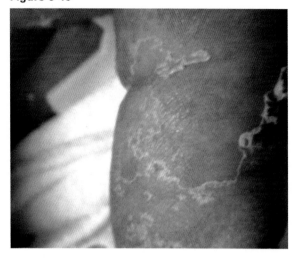

Typically, erythematous papulovesicles and macules evolve into pustules and areas of superficial desquamation over a period of 6 to 8 days.

Figure 6-47

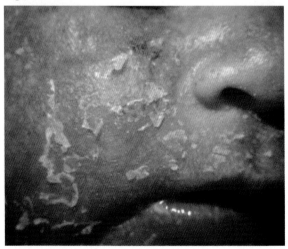

Congenital cutaneous candidiasis If congenital candidiasis involves only the skin, the disease follows a benign course. Infants with low birth weight may develop disseminated infection or respiratory distress and require systemic therapy.

Figure 6-48

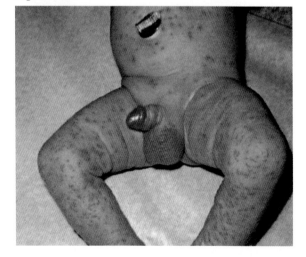

The characteristic lesions frequently involve the palms and soles and may be accompanied by paronychias and true nail involvement. In contrast to neonatal candidiasis (acquired during passage through an infected birth canal), the diaper area and oral mucosa tend to be spared.

Figure 6-49

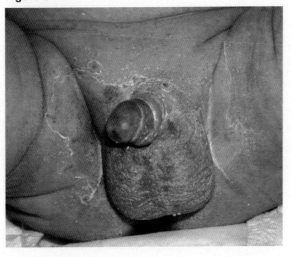

Candidiasis (moniliasis) Cutaneous infection with *C albicans* tends to occur in areas that are chronically moist, warm, and macerated. For this reason, *Candida* is among the most common causes of diaper dermatitis. Distinctive features sometimes include confluent, glistening, beefy-red erythema, and numerous small satellite lesions.

Figure 6-50

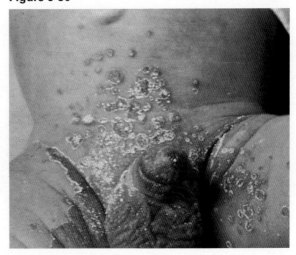

More extensive involvement is seen in Fig. 6-50; note the peripheral scaling and again the satellite lesions. On occasion, these peripheral pustules and papules will involve the entire abdomen and back. Diagnosis of cutaneous candidiasis can be confirmed by potassium hydroxide preparation or by fungal culture. Treatment consists of the use of imidazole creams, such as ketoconazole, or nystatin.

Figure 6-51

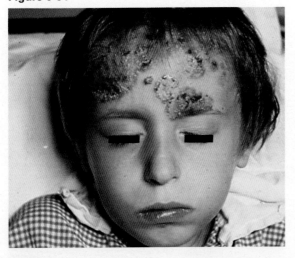

Chronic mucocutaneous candidiasis The immunologic inability to handle *C albicans* infection results in recurrent and severe infection of the mucous membranes, skin, and nails. Affected children have T-cell deficiencies due to a wide variety of underlying causes but manifest their mucocutaneous disease in similar fashion. Chronic mucocutaneous candidiasis may, in some patients, lead to granuloma formation in the areas of infection. The face is a common site for the formation of these indurated and hyperkeratotic plaques.

Figure 6-52

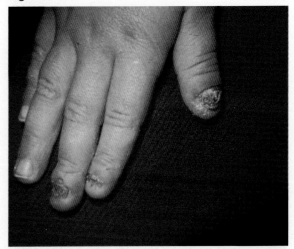

Figure 6-52 illustrates typical nail involvement in chronic mucocutaneous candidiasis. Patients develop swelling and tenderness of the proximal and lateral nail folds. Eventually, the nails become brittle and discolored and may be destroyed by the process. Chronic mucocutaneous candidiasis is sometimes part of an autoimmune polyglandular syndrome and such patients may suffer from a wide variety of endocrine abnormalities, along with vitiligo and alopecia areata.

Deep Fungal Infections

Figure 7-1

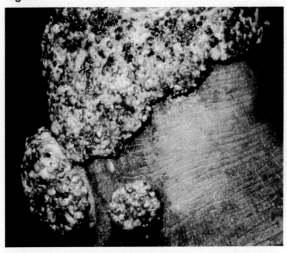

Chromoblastomycosis The granulomatous process shown in Fig. 7-1, which is variegated in color, is of 12 years' duration. It started as a small nodule, developed slowly into a verrucous mass, and acquired satellite extensions. The condition, so reminiscent of a tuberculous process, is a deep fungal infection caused by the species of *Phialophora*, *Fonsecaea*, and *Cladosporium*, which are indigenous to parts of South America and other regions with warm climates. Lesions that are too large for surgical excision are treated with combinations of systemic flucytosine, amphotericin B, and ketoconazole.

Figure 7-2

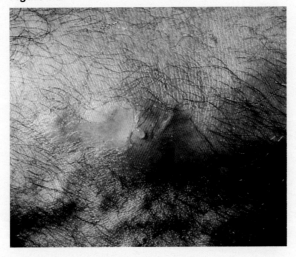

Coccidioidomycosis This disease, caused by the dimorphic fungus *Coccidioides immitis*, is endemic to the southwestern United States and parts of Central and South America. Most individuals in those areas develop the disease as an inconsequential upper-respiratory infection.

Figure 7-3

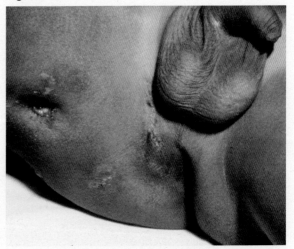

Severe disseminated disease can follow pulmonary infection and may involve the skin. In Figs. 7-2 and 7-3, the lesions are typically abscesses, nodules, or verrucous and inflammatory plaques. Primary infection of the skin, which is rare, is accompanied by regional lymphadenopathy. Amphotericin B, with or without itraconazole or fluconazole, is the customary treatment.

Figure 7-4

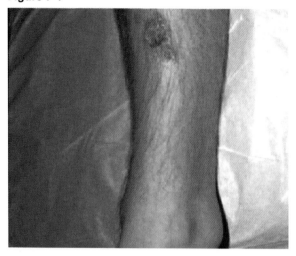

Sporotrichosis Cutaneous infection with *Sporothrix schenckii* is a disease with worldwide distribution. The majority of cases are seen in Central and South America but outbreaks occur in the United States. The disease affects both children and adults and occurs when the causative fungus, in either contaminated soil or plant materials, contacts traumatized skin.

Figure 7-5

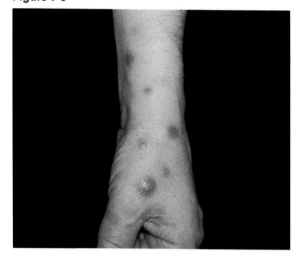

The thorn of a rose bush may provide both the organism and a site of entry, and there have been outbreaks among children playing among bales of hay. Pictured here is the most common form of sporotrichosis, the lymphocutaneous type. It causes an ulcerated lesion at the site of inoculation (Fig. 7-4) and a string of nodules or ulcerations along the lines of lymphatic drainage (Fig. 7-5).

Figure 7-6

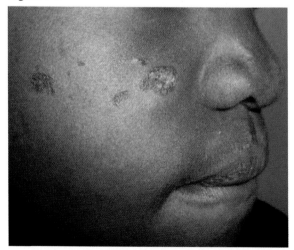

Sporotrichosis This is an example of fixed cutaneous sporotrichosis on the face. Lesions of this type are usually attributed to exposure during outdoor play. Specifically, acquisition of *S schenckii* has been attributed to playing in bales of hay or in sphagnum moss. Transmission from a cat has also been described.

Figure 7-7

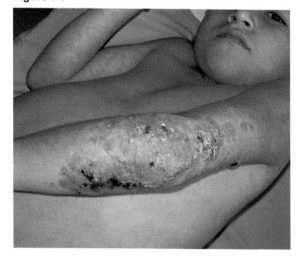

These tender secondary lesions may become chronic and extend into subcutaneous tissues. Very rarely, and especially in the immunocompromised host, disseminated or systemic sporotrichosis follows cutaneous infection. Diagnosis of sporotrichosis can be confirmed by culture of exudate or tissue from the skin lesions on Sabouraud agar.

Figure 7-8

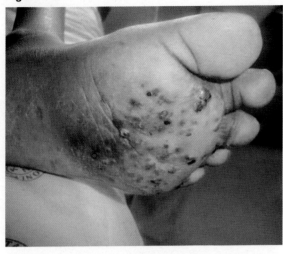

Mycetoma Also known as Madura foot, this is a chronic gran-ulomatous infection which results in swelling, discharge, and an exudate that contains characteristic grains. It is most com-mon in India and Africa, and is also seen in Brazil, Mexico, and Venezuela.

Figure 7-9

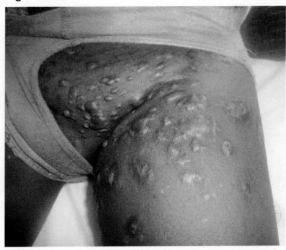

Mycetoma caused by microaerophilic actinomycetes (such as *Nocardia* and *Streptomyces*) is referred to as actinomycetoma. Mycetoma that is caused by true fungi (*Fusarium, Exophiala, Madurella,* and others) is called eumycetoma. The choice of treatment depends on the cultured organism, and lesions often resolve with scarring, as shown in Fig. 7-9.

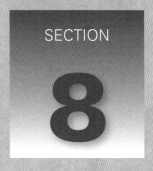

SECTION

8

Bites and Infestations

Figure 8-1

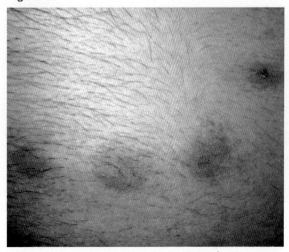

Figure 8-2

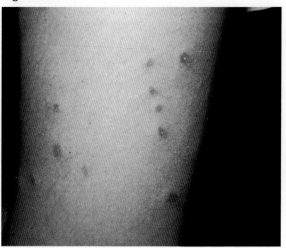

Insect "bites" Many effects of metazoal parasitism are attributed to bites. Some metazoa (insects in a loose sense) do indeed bite, and others sting, but what we frequently designate as insect bite is attachment for feeding. The result of such attachment looks like a bite and is sooner or later attended by pain, itching, or stinging. True bites and stings, however, are instantly painful; many have immediate or late, more baleful effects; and most are generally inflicted in self-defense or seemingly wanton offense, not for feeding.

Attachment for feeding is parasitism that may be silent for a while and then variably symptomatic. In a given region, common indigenous metazoa that cause cutaneous effects by a bite, sting, or attachment for feeding may be recognized or guessed from signs and symptoms. These two illustrations are representative. Figure 8-1 may be guessed with reasonable correctness to be mosquito "bites," and Fig. 8-2, clustered on the lower leg and ankle, to be flea bites. Because different family members may have different degrees of sensitivity, it is possible that only one or several in the household will develop these lesions, and others will be spared.

Figure 8-3

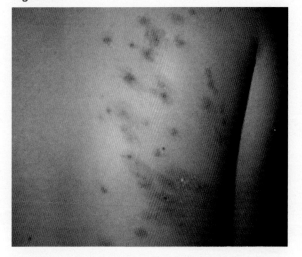

Figure 8-4

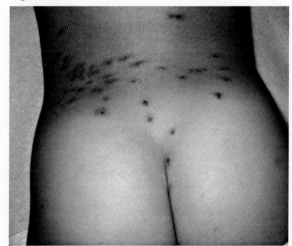

Insect "bites" The location of bites gives important clues to the causative insects. Those pictured in Figs. 8-3 and 8-4 are unlikely to be from mosquitoes (which tend to bite on exposed areas of skin) or fleas (which tend to bite the ankles and lower legs). A variety of crawling insects and mites can cause lesions of this sort, including chiggers.

Chigger bites are caused by trombiculid mites. These mites live in tall grasses and weeds and are most active in summer and fall. They attach to the skin as one walks by and brushes up against the vegetation. Lesions tend to occur in areas that are warmer, moister, or covered by tight clothing. The intense itching may last for several days.

Figure 8-5

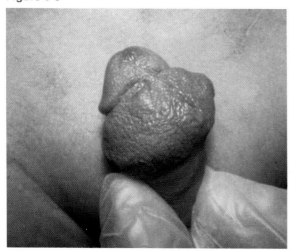

Insect "bites" Certain insects creep under clothes and bite when they reach a point of restriction such as a sock or belt. Figure 8-5 shows bite marks and vast edema on the penis. The assaulting insect may have been an ordinary one that merely took advantage of a child left undressed and unguarded.

Figure 8-6

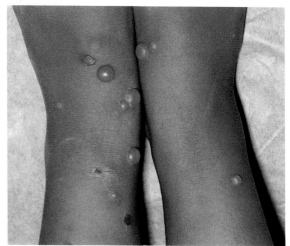

When a subject has been bitten, stung, or fed upon, the consequent lesion may be typical at the time and in its course to resolution or may be modified by scratching, secondary infection, or idiosyncratic host response. In the case of the mosquito, the lesions may be one, few, or many, depending on the insensitivity, foolhardiness, or defenselessness of the subject assailed.

Figure 8-7

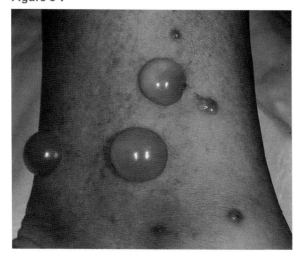

Insect "bites" The vesicular lesions in Fig. 8-6 and the bullous lesions in Fig. 8-7 are evidence of a strong hypersensitivity reaction to the offending insect.

Figure 8-8

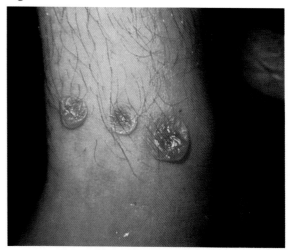

Dermatitis caused by the common carpet beetle The common carpet beetle is not common in modern well-sanitized homes, and even where it is abundant, effects from it are not common. Nevertheless, on occasion, the crawl of the insect on an unwary individual leaves its marks as wheals, papulovesicles, or bullae. Figure 8-8 shows just such an event in the form of large, flaccid blisters. The three lesions in a line record the walk of a creature and the deposition of its irritant principle.

Figure 8-9

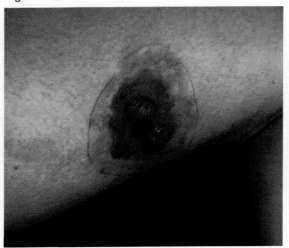

Spider bites Spiders, timid creatures for all their fierce looks, would rather entertain insects in their parlors than attack humans. The tarantula is more dangerous in fable than in fact. Two spiders can deliver painful bites and serious veneration if frightened or cornered: the black widow spider *(Latrodectus mactans)* and the brown recluse spider *(Loxosceles reclusa)*. The bite of the latter is illustrated in Fig. 8-9. It is a hemorrhagic bleb; in time it will become a necrotic ulcer. The patient will be severely sickened.

Figure 8-10

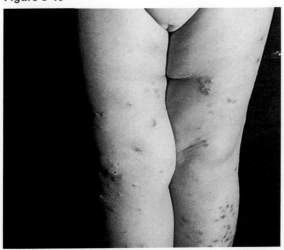

Papular urticaria This is a pruritic dermatosis that is causally related to bites by mosquitoes, fleas, or other insects. Children with this common disorder tend to have recurrent episodes during the spring and summer months. The lesions consist of firm erythematous papules, sometimes with surrounding wheals. They favor exposed areas, especially the anterior lower extremities and lower arms. The individual papules are often excoriated and are sometimes impetiginized.

Figure 8-11

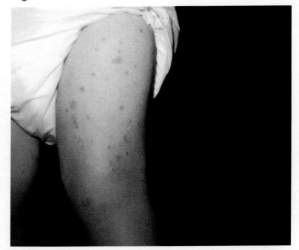

The lesions tend to last for several days to weeks but will persist longer if chronically scratched or rubbed. Papular urticaria is more common among children with atopic diathesis and represents a hypersensitivity reaction to the assaulting arthropod. Treatment consists of lotions, topical steroids, and antihistamines. The elimination of the offending insect from the household environment is helpful but will not prevent encounters during outdoor play.

Figure 8-12

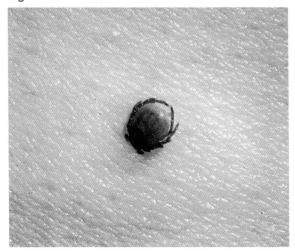

Figure 8-13

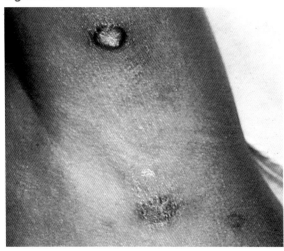

Ticks Figure 8-12 shows an engorged deer tick attached to its human host. Ticks of the *Ixodes* species are vectors of Lyme disease as well as hemorrhagic fevers and viral encephalitis. Most tick bites are not painful and therefore may go unnoticed by patients for variable periods of time. A tick bite may appear as a red papule or may progress to erythema with local swelling, blistering, or ecchymosis. Chronic tick bite granulomas can develop and last for months to years.

Tick "bite" Tick infestation occurs when the female soft or hard tick inserts her proboscis into the skin in order to withdraw blood. The site of attachment may develop into an erythematous nodule, and persistent pruritus may result if tick parts are left within the skin. Although most tick bites are insignificant, these insects are the vectors of tick bite fever, Rocky Mountain spotted fever (Figs. 4-34 and 4-35) and erythema chronicum migrans (Lyme disease) (Figs. 4-8 to 4-11).

Figure 8-14

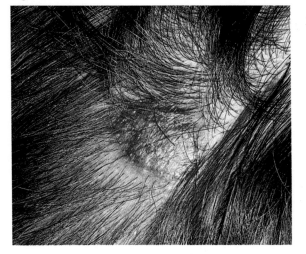

Tick bite granuloma Sometimes at the site of a tick bite, a persistent firm papulonodular lesion may develop. A common site for this reaction to develop is in the scalp. This area may be very pruritic and with excoriation may result in secondary infection.

Figure 8-15

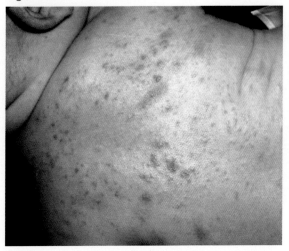

Scabies Infection of the skin by the human scabies mite *(Sarcoptes scabiei* var. *hominis)* is an extremely common skin disease of childhood. Figure 8-15 shows a child with multiple intensely pruritic lesions on the trunk. Examination of adult family members for lesions in the finger webs, waist line, and wrists provide a clue to the diagnosis in the child.

Figure 8-16

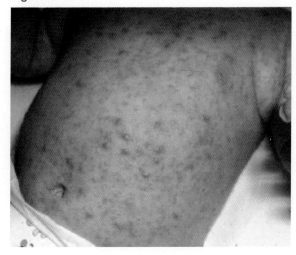

Figure 8-16 shows another severe case of scabies. The infant with scabies illustrated here has numerous excoriated papules and a diffuse eczematous dermatitis. In infants, scabies frequently involves the entire cutaneous surface including the face and scalp. Young infants without apparent pruritus may manifest extreme irritability.

Figure 8-17

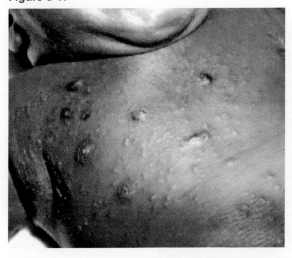

Scabies Inflammatory nodular lesions involving the axillae and the diaper area are particularly typical of scabies in the very young child. These lesions may coexist with burrows, papules, vesicles, pustules, and areas of crusting.

Figure 8-18

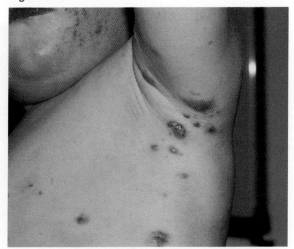

The nodules may persist for quite some time after the infestation is treated with a medication such as topical permethrin, and their presence does not reflect a persistent infestation. If no new lesions are developing, the persistent nodules can be treated with topical corticosteroids.

Figure 8-19

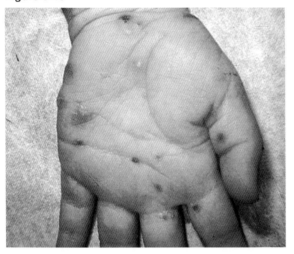

Scabies The location of primary lesions is often helpful in establishing the diagnosis of scabies. In young children, the palms and soles are sites of predilection. In older children and adolescents, the most common sites for the intensely pruritic lesions are the anterior axillary lines, the inner aspect of the upper arm, the areolae, the penis, the wrists and interdigital webs, and the ankles (Figs. 8-19 to 8-21).

Figure 8-20

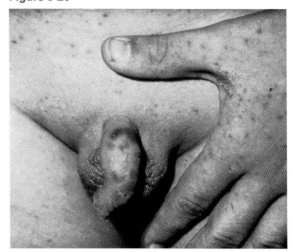

The preferred treatment of scabies is a single overnight application of a 5 percent permethrin cream, repeated 1 week later. The application of any scabicide must be accompanied by a thorough laundering of all recently worn clothing and of bed linen, which may still contain mites or eggs. All close contacts should be treated.

Figure 8-21

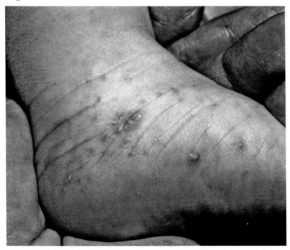

Scabies Figure 8-21 illustrates the presence of numerous papulovesicular lesions on the sides of the feet in a child with scabies.

Figure 8-22

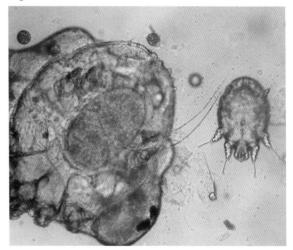

Figure 8-22 shows a scabies mite. The mite has an ovoid body with four pairs of short legs. Eggs and feces (scybala) are deposited in the burrows by the female mite, and it is common to find all or some of these elements in a scraping of a burrow.

Figure 8-23

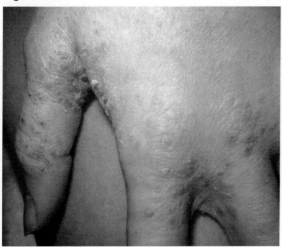

Scabies Children and adolescents often develop lesions on the dorsum of the hands and between the fingers. This is an area where burrows are commonly seen.

Figure 8-24

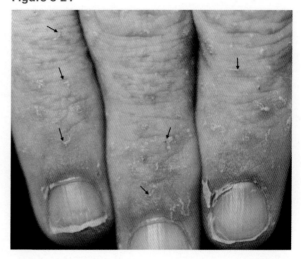

Figure 8-24 illustrates numerous burrows on the dorsal fingers. The black arrows are only pointing to a few of the burrows that are present.

Figure 8-25

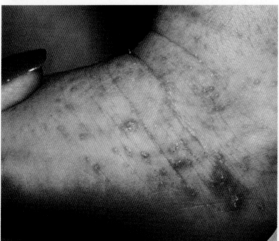

Scabies Figure 8-25 illustrates burrows that are diagnostic of scabies. Burrows are represented by slightly raised white to light-brown linear lesions. The superficial part of the burrow has a scaly appearance, and at the distal end there may be a tiny black dot representing the mite, eggs, and/or fecal material (scybala) in a small vesicle.

Figure 8-26

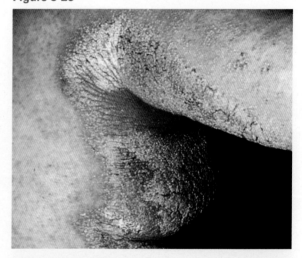

Scabies This is a photograph of what is called crusted or Norwegian scabies. Individuals with this form of disease develop thick areas of heavy crusting. Favored locations for the hyperkeratotic plaques include the elbows, knees, scalp, and buttocks. Norwegian scabies occurs most commonly in patients with Down syndrome and among those who are debilitated or who suffer from an immune deficiency. In crusted scabies, the areas of involvement contain numerous mites, and therefore the disease is highly contagious.

Figure 8-27

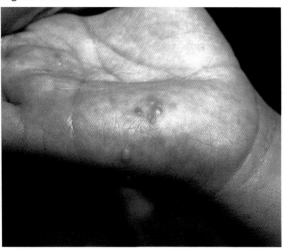

Postscabetic acropustulosis Infants and children who are successfully treated for scabies may subsequently develop recurrent crops of intensely pruritic papules and pustules on the hands and feet. If persistent scabies infestation has been ruled out, this form of id reaction should be treated with topical corticosteroids. This persistent dermatitis appears to be most common in developing countries, and also in the context of international adoption.

Figure 8-28

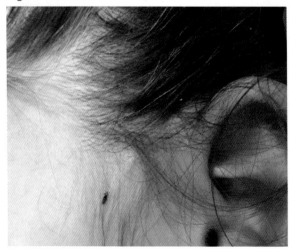

Pediculosis capitis (head lice) The head louse is a wingless six-legged insect that is the smallest of the three human lice. It is adapted to live in the hair of the scalp only and lives by feeding on blood. The female louse lays approximately four eggs per day and has a life span of 2 to 4 weeks.

Figure 8-29

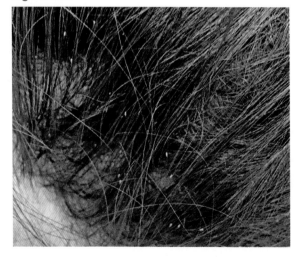

It uses a gluey substance to attach the egg cases or nits to the hair. Note the live louse in Fig. 8-28 with some nits in the scalp above the ear. Numerous nits are noted in the occipital scalp in Fig. 8-29.

Figure 8-30

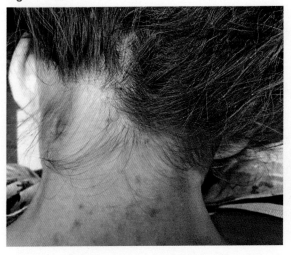

Pediculosis capitis (head lice) The diagnosis of pediculosis capitis is suggested by the presence of itching in the posterior scalp or signs of redness, a papular eruption as noted in Fig. 8-30, or folliculitis at the nape of the neck. Note the numerous nits in the scalp above the papular neck eruption.

Figure 8-31

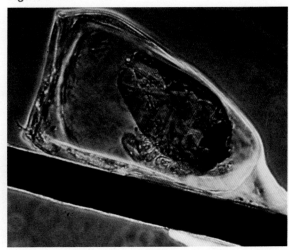

The diagnosis of head lice is confirmed by the presence of nits, which, even when sparse, are easily recognized with hand-lens magnification. The nit can be recognized by examining an infested hair under the microscope; a close-up is shown in Fig. 8-31.

Figure 8-32

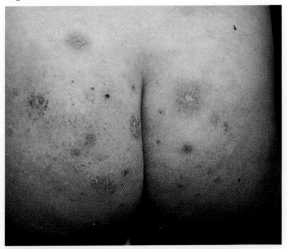

Pediculosis corporis The body louse belongs to the genus *Pediculus*; it is larger and broader than the head louse. While the head louse infests the skin of the scalp, the body louse does not live on the body. It lives in the seams of undergarments and comes onto the body only to feed. Clinically, one sees marks of feeding and excoriations; the lice themselves can be found in the clothes. Treatment consists of disinfestation of clothing and bedding and the application of a pediculicide to the patient.

Figure 8-33

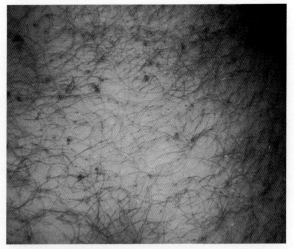

Pediculosis pubis The pubic louse *(Phthirus pubis)* is aptly called the crab louse. Examined under the microscope, this insect is broad like a crab and has legs that look like claws. On the skin, the louse looks like a brown fleck and may be mistaken for a freckle. Nits are also easily seen grossly and better by hand-lens magnification. Figure 8-33 is a good representation. Infestation may also occur in the eyelashes and axillary hair.

Figure 8-34

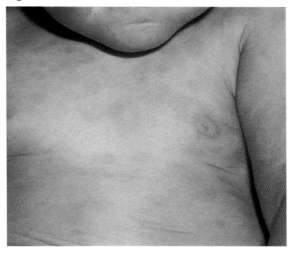

Macula ceruleae These bluish macules are the result of the bite of *Pthirus pubis*, the pubic or crab louse. Most likely, the color results from an anticoagulant that is contained in the saliva of the organism. In sexually active adolescents, pubic lice may probably be acquired from an infested partner. Young children may acquire this infestation from innocent contact with an affected adult, but the possibility of sexual abuse should also be considered.

Figure 8-35

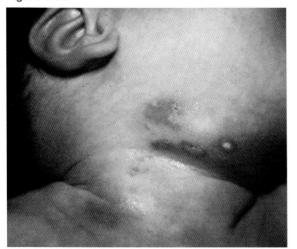

Myiasis The term for infestation with the larvae of flies is pronounced mī'yĕ-sĭs or mī-ī' ĕ-sĭs. In this condition, flies deposit fertilized ova upon neglected wounds or under onycholytic nails. The infestation is usually a sign of poor hygiene. *Dermatobia hominis, Wohlfahrtia vigil*, and several other species of botflies and warble flies may foster their young in this way. Antibiotics may be needed to treat secondary infection.

Figure 8-36

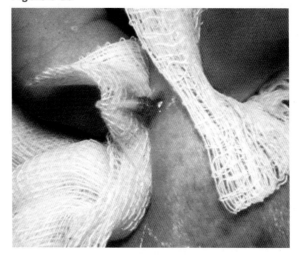

Figure 8-35 shows a cutaneous lesion but does not reveal the larvae, which can be better seen in movement in vivo by the naked eye. Figure 8-36 shows a larva clearly. In most cases, the larvae can be easily removed mechanically under local anesthesia.

Figure 8-37

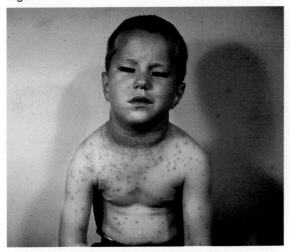

Caterpillar dermatitis The hair of caterpillars and moths may produce pruritic or painful inflammatory skin lesions. The puss caterpillar and the brown-tail moth are the most common offenders. The toxin on the spines and hair of these insects causes an irritant dermatitis. The resultant lesions, which are sometimes seen in linear array, may be papular or urticarial and are accompanied by itching or stinging. Systemic symptoms are rare but may occur. The hair may be seen microscopically in skin scrapings. Treatment is purely symptomatic.

Figure 8-38

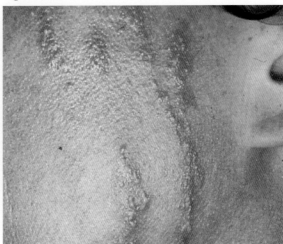

Dermatitis caused by blister beetles There are several species of beetles (order Coleoptera) that secrete cantharidin or some other vesicant substance onto their bodies. The crawl of the so-called blister beetles smears their irritant substances on the skin, causing the edema and blistering illustrated in Fig. 8-38. Treatment with cool compresses and topical antibiotics to prevent superinfection is usually adequate.

Figure 8-39

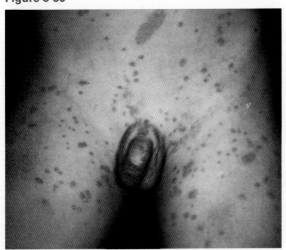

Seabather's eruption This eruption is an acute, pruritic dermatitis that occurs under covered areas after one bathes in seawater. Pruritus begins shortly after leaving the water, with the subsequent development of erythematous macules, papules, or urticarial lesions. Children may present with fever and chills. These intensely itchy lesions tend to resolve spontaneously over a period of 1 to 2 weeks. Recent reports have linked this eruption to the larvae of the phylum Cnidaria, which comprises jellyfish, corals, hydroids, and sea anemones.

Figure 8-40

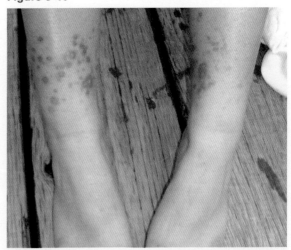

Swimmer's itch This is an acute dermatitis produced by the cercarial forms of schistosomes and primarily occurs in uncovered areas of the body. When occurring on the ankles, this is sometimes called "clamdigger's itch." The eruption may be acquired in fresh water or saltwater. Like any intensely pruritic condition, excoriations and secondary infection are complications. Treatment consists of antipruritics and antibiotics when superinfection occurs.

Figure 8-41

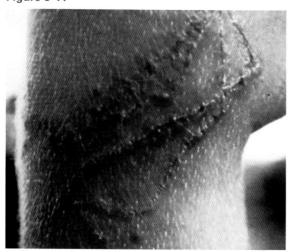

Figure 8-42

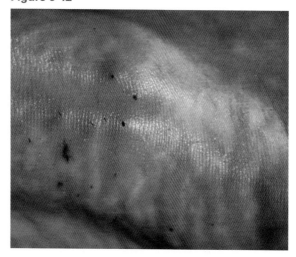

The sting of the Portuguese man-of-war One of the most painful effects on skin is the consequence of attack by oceanic hydrozoans known as Portuguese men-of-war, which are amazing for their size, brilliant color, and power to induce whealing. They have a small float that buoys them up and from which hang long tentacles. The wrap of these tentacles results in linear stripes, which look like whiplashes, caused not by the force of their swing but from deposition of urticariogenic and irritant substances.

The effect of contact with a sea urchin Sea urchins are a gastronomic delight when prepared properly, but a cutaneous torture when stepped on unprepared. The echinoids have spines that in some species are several inches long. Driven into skin when one steps or falls on or brushes against the creatures, the hard spines break and lodge in skin. Pain is inevitable, and secondary infection is nearly inevitable if they are left in (Fig. 8-42). Nothing but tedious and meticulous extraction of every one of dozens, possibly scores, of spines is required for relief.

Figure 8-43

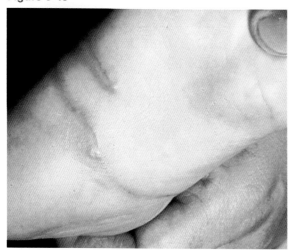

Figure 8-44

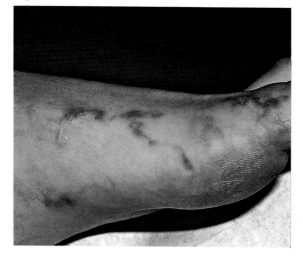

Larva migrans (creeping eruption) Infestation of the skin with larvae of certain helminths, notably *Ancylostoma braziliense*, is common on the southern coast of the United States as well as in some other parts of the world. Helminths such as *A braziliense* infest the intestines of animals, particularly the dog, whose excreta contain larvae that have remarkable capacity to enter the unbroken skin.

Attaining the interior just below the stratum corneum, the immature forms move in a serpentine, erratic way, creating long channels. The larvae are sometimes barely discernible at the ends of the channels in the direction of travel. The feet, buttocks, arms, hands, and back are the common sites of lodgment and lesions. Treatment consists of a topical application of thiabendazole.

Figure 8-45

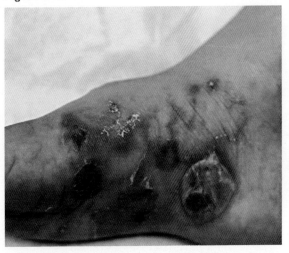

Larva migrans (creeping eruption) Figure 8-45 illustrates the typical linear lesions, along with vesicles and bullae.

Figure 8-46

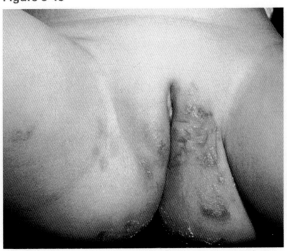

These characteristic linear lesions, shown in Fig. 8-46, on the buttocks and labia occurred in an infant who was unwittingly placed on a contaminated beach or lawn.

Figure 8-47

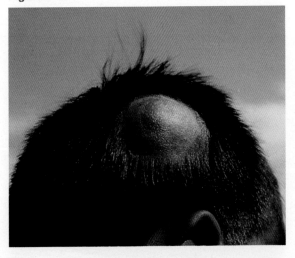

Onchocerciasis *Onchocerca volvulus*, such as *Tunga penetrans, Dracunculus medinensis, Wuchereria bancrofti*, and *Loa loa*, is limited to parts of the developing world. All these metazoa infest deeply and are difficult to eradicate. The filarial elephantiasis caused by *W bancrofti*, the edema (Calabar swellings) around the eyes caused by the "African eye worm" *(Loa loa)*, and the interdigital nodule, usually between toes, that harbors yards of the guinea worm *(D medinensis)* are endemic to varying regions of Africa, South America, and Asia.

Figure 8-48

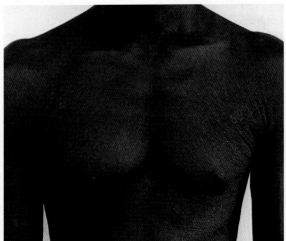

Onchocerciasis is seen commonly in parts of Mexico. The metazoan that causes this disease is often found in the scalp and around the eyes where infection may have serious consequences. Figure 8-47 is a lumpy lesion on the scalp caused by the adult worm. Figure 8-48 shows less discernible lesions on the chest. These are caused by the organism in its microfilarial phase.

Atopic Dermatitis

Figure 9-1

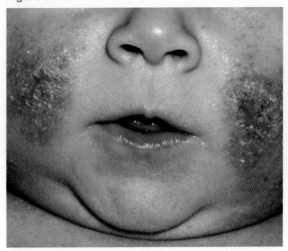

Atopic dermatitis This condition is the most common of all pediatric dermatoses. For the majority of patients, the onset occurs during infancy. The classic facial appearance in this age group is illustrated in Figs. 9-1 through 9-4.

Figure 9-2

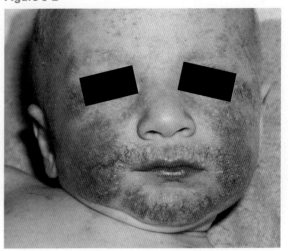

There are symmetrical patches of erythema, exudation, and scale involving the cheeks and chin. It is not unusual also to see widespread involvement of the trunk and extensor extremities during infancy; the diaper area is most often spared.

Figure 9-3

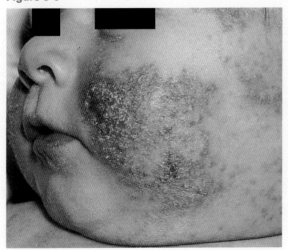

Atopic dermatitis Pruritus is a cardinal feature of atopic dermatitis and may be evidenced in the infant by irritability, scratching, and rubbing against nearby objects.

Figure 9-4

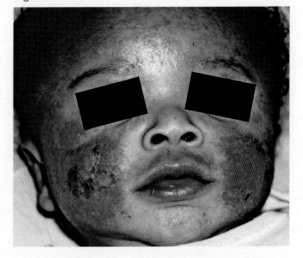

Atopic dermatitis is an inherited disorder. Children with the disease most often have a family history of the atopic diathesis (atopic dermatitis, asthma, or allergic rhinitis) and may themselves manifest asthma or allergic respiratory disease.

Figure 9-5

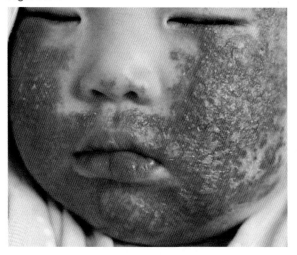

Atopic dermatitis Figure 9-5 shows a severe case of atopic dermatitis with early evidence of impetiginization.

Figure 9-6

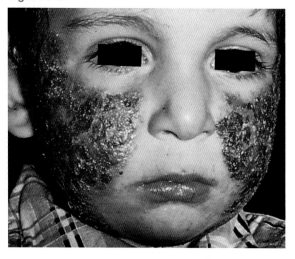

Figure 9-6 shows a similar distribution in an older child. In this case, also, impetiginization may be contributing to the crusted appearance of the lesions.

Figure 9-7

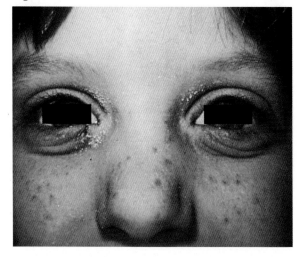

Atopic dermatitis When the diagnosis of atopic dermatitis is in doubt, the search for associated clinical findings is often helpful. The Dennie-Morgan line is a double fold under the eye, which is seen in many children with atopic dermatitis.

Figure 9-8

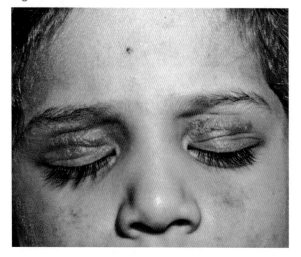

Pictured here is another child with periocular involvement. Children who suffer from seasonal allergies with associated conjunctivitis and itching may have worsening of the erythema, scale, and lichenification around the eyes during "allergy season".

Figure 9-9

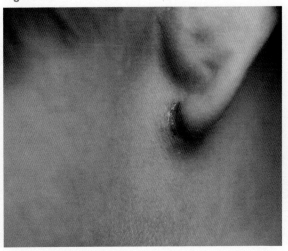

Atopic Dermatitis Figure 9-9 shows another telltale sign: a fissure at the junction of the pinna of the ear and the face. Other associated findings related to atopic dermatitis include lichen spinulosus (Fig. 9-23), pityriasis alba (Figs. 9-24 and 9-25), ichthyosis vulgaris (Figs. 15-1 to 15-4), and keratosis pilaris (Figs. 15-63 and 15-64). Children with atopic dermatitis are also frequently noted to have hyperlinear palms and soles. Keratoconjunctivitis and cataracts may occur in the child with atopic dermatitis.

Figure 9-10

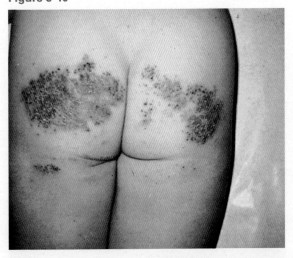

Atopic dermatitis During childhood, the most common locations of atopic dermatitis are the antecubital and popliteal fossae and the posterior neck. Figures 9-10 and 9-11 show children in whom the involvement is more widespread. The lesions show the characteristic erythema, oozing, and crusting of acute atopic dermatitis.

Figure 9-11

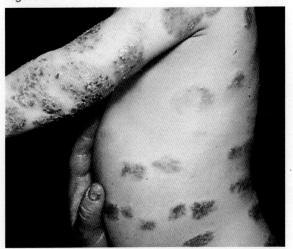

The exact pathogenesis of atopic dermatitis remains a mystery. Patients with the disease seem to have altered autonomic function and increased plasma histamine levels. Many have elevated levels of IgE, but some are completely normal in this respect. However, none of these observations has yet provided a basis for understanding the chronic and recurrent skin lesions of atopic dermatitis. An inherited abnormality in filaggrin expression affects barrier function and seems to be associated with this disease in some children.

Figure 9-12

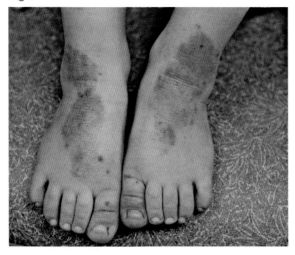

Figure 9-13

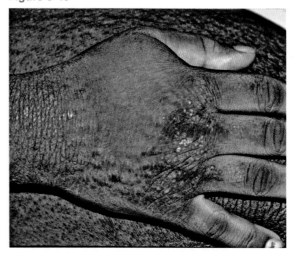

Atopic dermatitis Figures 9-12 and 9-13 are illustrations of atopic dermatitis on the dorsum of the feet and the hand. These are among the common sites of involvement in somewhat older children. The majority of children with atopic dermatitis experience improvement of their disease and many have normal skin as adults. However, the severe pruritus and the unpleasant appearance of the skin that accompany the exacerbations of this condition can be extremely troubling to the parent and child alike.

Food allergies sometimes play a role in severe eczema in infants. The role of diet in the treatment of atopic dermatitis in older children remains controversial. Despite evidence that some children with atopic dermatitis display a significant histamine response to some foods, it is fair to say that the majority of children with the disease do not respond to modifications of their diet. However, any foods that cause an obvious worsening of the condition should be avoided. Occasionally, food allergy in the atopic child may even be manifested by the rapid evolution of contact urticaria on the face and hands.

Figure 9-14

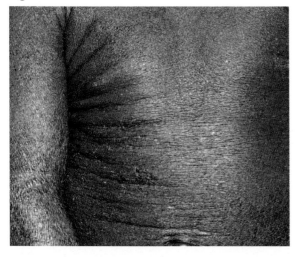

Figure 9-15

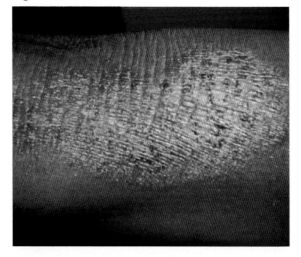

Atopic dermatitis Figures 9-14 and 9-15 illustrate skin that is scaly and lichenified. The treatment of atopic dermatitis should include the establishment of a routine of skin care that maintains adequate hydration of the skin.

Parents should be encouraged to apply a lubricating ointment to the child's skin several times a day. Topical corticosteroid ointments are currently the mainstay of medical management. Many children do well with proper use of the milder, nonfluorinated ointments, but some require stronger preparations for brief periods of time.

Figure 9-16

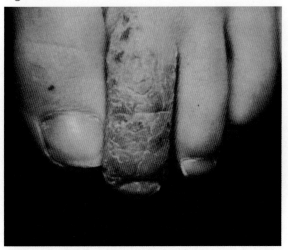

Figure 9-17

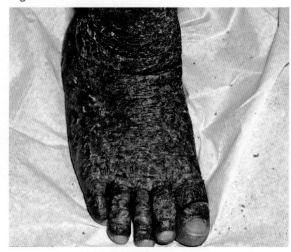

Atopic dermatitis Figure 9-16 shows atopic dermatitis involving one toe. Figure 9-17 shows scaling and lichenification of the entire foot and ankle flexure. The dangers of local atrophy and stria formation and of systemic absorption must be considered carefully with the use of the stronger topical corticosteroids. Important adjuncts to therapy include topical calcineurin inhibitors, oral antihistamines and, occasionally, a brief course of oral antibiotics to reduce skin colonization with *Streptococcus* and *Staphylococcus*.

Important adjuncts to therapy include topical calcineurin inhibitors (tacrolimus and pimecrolimus), oral antihistamines, and, occasionally, a brief course of oral antibiotics to reduce skin colonization with *Streptococcus* and *Staphylococcus*. Very rarely, children with extremely severe disease require systemic therapy with drugs such as methotrexate, cyclosporine and azathioprine.

Figure 9-18

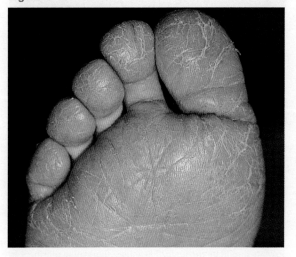

Figure 9-19

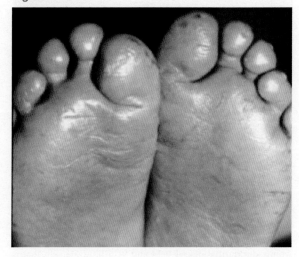

Juvenile plantar dermatosis Figures 9-18 and 9-19 show erythema and fissuring on the weight-bearing surface of the foot. This disorder, which tends to be worse in the winter months, is called *juvenile plantar dermatosis*. It is much more common in children with atopic dermatitis.

Juvenile plantar dermatitis, which has also been called *wet-dry foot syndrome*, is caused by excessive sweating of the feet in occlusive footwear and rapid drying in a low-humidity environment. The use of emollient ointments is extremely helpful.

Figure 9-20

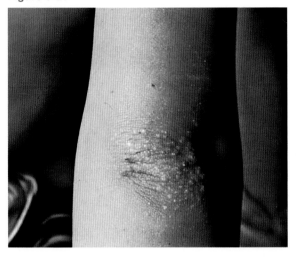

Figure 9-21

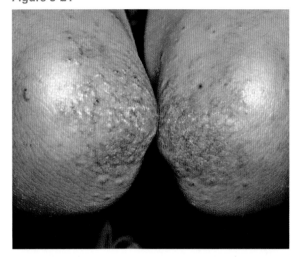

Frictional lichenoid dermatitis Figures 9-20 and 9-21 illustrate fine, erythematous, and flesh-colored papules on the elbows. This pruritic eruption, also termed as *summer prurigo* or *summertime pityriasis,* occurs most commonly but not exclusively in children with the atopic diathesis.

The rash is seen most frequently between the ages of 4 and 10 years and tends to recur seasonally in the late spring or early summer. Some children also have lesions on the knees and dorsa of the hands. Children with allergic contact dermatitis from nickel may develop a very similar rash as an id reaction.

Figure 9-22

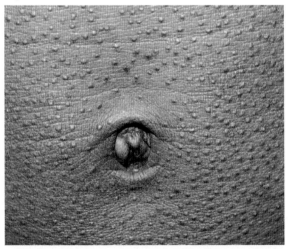

Figure 9-23

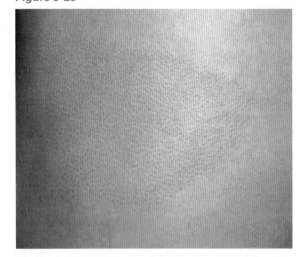

Atopic dermatitis with follicular accentuation In children with skin of color, it is common for atopic dermatitis to present as clusters of small papules located at each of the vellus hair follicles. This form of eczema is also pruritic, and treatment for this condition is the same as for other causes of eczema.

Lichen spinulosus This condition consists of a small aggregation of keratotic papules at the openings of the hair follicles. The follicular hyperkeratosis is so marked that the involved area has an appreciable spiny texture, but the areas do not itch (Fig. 9-23). The typical circular or oval plaque is present in Fig. 9-23. Lichen spinulosus is probably most common among children with atopic dermatitis. Effective treatment may be achieved by the use of topical preparations containing keratolytics, such as small percentages of salicylic acid (2%-3%), urea (10%-20%), and alphahydroxy acids.

Figure 9-24

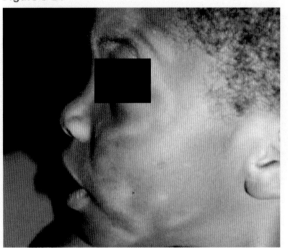

Figure 9-25

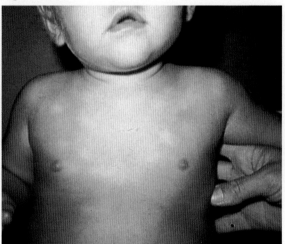

Pityriasis alba This is a condition that is characterized by blotchy areas of hypopigmentation with or without scale. The lesions are usually asymptomatic. In older children, the cheeks are a favored location, but in infants, the process may be more generalized (Figs. 9-24 and 9-25). Both figures illustrate how the borders of the lesions tend to fade into the surrounding normal skin. This contrasts with vitiligo (Figs. 27-12 through 27-17), another common cause of pigment loss. In vitiligo, the areas of involvement tend to be a whiter white and are more sharply demarcated.

Pityriasis alba is more common among children with atopic dermatitis and may represent a form of postinflammatory hypopigmentation. There may or may not be a preceding inflammatory dermatosis in the same area. It is important to reassure the parent and child that the loss of pigment is temporary and that complete restoration of normal skin color will occur. The use of a mild topical steroid or topical tacrolimus or pimecrolimus may speed the process.

Figure 9-26

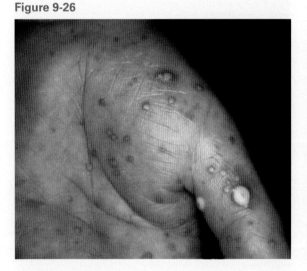

Figure 9-27

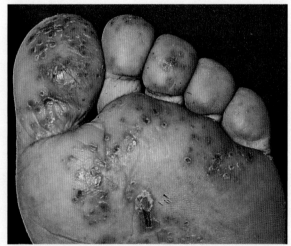

Pompholyx (dyshidrotic eczema) This is a chronic, recurrent eruption of the hands and feet that is often accompanied by severe pruritus. It is considerably more common among individuals with an atopic history or with a family history of atopic disease. Figures 9-26 and 9-27 show a number of deep-seated vesicles and pustules on the palm and sole.

Small, firm vesicles along the sides of the fingers are a particularly common clinical sign. At times, bullae may occur. Patients who develop pompholyx often tend to have hyperhidrosis of the hands and feet. Some observers note that episodes of the disease are brought on by stress. Management of this condition is best achieved by the use of topical corticosteroid creams or ointments.

Allergic and Irritant Contact Dermatitis

Figure 10-1

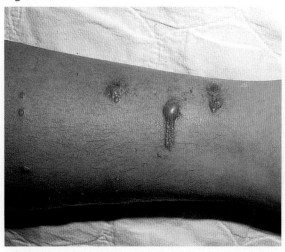

Allergic contact dermatitis (Poison ivy) Contact dermatitis is a T cell-mediated delayed hypersensitivity response to a variety of different antigens. Acute lesions are characterized by erythema, vesiculation, and oozing, whereas chronic areas of involvement may be dry and lichenified.

Figure 10-2

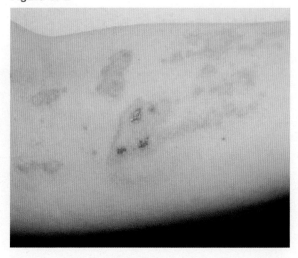

The diagnosis of allergic contact dermatitis (ACD) is a simple one when there is a clear history of exposure to an allergen or when the distribution of the lesions provides a strong clue. At other times, the identification of the causative agent can be very difficult.

Figure 10-3

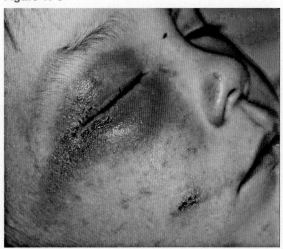

Allergic contact dermatitis (Poison ivy) A number of different plants are capable of causing contact dermatitis. By far, the most common are members of the genus *Toxicodendron*: poison ivy, oak, and sumac. Figures 10-3 and 10-4 are illustrations of contact dermatitis from poison ivy, the most common single cause of contact dermatitis in childhood.

Figure 10-4

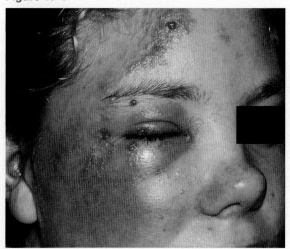

The linear array of vesicles and bullae in Figures 10-1 and 10-2 reflects the pattern in which the resin was transferred from leaf to skin. Figures 10-3 and 10-4 show severe facial involvement and a more diffuse reaction. Children who experience recurrent episodes of this phytodermatitis should be encouraged to learn to recognize the causative plants.

Figure 10-5

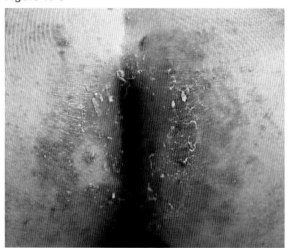

Allergic contact dermatitis (wet wipes) Wet wipes containing the preservative methylisothiazolinone are a cause of ACD. This form of ACD can be misdiagnosed as psoriasis, eczema, or impetigo. Discontinuation of wet wipes results in a complete resolution of this dermatitis.

Figure 10-6

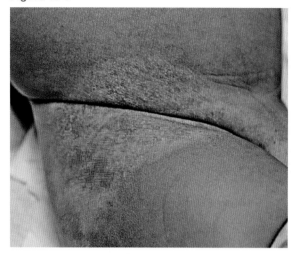

Allergic contact dermatitis (disposable diapers) Allergic reactions to the chemical components of a disposable diaper, including dye, may present as pictured in Fig. 10-6. "Lucky Luke" or "cowboy holster" dermatitis has the pattern of a cowboy's gunbelt, with triangular-shaped erythema beneath the side bands of the diaper on the lateral buttocks, flanks, and upper lateral thighs.

Figure 10-7

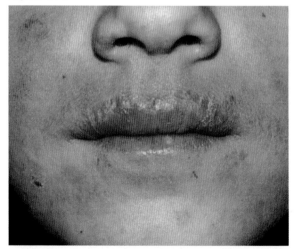

Allergic contact dermatitis (mango) Contact dermatitis to mango may present as a chronic rash on the lips and around the mouth. Mango is a member to the Sumac family, and its sap contains the oil Urushiol. It is important to inquire about recent mango consumption when diagnosing an eruption like the one pictured in Fig. 10-7.

Figure 10-8

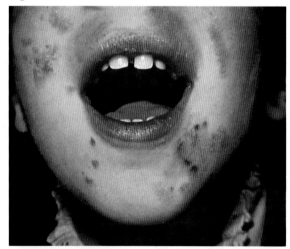

Allergic contact dermatitis (neomycin) The child in Fig. 10-8 has an ACD resulting from the repeated application of a preparation containing neomycin. The development or worsening of an eczematous eruption after the use of a topical medication, either prescribed or over-the-counter, should alert the physician to the possibility of a contact dermatitis (dermatitis medicamentosa). In addition to neomycin, common offenders are the stabilizer ethylenediamine and the paraben preservatives.

Figure 10-9

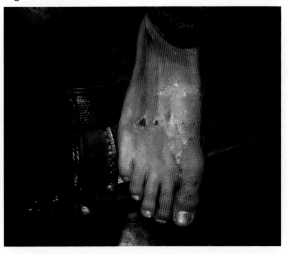

Figure 10-10

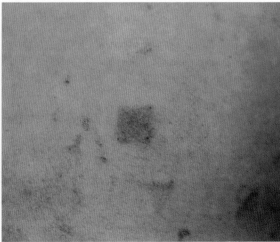

Allergic contact dermatitis (shoes) The allergic contact dermatitis Fig. 10-9 was caused by a sandal. Note how the eruption conforms, like a patch test, to the design of the thongs. Shoe dermatitis should be considered in any eczematous eruption on the dorsum of the foot in a child. The agent responsible for the rash in this photograph was a tanning agent or dye. The other common causes of shoe dermatitis are rubber and rubber accelerators, adhesives, and leather. If the allergen is correctly identified by patch testing, it is possible to select the footwear that is tolerable.

Allergic contact dermatitis Figure 10-10 demonstrates the use of patch testing done for determining the cause of an ACD and illustrates a positive reaction in the form of erythema at 48 hours in a person who has been sensitized to the offending agent.

Figure 10-11

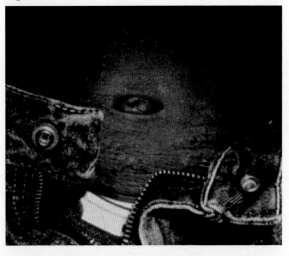

Figure 10-12

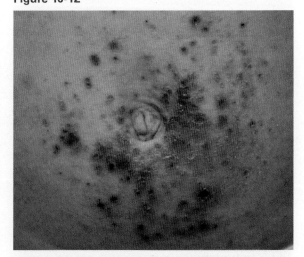

Nickel contact dermatitis The development of an itchy eczematous eruption near the umbilicus is virtually pathognomonic for contact dermatitis to nickel. The source is the small metal snap in the blue jeans or the metal belt buckle. The simultaneous occurrence of an id reaction, sometimes with small lichenoid papules on the elbows and knees, is very common.

Lesions can be treated effectively with topical corticosteroids, but the only cure results from strict avoidance of nickel. This is easier said than done. Parents must buy jeans without nickel snaps or sew in a small piece of fabric to protect the underlying skin. Families should be reminded that wearing jeans with a nickel snap for just several hours out of the month would reactivate the entire process.

Figure 10-13

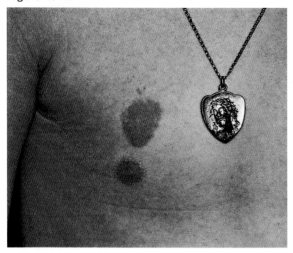

Nickel contact dermatitis Children with contact dermatitis to nickel should also avoid metal jewelry and should be advised against ear piercing. Infants may present with skin lesions corresponding to the location of snaps on their pajamas or other garments.

Figure 10-14

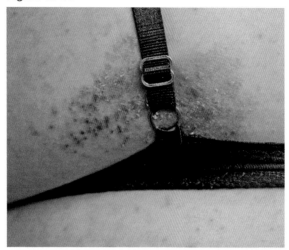

Nickel contact dermatitis Allergy to nickel is one of the most common causes of contact dermatitis. Older children and adolescents may show reactions to watches, chains, belt buckles, or earrings. Figure 10-14 shows an example of contact dermatitis in the metal clasp of a bra. It is possible to test for the presence of nickel by using a spot test kit, which is a liquid containing 1% dimethylglyoxime and 10% ammonium hydroxide.

Figure 10-15

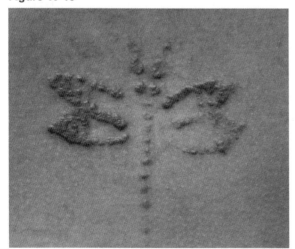

Allergic contact dermatitis (Reaction to temporary tattoo) Contact allergy to temporary tattoos has become an increasingly common phenomenon. In most cases, the tattoo material does not contain pure henna, but is a mixture of brown henna with paraphenylenediamine (PPD) called *black henna*. The patient shown in Fig. 10-15 is allergic to PPD in the tattoo.

Figure 10-16

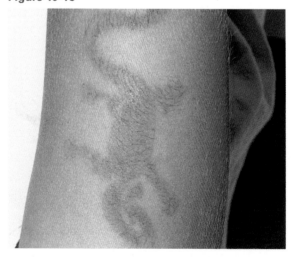

In fact, the concentration of PPD in black henna is higher than that seen in commercial hair dyes. After resolution of the eczematous skin eruption, postinflammatory hyperpigmentation may persist for a considerable period of time.

Figure 10-17

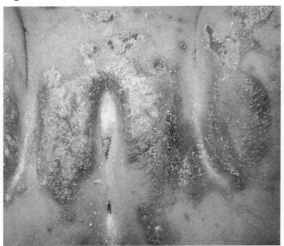

Irritant diaper dermatitis The most common form of diaper dermatitis is related to the combination of moisture and friction. The result is illustrated in Fig. 10-17. Note that the areas of involvement are folds of skin that are in direct apposition to the diaper itself; the skin creases tend to be spared. The bright erythema and shiny appearance of the involved skin are typical. Rashes of this type must be differentiated from candidiasis, seborrheic dermatitis, diaper contact dermatitis, and psoriasis.

Figure 10-18

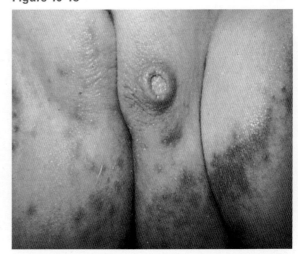

Erosive diaper dermatitis (dermatitis of Jacquet) Inflammation that results from the precipitating factors of wetness, heat, friction, and debris in intertriginous places varies directly with the intensity and duration of those precipitating factors. The inflammation may be merely a slight erythema, a tumid, beefy redness with serous exudation, or an area of ulceration. The punched-out ulcers illustrated in Fig. 10-18 are typical of the erosive diaper dermatitis of Jacquet.

Figure 10-19

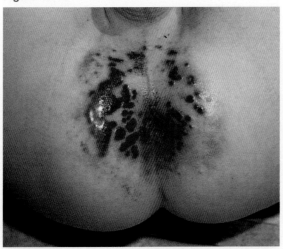

This severe irritant dermatitis responds to the use of barrier creams, mild topical steroids, and frequent diaper changes (Fig. 10-19). Evaluation for candidiasis or bacterial infection should be considered in those who do not respond to treatment.

Figure 10-20

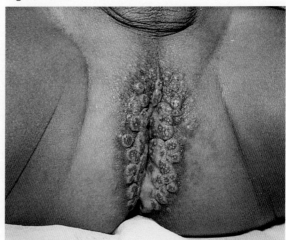

Pseudoverrucous papules and nodules This unique diaper dermatitis was originally described in the skin surrounding urostomies, but can occur as a result of chronic diarrhea (sometimes from Hirschsprung disease), encopresis, or urinary incontinence. The flat topped or round lesions are shiny, erythematous, and moist (Fig. 10-20). They resolve completely when the problem causing chronic irritation in the diaper area has been corrected.

Figure 10-21

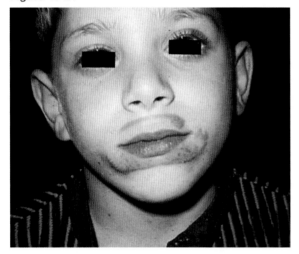

Figure 10-22

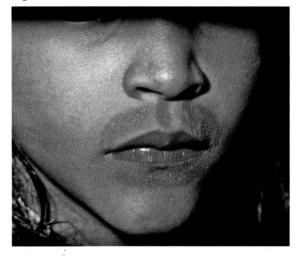

Lip licking dermatitis Irritant contact dermatitis is an eczematous eruption that results from the application of an irritating substance to the skin. Examples would include strong acids or alkalis, harsh soaps, and bleaches. In these cases, T cell–mediated allergy is not involved. The irritant in Fig. 10-21 is saliva. The child pictured here has developed a habit of licking his lips.

Some children do this as compulsively as others suck their thumbs or bite their nails. Notice how the design of the inflammatory lesions conforms to the extent to which the lips can be drawn into the mouth or licked by the tongue. In Fig. 10-22, postinflammatory hyperpigmentation is shown in a child who has recovered from inflammation induced by chewing and blowing bubble gum.

Figure 10-23

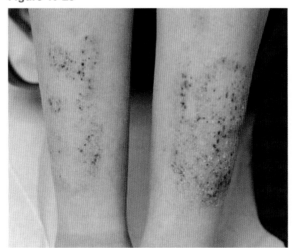

Shin guard dermatitis There is controversy as to whether this is an allergic contact dermatitis or an irritant contact dermatitis. This condition is seen in patients who play a sport, such as soccer, where a shin guard is commonly used (Fig. 10-23). Some patients have a positive patch test but most do not. The entity may just represent irritation from friction and sweating under the shin guard. Treatment is aimed at decreasing the inflammation with a topical steroid and protecting the area with a barrier under the shin guard.

Photodermatoses

Figure 11-1

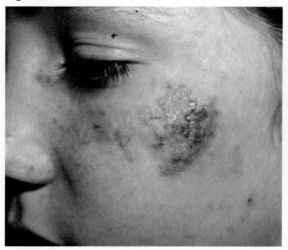

Polymorphous light eruption Patients with this condition develop papules, papulovesicles, or erythematous plaques in response to sun exposure. The lesions erupt a few hours to several days after the subject has been exposed to sunlight. Lesions are most often located on the face, upper chest, and exposed parts of the extremities. Ocular inflammation and cheilitis may also occur.

Figure 11-2

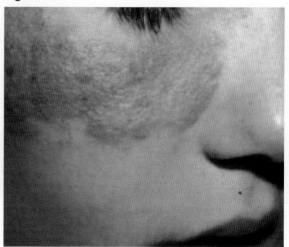

Among Native Americans and the indigenous populations of Latin America, polymorphous light eruption tends to be a familial disease with childhood onset. Figures 11-1 and 11-2 show patients with areas of erythema and edema.

Figure 11-3

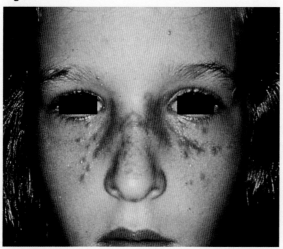

Polymorphous light eruption The "butterfly rash" illustrated in Fig. 11-3 gives a sense that polymorphous light eruption can sometimes be difficult to differentiate from the cutaneous findings in systemic lupus erythematosus. Both immunofluorescence and serology are useful techniques in differentiating the two diseases.

Figure 11-4

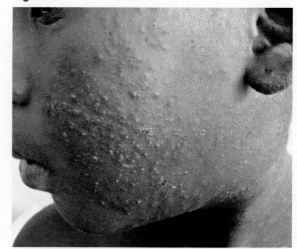

Sunscreens, antimalarial medications, topical corticosteroids, and, in older children, psoralens with ultraviolet light (PUVA) are among the treatments used for polymorphous light eruption.

Figure 11-5

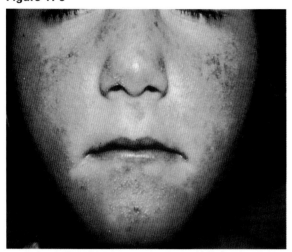

Photoallergic dermatitis In addition to sunburn and polymorphous light eruption, there are several other abnormal cutaneous reactions in which sunlight is a part of the causative mechanism. In photoallergic dermatitis, sensitization and subsequent clinical reactions develop to a topically applied or internally administered substance that has been activated to allergenicity by sunlight. Sulfonamide antibiotics, phenothiazines, and halogenated salicylanilides are among the most common causative agents in photoallergy.

Figure 11-6

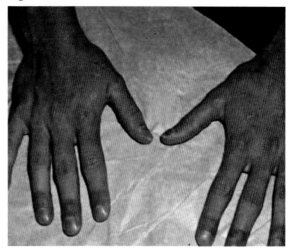

Photoxic dermatitis In phototoxic reactivity, no immunologic mechanism is involved, and the patient reacts as anyone would to a primary irritant. Phototoxic drugs and chemicals include some dyes, coal tar derivatives, and psoralens. Drugs that may cause a phototoxic reaction include the sulfonamides, tetracyclines, and thiazides. Pictured in Fig. 11-6 is a teenager who developed erythema on the backs of his hands from sun exposure while taking doxycycline for his acne.

Figure 11-7

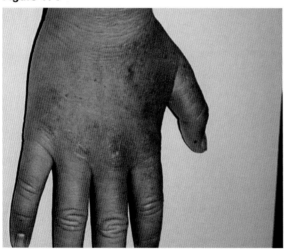

Erythropoietic protoporphyria We have included this metabolic disorder among the photodermatoses because it must always be considered in children who develop a rash after sun exposure. This is among the more common porphyrias; onset is usually during early childhood. The typical presentation of this disease features the development of pruritus and burning of the skin in areas of recent sun exposure. These sensations may be accompanied by erythema, edema, and vesiculation.

Figure 11-8

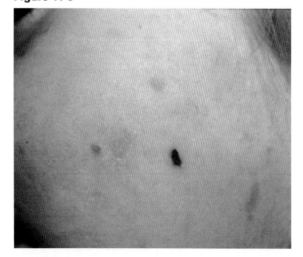

Over time, superficial scarring and a waxy thickening of the involved areas develop. These changes, as seen on the face, are illustrated in Fig. 11-8. The bridge of the nose is another common area of involvement. Children with erythropoietic protoporphyria have inherited a deficiency of the enzyme ferrochelatase, which normally converts protoporphyrin to heme. The disease can be readily diagnosed by testing for elevated free erythrocyte protoporphyrin level. The most serious complication is the development of hepatic involvement. Treatment of the skin disease consists of avoidance of the sun and oral therapy with beta-carotene.

Figure 11-9

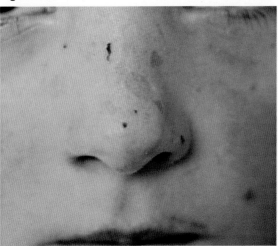

NSAID-induced pseudoporphyria Patients being treated with nonsteroidal anti-inflammatory medications (NSAIDs), such as naproxen, oxaprozin, and nabumetone, may experience an eruption characterized by the development of erythema, vesicles, and shallow atrophic scars after sun exposure.

Figure 11-10

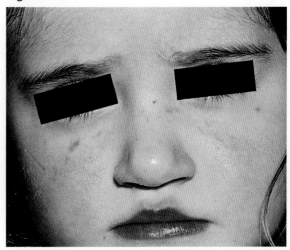

In many patients, frank vesicles are not appreciated. The acute eruption may persist for a few weeks after the medication has been stopped.

Figure 11-11

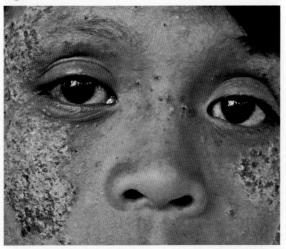

Actinic prurigo Actinic prurigo is a chronic skin disorder caused by an abnormal reaction to sunlight. It is most common in indigenous populations in Central and South America. Lesions develop hours or days after exposure to sunlight, and are pruritic. Many children with actinic prurigo also develop conjunctivitis and swelling and inflammation of the lower lip.

Figure 11-12

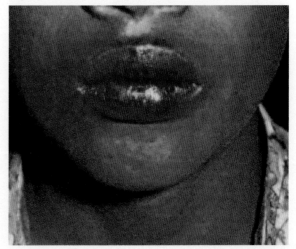

Actinic prurigo cheilitis Cheilitis, particularly of the lower lip, may be the sole manifestation of actinic prurigo. The swelling may be accompanied by itching, tingling, or pain. Treatment of actinic prurigo and of the associated cheilitis is mostly based on various methods of sun protection. Topical steroids are also of some benefit and for severe cases, thalidomide is sometimes prescribed.

Figure 11-13

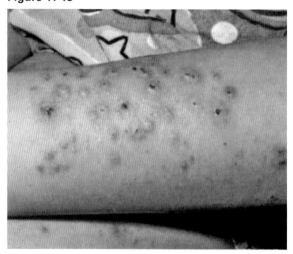

Figure 11-14

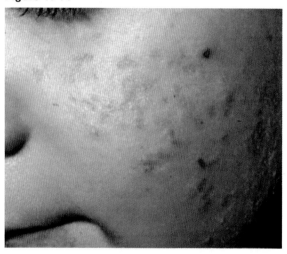

Hydroa vacciniforme This is a rare blistering eruption of sun-exposed skin. It most often occurs during childhood and resolves spontaneously over time. The itching and burning papules develop within hours after sun exposure and rapidly progress to vesicles or blisters. The eyes may also be involved with a mild keratoconjunctivitis.

Some active lesions, and some areas of scarring on the face are shown in Fig. 11-14. Sun avoidance, the proper applications of high sun protection factor (SPF) sunscreens, and sun protective clothing are strongly advised.

Figure 11-15

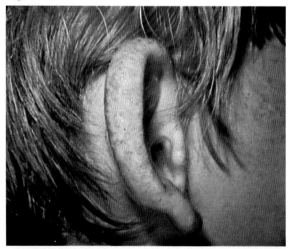

Figure 11-16

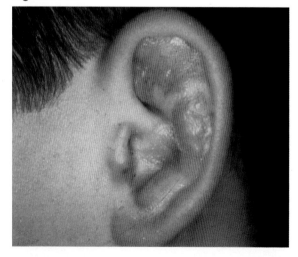

Juvenile spring eruption This term refers to a disease with its onset in early childhood. Patients develop an intensely pruritic eruption in response to sunlight. The papules, vesicles, and crusted plaques tend to favor areas of exposed skin but may become generalized. The disease process is most severe during

the late spring and summer. Illustrated in Figs. 11-15 and 11-16 is the inflammatory pruritic dermatitis on a common location, the pinnae of the ears. Treatment for children with this clinical syndrome consists of maximal protection from sunlight. Topical steroids are of some benefit during exacerbations.

Figure 11-17

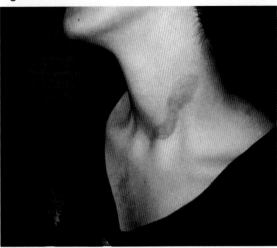

Photodermatitis (berloque dermatitis) This condition is a special kind of photoreaction in which the skin becomes slightly inflamed and quickly develops hyperpigmentation. The cutaneous changes are the result of contact with a photosensitizing chemical, followed immediately by sunlight. Figure 11-17 illustrates the form of this condition that results from the application of a psoralen-containing perfume, such as oil of bergamot. Note that the hyperpigmentation follows the exact distribution in which the perfume was applied.

Figure 11-18

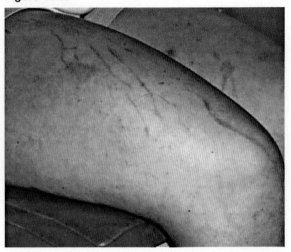

Phytophotodermatitis In addition to perfumes, a number of plants, grasses, fruits, and vegetables contain psoralen as a photosensitizer. The linear lesions pictured Figs. 11-18 and 11-19 resulted from the dripping of lime juice on to the legs, followed by sun exposure.

Figure 11-19

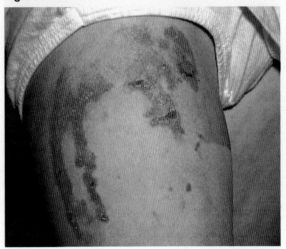

Phytophotodermatitis The child who helps mother or father slice limes before a trip to the park may develop an identical eruption on the hands. Celery and parsley may present similar problems.

Figure 11-20

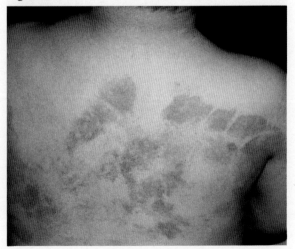

It is important to recognize this entity since some affected infants and children have been mistakenly thought to have bruising from child abuse.

Papulosquamous Diseases

Figure 12-1

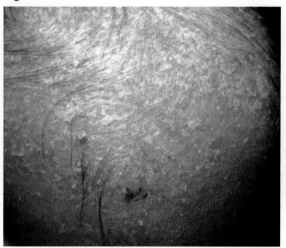

Seborrheic dermatitis This term refers to a scaly, crusting, and erythematous eruption that is most common in infancy (ages 2-12 weeks), where it tends to favor the scalp, diaper area, and intertriginous folds. Figure 12-1 is an illustration of the process in the scalp where it is often referred to as *cradle cap*.

Figure 12-2

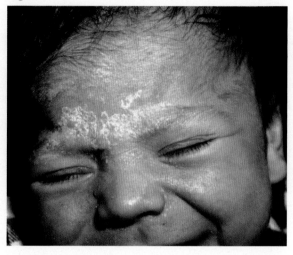

Figure 12-2 illustrates severe involvement in the eyebrows, a common area of involvement. A subset of infants with seborrheic dermatitis will go on to develop atopic dermatitis and it sometimes may be difficult to differentiate between these two conditions.

Figure 12-3

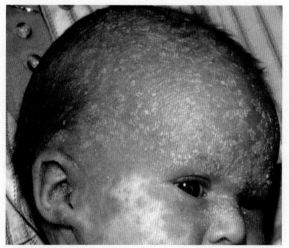

Seborrheic dermatitis Figure 12-3 shows very severe facial and scalp involvement. Some basic principles are that the lesions of seborrheic dermatitis are usually well circumscribed, do not itch, and localize toward the face, scalp, and intertriginous areas. The greasy red-orange scaliness of seborrheic dermatitis is somewhat helpful in differentiating this disorder from atopic dermatitis.

Figure 12-4

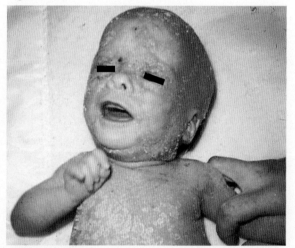

Figure 12-4 shows a more extensive process that is nearly generalized, dry, and scaly. Seborrheic dermatitis has its onset early in infancy and usually resolves by 1 year of age; atopic dermatitis tends to be more persistent.

Figure 12-5

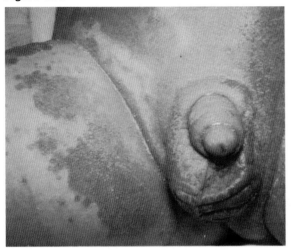

Seborrheic dermatitis The cause of this very common condition remains unknown. Although it favors areas with an increased number of sebaceous glands, there is no evidence that seborrheic dermatitis is a disease of sebaceous glands or is related to excessive sebum production.

Figure 12-6

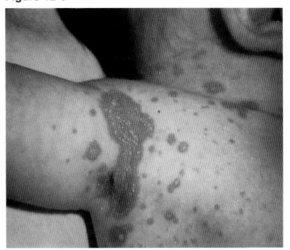

Some studies have suggested that the lipid composition of sebum in seborrheic dermatitis may be abnormal. Bacteria and yeasts are often present in areas of involvement, but neither *Candida albicans* nor *Pityrosporum ovale* has been shown to be an etiologic agent.

Figure 12-7

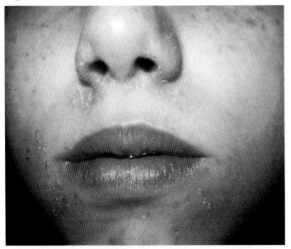

Seborrheic dermatitis Seborrheic dermatitis, common during infancy, is relatively unusual during later childhood. It resurfaces as a problem during adolescence and then seems to become progressively more common through adult life. The adolescent variant primarily involves the scalp, forehead, tarsal margins of the eyelids (blepharitis), ears, and nasolabial folds. Seborrheic dermatitis is easily controlled but not curable. Treatment may consist of the topical application of ketoconazole cream or a mild topical steroid. The frequent use of tar shampoos is particularly helpful in the control of seborrheic dermatitis of the scalp.

Figure 12-8

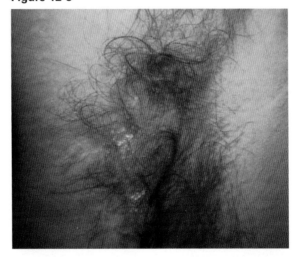

During puberty and in adulthood, seborrheic dermatitis occurs not only on the scalp and face but also on the chest, on the back, and in intertriginous spaces such as the axillae (illustrated in Fig. 12-8), inframammary areas, groin, and intergluteal folds. Lesions on the chest and back are described as *petaloid,* that is, flat and demarcated like petals; in intertriginous spaces, the appearance can be glistening red.

Figure 12-9

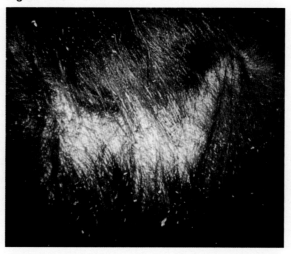

Tinea amiantacea This term requires etymological explanation. The *tinea* does not mean superficial fungal infection but rather a condition that resembles a superficial mycosis. *Amiantacea* means asbestos-like. The combination describes a superficial scaly process that recalls the crumbling exfoliation of asbestos. Such an appearance occurs in the scalp in some cases of seborrheic dermatitis, psoriasis, tinea capitis, and pityriasis sicca (dandruff). The term is discarded as soon as a better diagnosis is made.

Figure 12-10

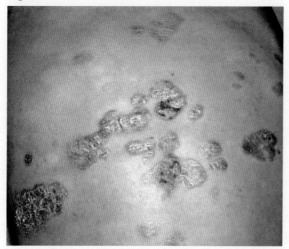

Figure 12-11

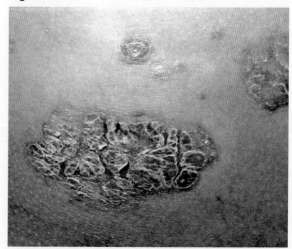

Psoriasis More than one-quarter of all individuals with psoriasis develop their disease during childhood or adolescence. The degree of involvement is extremely variable; some children develop only a few localized plaques, while others suffer from generalized skin disease and severe arthritis.

Pictured in Figs. 12-10 and 12-11 are the typical lesions of psoriasis; the plaques have a red-to-orange hue, are scaly, and are sharply demarcated from the surrounding skin.

Figure 12-12

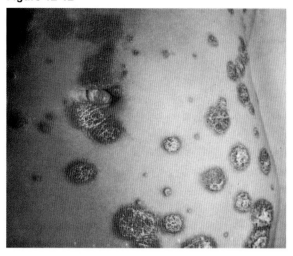

Figure 12-13

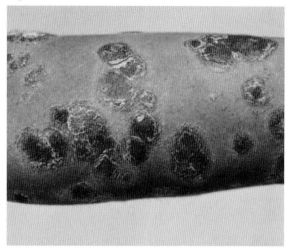

Psoriasis The distinctive character of the scale is appreciated in these figures. The scale is usually described as silvery or micaceous (resembling the mineral mica). When the scale is removed, pinpoint areas of bleeding (Auspitz sign) are uncovered.

Each lesion of psoriasis represents an area of rapid epidermal cell turnover. The thickening of the involved epidermis and the overlying parakeratosis translate into the raised and scaly appearance of the involved skin.

Figure 12-14

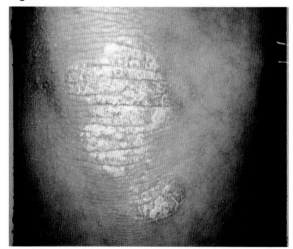

Figure 12-15

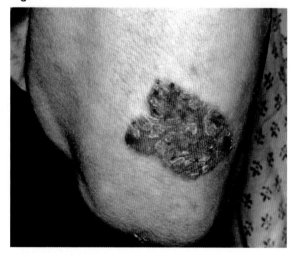

Psoriasis The symmetrical involvement of the knees is a common pattern; elbows and buttocks are other favored locations for plaques like these.

A typical sharply demarcated plaque with micaceous scale on the knee is shown in Fig. 12-14 and on the elbow in Fig.12-15.

Figure 12-16

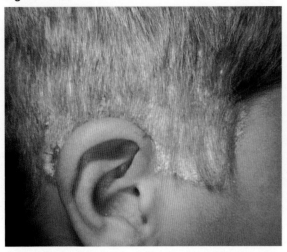

Figure 12-17

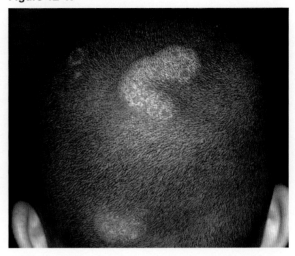

Psoriasis In Fig. 12-16 and 12-17, we see plaques of dense adherent scale in the scalp. Circumscribed areas of micaceous scale in the scalp are a common presenting sign of psoriasis. This disorder can usually be differentiated from tinea capitis by the character of the scale, the sharp demarcation, and, usually, the absence of hair loss.

Lesions in the scalp tend to cause pruritus. When treating the scalp, it is important to decrease the scale so that the topical medications become more effective. Preparations containing salicylic acid, a keratolytic, are especially useful for the treatment of scalp psoriasis.

Figure 12-18

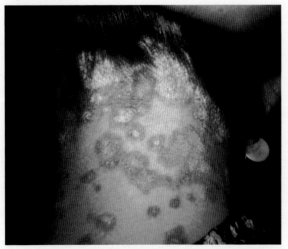

Figure 12-19

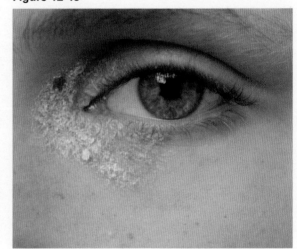

Psoriasis In Fig. 12-18, we see typical involvement of the glabrous skin of the neck, with extension into the scalp. This is a common location, and, in some cases, psoriasis may develop over a persistent nevus simplex (stork bite) in that area.

Unilateral, or, more commonly, symmetrical involvement of the skin around the eyes may occur in psoriasis. The involvement of the medial aspect, as shown in Fig. 12-19, is particularly common.

Figure 12-20

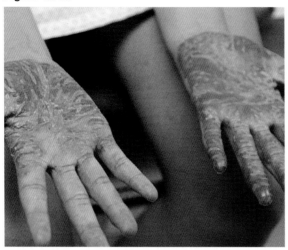

Psoriasis Figures 12-20 to 12-23 show the erythema, scaling, and thickening of portions of the palms and soles that are very common in both children and adults with psoriasis. Therapy of psoriasis is based on the skillful use, either alone or in combination, of a number of therapeutic agents.

Figure 12-21

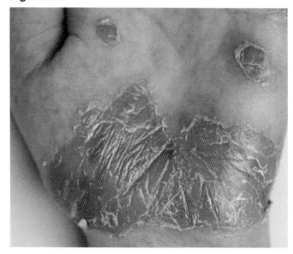

The most common topical treatments include topical steroids, tars, keratolytics, ultraviolet light, and topical calcipotriol and tazarotene in older patients. Children with simple plaque psoriasis can sometimes be managed with short-contact anthralin preparations.

Figure 12-22

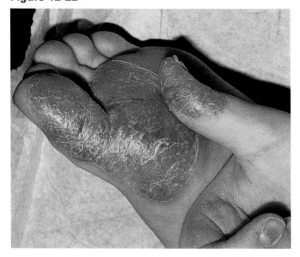

Psoriasis When topical steroids are used, it is important to employ the least potent preparation that is effective and to avoid the use of fluorinated steroids on the face and in intertriginous areas. Careful exposure to sunlight during the summer months and artificial ultraviolet light at other times is enormously beneficial in selected patients with extensive involvement.

Figure 12-23

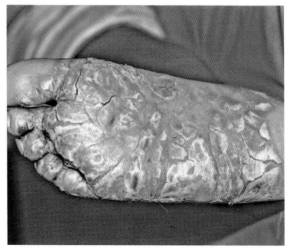

Thickening and fissuring of the palms or soles can become extremely painful. Patients with severe involvement like this, and those with severe generalized involvement may sometimes require systemic therapy. Treatments include methotrexate, acitretin, and biologic agents.

Figure 12-24

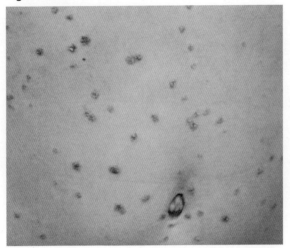

Figure 12-25

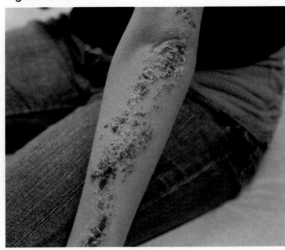

Psoriasis In Fig. 12-24, the lesions consist of numerous papules, each covered with the typical silvery scales of psoriasis. This form of the condition, termed *guttate psoriasis*, is more common in childhood and may have an explosive onset. There is often a history of an antecedent upper-respiratory infection, and streptococcal disease is of particular importance in triggering this eruption. The use of oral antibiotics that are effective against *Streptococcus* sometimes hastens the resolution of guttate psoriasis. The use of mild topical corticosteroids is of benefit.

Rarely, patients develop psoriasis in a linear distribution. In some cases, this is a simple result of Koebnerization, the development of lesions in areas that are being scratched or traumatized in some other way. In other cases, the development of linear psoriasis follows the lines of Blaschko, and may indicate a somatic mutation in the skin.

Figure 12-26

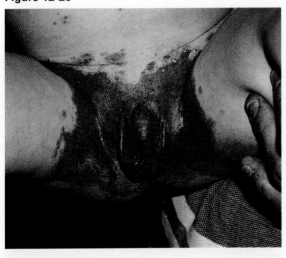

Figure 12-27

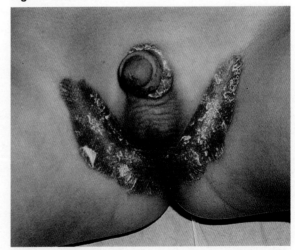

Psoriasis Pictured here are two representations of psoriasis in the diaper area. In Fig.12-26, the entire diaper area is involved with a sharply demarcated erythematous scaling eruption. Figure 12-27 shows the sharply demarcated eruption with minimal involvement of the scrotum but involvement of the prepuce of the penis. When onset of the disease occurs during infancy, this is a very common area of involvement.

It is postulated that the repeated irritation in this area constitutes a type of Koebner phenomenon. Scales are less in evidence in Fig. 12-26 because of the maceration that is inevitable in this location. Note the sharp demarcation of the lesions. Treatment of psoriasis in the diaper area can be difficult. Low-potency topical corticosteroids should be used judiciously with the use of barrier creams.

Figure 12-28

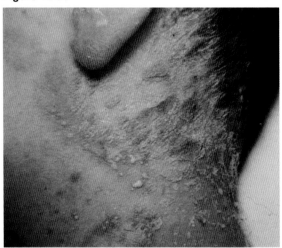

Figure 12-29

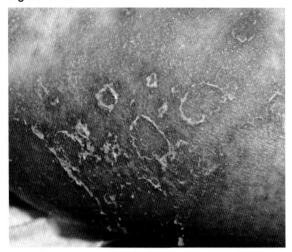

Pustular psoriasis Figures 12-28 and 12-29 illustrate pustular psoriasis. Both are examples of the disease in relatively mild form, but even in these the suppurative quality of the lesions can be appreciated. Severe pustular psoriasis, also known as the *von Zumbusch form,* is a rare and potentially life-threatening disease.

Pustular psoriasis may be triggered by physical or emotional stress, a number of medications, or the abrupt discontinuation of steroid therapy, and must be differentiated from other disorders, including pustular drug eruptions.

Figure 12-30

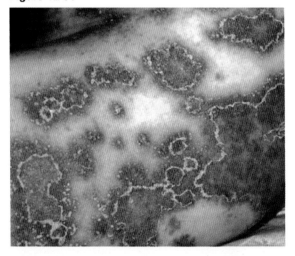

Figure 12-31

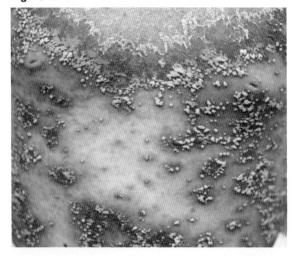

Pustular psoriasis Patients with this form of disease can develop shaking chills, fever, and leukocytosis. Numerous superficial pustules develop on psoriatic plaques and on uninvolved skin. Over a brief period of time, the pustules enlarge and become confluent; lakes of pus form. The process may eventuate in an exfoliative erythroderma. Hospitalization and careful supportive therapy are important aspects of treatment.

Pustules with identical appearance may be seen in a deficiency of interleukin 1 receptor antagonist (DIRA), and this disorder may also cause lytic lesions in the bones. Treatment for this disorder is anakinra, a recombinant form of the human interleukin-1 receptor antagonist.

Figure 12-32

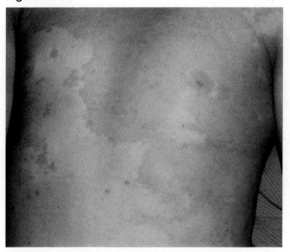

Figure 12-33

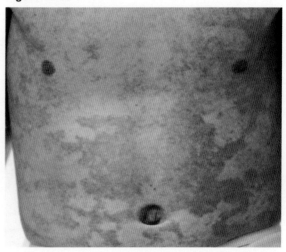

Pityriasis rubra pilaris This is a chronic and often severe cutaneous disorder that may sometimes begin during childhood. Depending on the stage and location of the disease process, the appearance varies. The most unique distinguishing manifestation of this disease is the red-orange perifollicular keratotic papules that are usually located on the dorsal surfaces of the fingers and hands. The "nutmeg grater" appearance in these areas is pathognomonic of pityriasis rubra pilaris.

Figures 12-32 and 12-33 illustrate the disease process as it appears on the trunk. Follicular localization may be apparent early in the condition, but later, orange-red plaques with scaling are more usual. The condition may become generalized, but usually some islands of normal-appearing skin remain interspersed between involved areas.

Figure 12-34

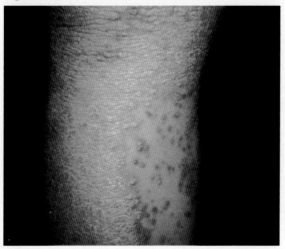

Figure 12-35

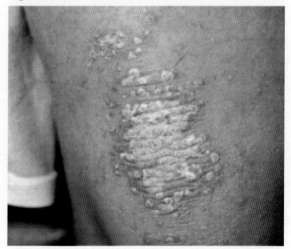

Pityriasis rubra pilaris Figure 12-34 and 12-35 show both discrete follicular papules and larger confluent, psoriasiform plaques on the leg.

The circumscribed collection of scaly papules, which become confluent, is characteristic, but may, at times, be difficult to differentiate from psoriasis.

Figure 12-36

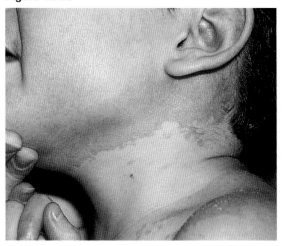

Pityriasis rubra pilaris Erythema and scaling of the face and scalp may represent the initial presentation of pityriasis rubra pilaris. Pityriasis rubra pilaris in children has been divided into subtypes based on natural history and clinical appearance. The *classic* juvenile form affects children in the first 2 years of life and often tends to become generalized and severe. The *circumscribed* juvenile type presents with patches of follicular papules and displays a lesser tendency toward progression to generalized disease. Finally, the *atypical* juvenile form is the rarest, has the poorest prognosis, and tends to be familial.

Figure 12-37

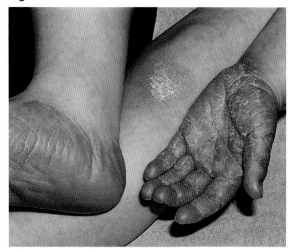

Figure 12-37 illustrates the highly characteristic appearance of the condition on the palm, knee, and sole. There is a diffuse hyperkeratosis that is symmetrical and covers the entire palmar surface. Dystrophy of both fingernails and toenails may be prominent. Palmoplantar involvement in pityriasis rubra pilaris is very common and can be disabling.

Figure 12-38

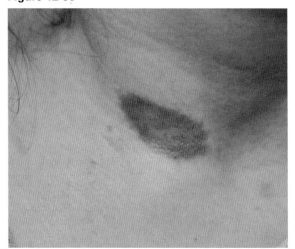

Pityriasis rosea This benign and self-limited eruption occurs most often in spring and autumn. Most patients are adolescents and young adults, but the disorder is not unusual in children and may even occur during infancy. In its classic form, pityriasis rosea follows a specific and predictable clinical course. The first solitary lesion is a circle or oval of erythema and scaling. As it develops to its full size of up to 2 to 3 cm, this so-called herald patch may easily be mistaken for a lesion of tinea corporis. The chest and upper thigh are common locations for the herald patch but any area may be involved.

Figure 12-39

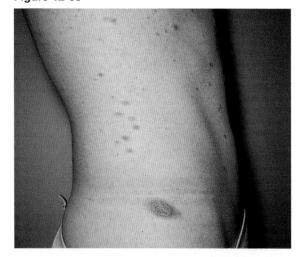

A typical herald patch is shown in Fig. 12-38 and the lower edge of Fig. 12-39. Within a period of 5 to 15 days, additional lesions begin to develop. Patients develop numerous round-to-oval pink-orange macules and papules that are 3 to 10 mm in diameter. Each has a trailing edge of fine scaling, the characteristic "collarette." Larger, round-to-oval patches may also be present. The lesions of pityriasis rosea tend to cluster on the trunk and proximal extremities and often are most numerous in the axillae. The generalized process is illustrated in Fig. 12-39. The duration of the total process is 6 to 9 weeks.

Figure 12-40

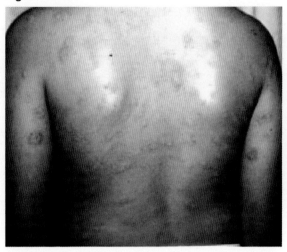

Figure 12-41

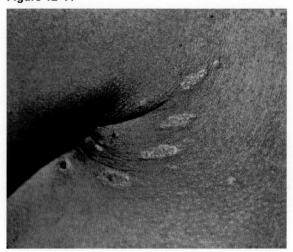

Pityriasis rosea Figures 12-40 and 12-41 illustrate well-developed lesions of pityriasis rosea in the midcourse of the condition. One can appreciate the parallel array of the individual macules. On the back and chest, this tendency of the lesions to follow skin lines (the so-called Christmas tree distribution) is usually most obvious.

A number of atypical forms of pityriasis may occur and these variations in both morphology and distribution seem to be more common during childhood. In particular, papules, pustules, and even vesicles may occur and their presence may suggest a number of other cutaneous disorders. However, a careful search will usually lead to one or several of the typical papulosquamous lesions. In addition, lesions may extend to involve the face and there may be relative sparing of the trunk. In some cases, the process is confined to intertriginous areas, as seen in Fig. 12-41.

Figure 12-42

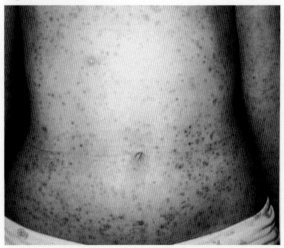

Figure 12-43

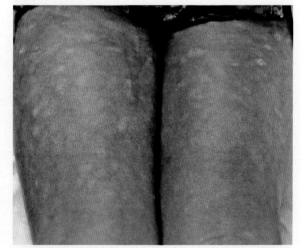

Pityriasis lichenoides chronica Pityriasis lichenoides chronica is a chronic disorder that consists of superficial lesions that evolve from papules into oval pink-brown papulosquamous lesions. There may be an adherent scale overlying the individual lesions, and there is sometimes mild pruritus. Involvement tends to favor the trunk and proximal extremities, although it may become more widespread.

Many cases of pityriasis lichenoides chronica are initially diagnosed as pityriasis rosea. However, the persistent course of this disease, with remissions and exacerbations, eventually distinguishes it. Pictured in Fig. 12-43 is a child with both crusted papules and hypopigmented macules. Many children with pityriasis lichenoides chronica develop areas of hypopigmentation, and these may arise de novo on normal skin.

Figure 12-44

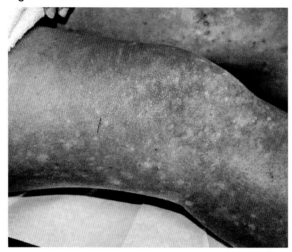

Pityriasis lichenoides chronica The widespread areas of hypopigmentation in this disorder may be persistent and disfiguring, involving also the face, as shown in (Fig. 12-45). In most cases, treatment with topical agents is of little value, and the most improvement is seen with narrow band ultraviolet B-light therapy. If this is unavailable, sun exposure may be helpful.

Figure 12-45

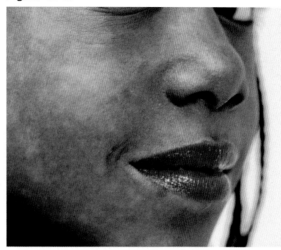

In our opinion, the relationship between this form of hypopigmentation and hypopigmented mycosis fungoides remains unclear. We do believe that children with this clinical phenotype usually show a good response to light treatment, and overall have an excellent prognosis.

Figure 12-46

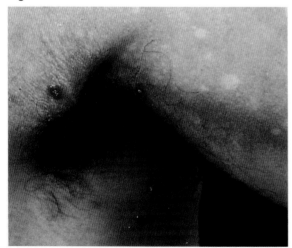

Pityriasis lichenoides et varioliformis acuta (PLEVA, Mucha-Habermann disease) This is a troubling papulosquamous disorder of acute onset that occurs in both children and young adults. Involvement tends to favor the anterior trunk and proximal extremities. Facial and palm and sole involvement is relatively rare, and pruritus is usually absent. Involvement of the axillae, as shown here, is common.

Figure 12-47

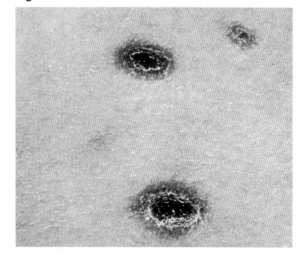

The individual lesions go through a distinctive process of evolution over a period of weeks. Lesions tend to occur in crops. Many patients are mistakenly labeled as having chickenpox; however, the typical dew drop on a rose petal lesion is not seen in PLEVA and the course of the disease is entirely different.

Figure 12-48

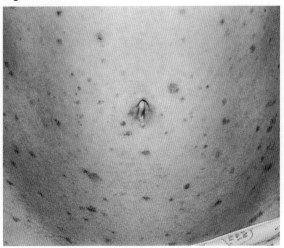

Pityriasis lichenoides et varioliformis acuta (PLEVA, Mucha-Habermann disease) Each lesion begins as an erythematous papule. The lesion enlarges to become a brownish 2 to 3 mm oval papule and then can develop a central area of hemorrhagic or necrotic crust. Lesions of this type are depicted in Figs. 12-48 and 12-49.

Figure 12-49

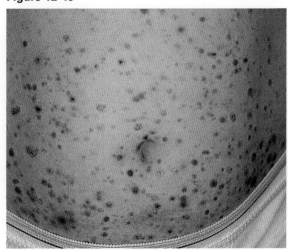

The condition generally has no systemic manifestations and tends to resolve gradually over a period of 4 to 6 months. However, some childhood cases last considerably longer and scarring and pigmentary changes frequently occur.

Figure 12-50

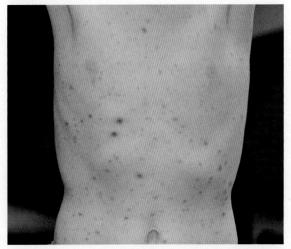

Pityriasis lichenoides et varioloformis acuta (PLEVA, Mucha-Haberman disease) Pictured in Fig. 12-50 is a child with numerous crusted papules on the abdomen. There is some evidence that resolution of this process can be hastened by a course of oral erythromycin or tetracycline (over age 9). The mechanism of action of the drug in this situation is not known.

Figure 12-51

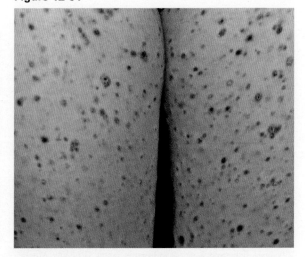

Figure 12-51 illustrates a severe case of PLEVA. Rarely, patients may develop a variant that is characterized by ulceronecrotic lesions, fever, and systemic symptoms.

Figure 12-52

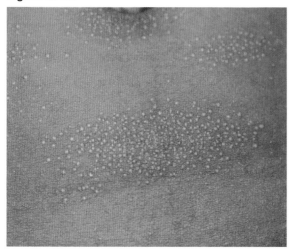

Lichen nitidus This is an unusual and distinctive dermatosis that has its peak incidence during childhood. The individual papules, as pictured in Fig. 12-52, are smaller than 1 mm in diameter. They are flat and shiny, with a round or polygonal shape.

Figure 12-53

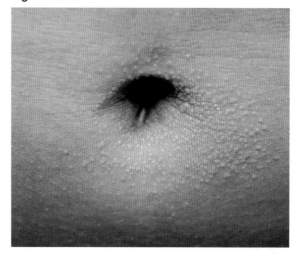

The lesions usually cluster, and an occasional linear grouping suggest that they occur in areas of trauma (the Koebner phenomenon) (Fig. 12-53). Lichen nitidus is occasionally seen in association with lichen planus. However, the marked differences in both histopathology and natural history indicate that they are different diseases.

Figure 12-54

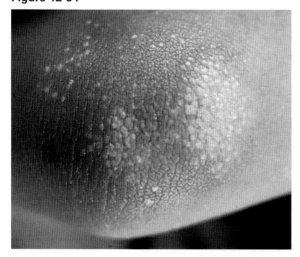

Lichen nitidus In Fig. 12-54, the shiny character of the lesions of lichen nitidus is more appreciable. The lesions of lichen nitidus are usually asymptomatic but pruritus may occur.

Figure 12-55

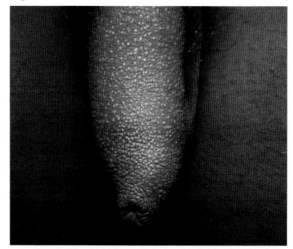

The penis is a site of predilection for this condition, as are the abdomen and upper extremities. They may clear spontaneously in a short period of time or they may last for months or years. There is no known effective treatment for the condition itself; itching can be treated symptomatically with antihistamines and mild topical steroids.

Figure 12-56

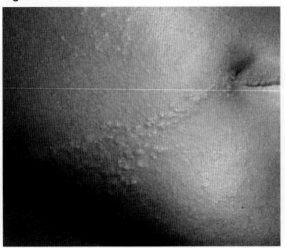

Lichen striatus This is a common and benign self-limited childhood dermatosis that is easily diagnosed from its classic appearance. Onset is usually between the ages of 3 and 10 years.

Figure 12-57

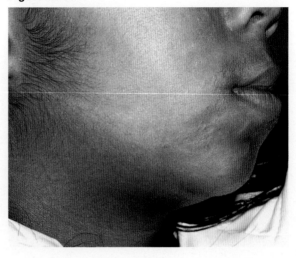

Lichen striatus is rare in young infants, adolescents, and adults. The lesions consist of pink, flesh-colored, or slightly hypopigmented flat-topped papules that evolve in a linear array following lines of Blaschko.

Figure 12-58

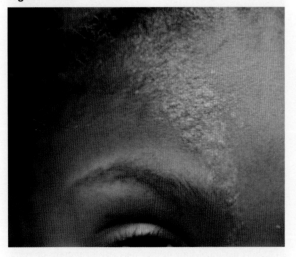

Lichen striatus Figure 12-58 illustrates a typical lesion of lichen striatus occurring in a different facial location. The area of involvement is often noted to become wider as it advances.

Figure 12-59

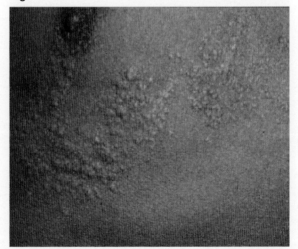

Figure 12-59 demonstrates lichen striatus following Blaschko lines on the trunk. The lesions of lichen striatus are usually asymptomatic but may last from months to years.

Figure 12-60

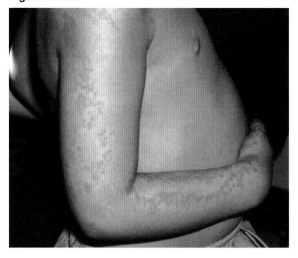

Lichen striatus The linear array of papules in this patient involves the entire arm. Because of the distribution along Blaschko lines, it is believed that lichen striatus represents inflammation of a group of cells which differentiated due to a somatic mutation during embryogenesis.

Figure 12-61

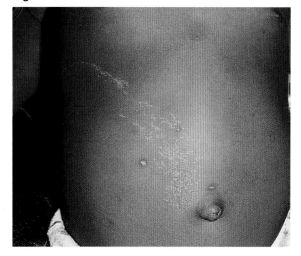

Postinflammatory hypopigmentation occurs following the initial inflammatory process. The etiology of the condition is unknown. Treatment is not strictly necessary, but mild topical steroids tend to speed the process of resolution.

Figure 12-62

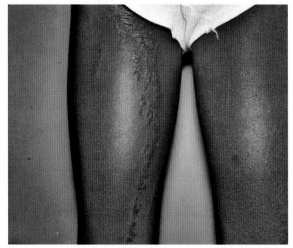

Lichen striatus Figure 12-62 illustrates another linear lesion of lichen striatus, in a typical lower extremity distribution.

Figure 12-63

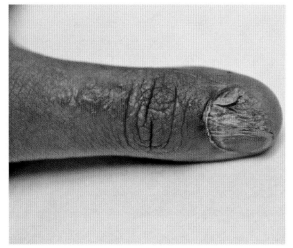

Lichen striatus may extend along the finger and then cause dystrophy of the associated fingernail or toenail. In some cases, distortion or destruction of the nail may be permanent.

Figure 12-64

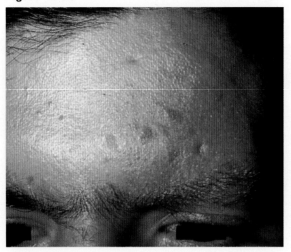

Figure 12-65

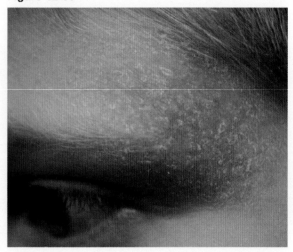

Follicular mucinosis This is an uncommon disorder of unknown etiology that affects both children and adults. The lesions, which are usually located on the head and neck, vary in clinical appearance. Most often, as illustrated in this figure, there are grouped flesh-colored papules.

This figure shows a patient with an erythematous scaly plaque and loss of eyebrow hair. When the disorder affects the scalp, it causes areas of permanent alopecia. In children, this disease tends to resolve spontaneously. Rarely, however, an association with lymphoma may occur. This can usually be diagnosed by careful examination of a skin biopsy at the time of disease onset.

Figure 12-66

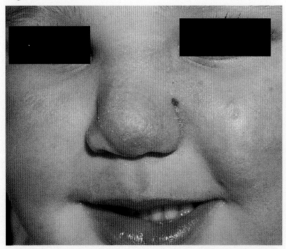

Figure 12-67

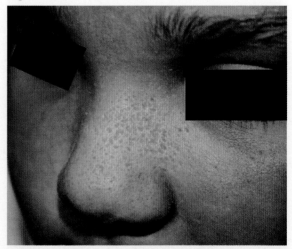

Follicular mucinosis In some cases, as illustrated in Fig. 12-66, there may also be erythematous plaques with follicular accentuation and scale. In this patient, the areas of involvement resolved with follicular atrophy, as illustrated in the second figure (Fig. 12-67).

In some children, only a few lesions develop and the condition resolves spontaneously over time. However, in others, the disorder is persistent and new lesions continue to develop.

Figure 12-68

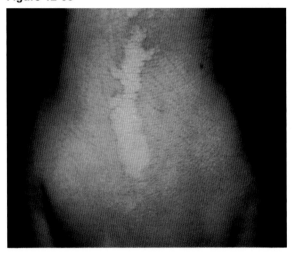

Porokeratosis This is a rare autosomal dominant dermatosis with unique clinical and histologic findings. Lesions usually develop during childhood and favor the hands, forearms, and face. Each lesion begins as a papule and evolves into an irregular atrophic plaque. A well-developed plaque is pictured in Fig. 12-68.

Figure 12-69

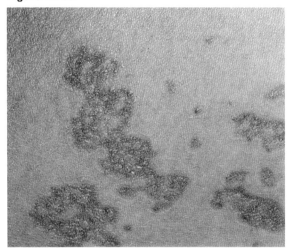

In Fig. 12-69 one can begin to appreciate the raised hyperkeratotic border that surrounds each circinate plaque. This border, which corresponds to the histologic finding cornoid lamella, is the most diagnostic clinical feature.

Figure 12-70

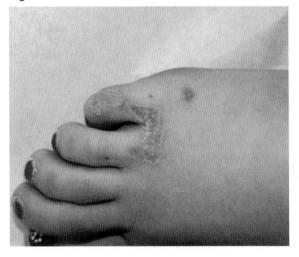

Porokeratosis (porokeratosis of Mibelli) Pictured in these figures are two variants of porokeratosis. The first is an isolated lesion, sometimes referred to as *porokeratosis of Mibelli*. Note the raised hyperkeratotic border and circinate plaque.

Figure 12-71

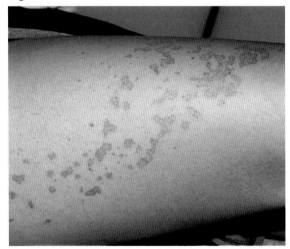

Linear porokeratosis The second case shows a linear array of lesions on the thigh. Linear porokeratosis, which follows the lines of Blaschko, is probably due to somatic mutation and resultant chromosomal mosaicism.

Figure 12-72

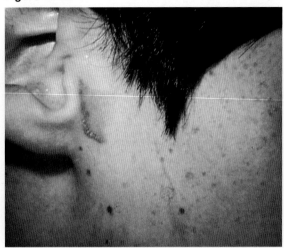

Elastosis perforans serpiginosa This rare disorder is characterized by small, cone-shaped, hyperkeratotic papules that are arranged in annular or circinate patterns. The lesions are usually localized but the process may also be disseminated. The underlying histologic process is the transepidermal elimination of elastic tissue.

Figure 12-73

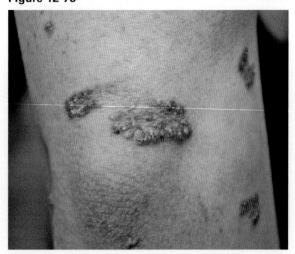

An association with heritable disorders such as Ehlers-Danlos syndrome, Marfan syndrome, pseudoxanthoma elasticum, osteogenesis imperfecta, Rothmund-Thomson syndrome, and Down syndrome has been reported. In most patients, there is no effective therapy. Attempts at surgical removal are complicated by the high incidence of recurrence and scar formation.

Figure 12-74

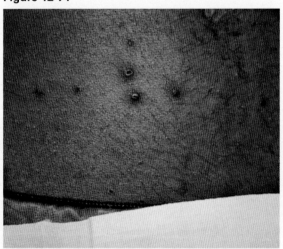

Perforating folliculitis This eruption consists of numerous small erythematous follicular papules with central keratotic plugging. The lesions, which vary in size from 2 to 8 mm, are usually located on the buttocks and thighs. The cause of this eruption is unknown; irritation of the hair follicle is probably the primary process. At various times, perforating folliculitis has been ascribed to the wearing of tight garments or to some chemical in clothing.

Figure 12-75

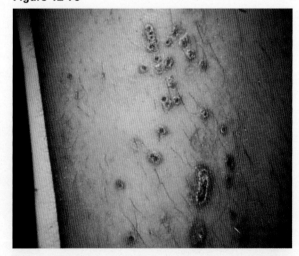

Reactive perforating collagenosis This rare disease usually has its onset during infancy and early childhood. Autosomal recessive, dominant, sporadic, and acquired forms have been reported. The lesions, as shown in Fig. 12-75, consist of small erythematous papules that gradually increase in size and develop a central hyperkeratotic plug. In some cases, the linear array of lesions suggests that they are induced by trauma—the so-called Koebner phenomenon. Pruritus is an occasional feature. Lesions usually last 6 to 8 weeks and then resolve, only to be followed by the eruption of fresh papules.

Figure 12-76

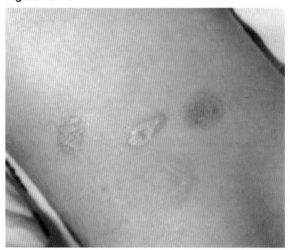

Lichen planus This condition is a pruritic eruption of unknown etiology. It is not uncommon in childhood. These illustrations are of the most representative lesions of lichen planus on a most common site, the wrists. The primary lesion consists of a flat-topped, polygonal, violaceous papule 2 to 6 mm in diameter. The characteristic shiny appearance of the individual papules is seen in these figures.

Figure 12-77

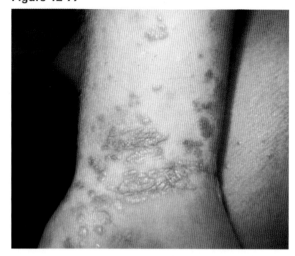

Figure 12-77 illustrates the tendency for the solitary lesions to form confluent plaques. Exaggerated surface markings in the overlying skin (Wickham striae) may also be evident but are difficult to appreciate from these figures. The forearms, the middle of the back, and the anterior surfaces of the lower extremities are other common locations.

Figure 12-78

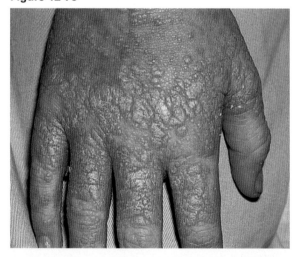

Lichen planus The clinical severity of lichen planus varies from a few mildly pruritic lesions in some cases to extensive and severe involvement of the skin and mucous membranes with intractable itching in others. Children with limited disease often respond well to the local application of topical corticosteroids. However, when the process is generalized, a short course of systemic steroids may be necessary and will sometimes yield a dramatic improvement.

Figure 12-79

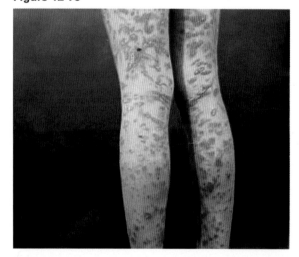

On the legs, lesions may become markedly hypertrophic and plaque-like. Lichen planus tends to be a problem of long duration, with periods of remission and exacerbation.

Figure 12-80

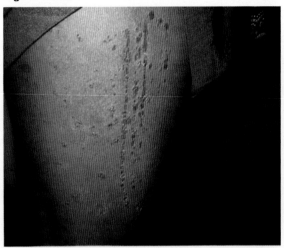

Lichen planus Figure 12-80 illustrates the tendency for new lesions to form in a scratch or abrasion. The so-called Koebner phenomenon is highly characteristic of lichen planus, and some evidence of "Koebnerization" is seen in almost every patient with this disorder.

Figure 12-81

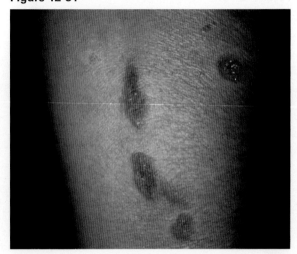

Most often, the lesions of lichen planus are small purplish papules, solitary or confluent, with exaggerated surface markings. There are, however, several variants. Some lesions develop adherent scales, sometimes vesiculation occurs, and rarely, necrosis and scarring may occur upon resolution. The lesions in Fig. 12-81 are larger and more inflammatory than usual; there is a suggestion of vesiculation and necrosis. The vesicular and bullous forms of lichen planus must sometimes be differentiated from other bullous disorders.

Figure 12-82

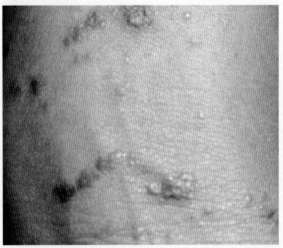

Lichen planus Although the etiology of lichen planus remains a mystery, the clinician must bear in mind that certain lichenoid drug eruptions may be clinically indistinguishable from true lichen planus. The most common agents are gold salts and antimalarial agents. Topical exposure to paraphenylenediamine may have the same result.

Figure 12-83

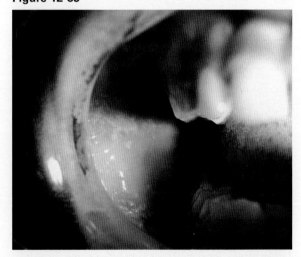

More than one-half of patients with cutaneous lesions will have oral mucosal involvement, and mucosal involvement may also occur without any skin lesions. The oral lesions are most commonly found on the buccal mucosa and the lips. The lesions are characteristically white reticulated patches, although bullae, erosions, and ulcers may be seen. Erosive lesions may be quite painful.

Figure 12-84

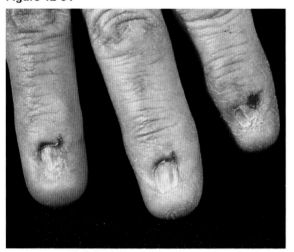

Lichen planus A small percentage of patients with lichen planus develop nail involvement. The severity varies. Some children develop only mild thinning or ridging of the nail plate. Others have a severe nail dystrophy, with pterygium formation and complete and permanent nail loss.

Figure 12-85

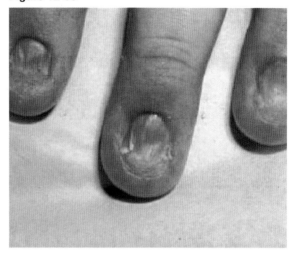

A case where the nails are destroyed is pictured in Fig. 12-85. Rarely, there may even be severe lichen planus of the fingernails and toenails without skin involvement. In any case, attempts to treat the severe forms of nail disease in lichen planus are rarely successful.

Figure 12-86

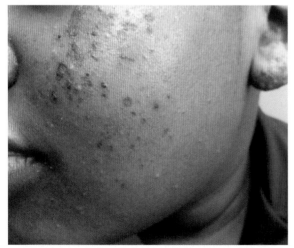

Actinic lichen planus This rare form of lichen planus occurs on sun-exposed areas and consists of either annular lesions, or, as pictured in Fig. 12-86, violaceous papules which coalesce to form plaques. Topical corticosteroids and antimalarials are among the effective treatments. Patients must also use topical sunscreens.

Figure 12-87

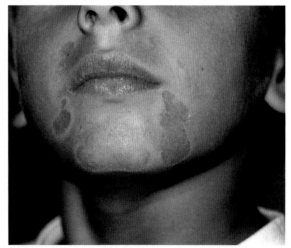

Annular lichen planus Figure 12-87 shows a patient with annular lesions on the face. This presentation is rare and overlaps with actinic lichen planus, in which the disease occurs on sun-exposed areas, most often the face. The lesions are usually round and well-defined. A central area of hyperpigmentation is surrounded by either erythema or hypopigmentation. The majority of cases seem to occur in India, Africa, and the Middle East.

Figure 12-88

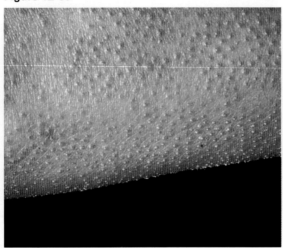

Figure 12-89

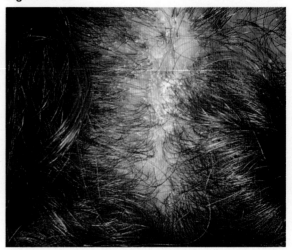

Lichen planopilaris (follicular lichen planus) This is a variant of lichen planus in which the primary involvement occurs around hair follicles. It is more common in females. Patients with this form of disease may have the more typical flat-topped papules and mucosal lesions as well. Pictured in Fig. 12-88 are numerous rough follicular papules on an extremity.

Lichen planopilaris can be a severe and disfiguring disorder when it involves the scalp. In such cases, either a temporary or permanent scarring alopecia may develop. Figure 12-89 shows a scalp with a scarring alopecia, follicular spines, and erythema. This condition is progressive and may be very difficult to treat, although the use of potent topical corticosteroids may be useful.

Nutritional, Metabolic, and Endocrine Diseases

Figure 13-1

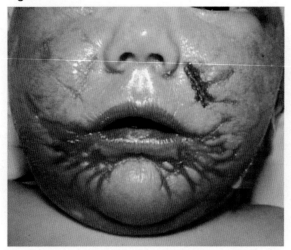

Figure 13-2

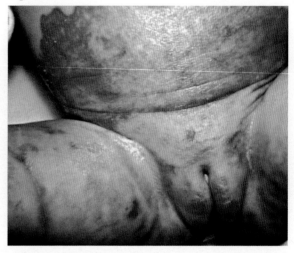

Acrodermatitis enteropathica This syndrome results from inadequate absorption or dietary intake of zinc. Figure 13-1 shows erythema, crusting, and fissuring of the perioral skin and cheeks. The eruption that is pictured here may be preceded by blisters. Other features of acrodermatitis enteropathica include stomatitis, paronychia, and alopecia.

The diaper area lesion that is seen in Fig. 13-2 is diffusely erythematous and has a sharply marginated border on the abdomen. Acrodermatitis enteropathica may be inherited in an autosomal recessive fashion. This form of the disease seems to be related to an inability to absorb zinc.

Figure 13-3

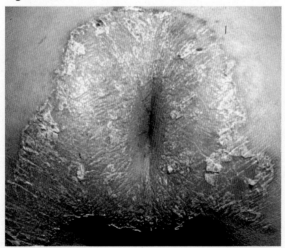

Figure 13-4

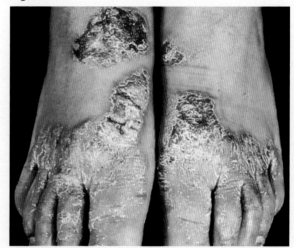

Acrodermatitis enteropathica Figure 13-3 shows a highly characteristic picture of the cutaneous changes of acrodermatitis enteropathica around the anus, the buttocks, and on the perineum. Note the psoriasiform appearance of this lesion and of those on the feet in Fig. 13-4. The full-blown picture of acrodermatitis enteropathica goes far beyond the typical changes of skin and hair. Affected children have severe diarrhea, growth

retardation, and irritability. Without treatment, the disease follows a progressive course and may even be fatal. The child with suspected acrodermatitis enteropathica should be evaluated for a low zinc level or a low alkaline phosphatase level when zinc levels are normal or below normal. Treatment with dietary zinc supplementation leads to a dramatic resolution of all symptoms and, in some cases, must be maintained indefinitely.

Figure 13-5

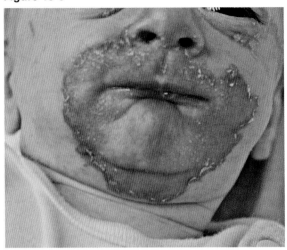

Acrodermatitis enteropathica Acquired acrodermatitis enteropathica is seen in infants who have received parenteral alimentation lacking sufficient zinc and, rarely, in breast-fed premature infants who have larger zinc requirements. Occasionally, acrodermatitis enteropathica in a full-term breast-fed infant may be the result of low levels of zinc in the breast milk.

Figure 13-6

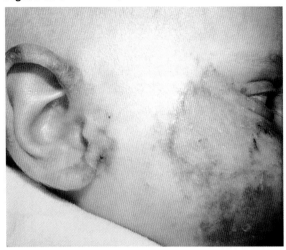

The patient with acquired acrodermatitis enteropathica requires temporary zinc replacement. The differential diagnosis of this eruption includes psoriasis, biotin and multiple carboxylase deficiencies, essential fatty acid deficiencies, and cystic fibrosis.

Figure 13-7

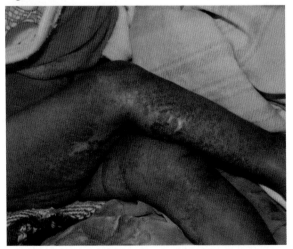

Kwashiorkor Kwashiorkor is a type of protein energy malnutrition. It is seen most commonly in developing countries, and onset tends to occur after weaning. At that time, the balance of protein and carbohydrate in breast milk is replaced by a diet that contains almost exclusively carbohydrates.

Figure 13-8

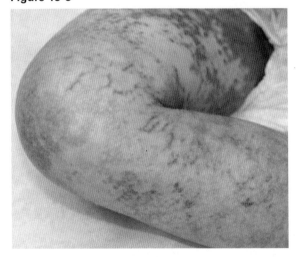

The initial signs are diarrhea, irritability, and edema of the hands and feet. Small dark patches appear at pressure points of the elbows, ankles, wrists, and knees, and then spread. The patches have a sharp border and tend to peel; the superficial desquamation in these areas is often likened to the appearance of flaking paint or enamel.

Figure 13-9

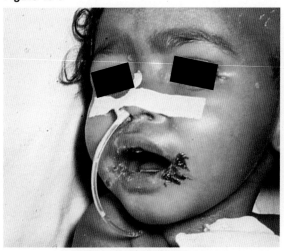

Kwashiorkor As the condition progresses, there develops a generalized red-brown discoloration. Other findings include fissuring at the edges of the mouth (Fig. 13-9) and the development of coarse, hypopigmented hair. Photosensitivity and easy bruising may also be present.

Figure 13-10

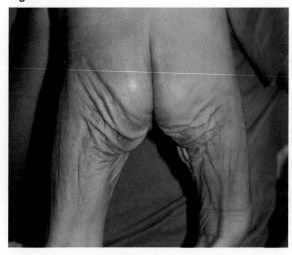

Marasmus Figure 13-10 illustrates the classic "baggy pants" appearance in protein-calorie malnutrition, also known as marasmus. Due to prolonged starvation, the child appears very thin, and has little subcutaneous fat or muscle mass. The child may also have a thin "old man" face. There is no associated edema of the lower extremities.

Figure 13-11

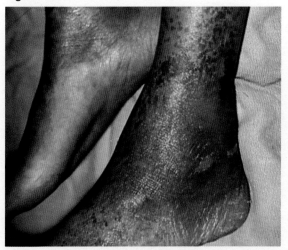

Pellagra Pellagra is a disease caused by inadequate dietary intake of niacin. It is now seen in parts of the world where dietary intake of tryptophan, an amino acid precursor of niacin, is inadequate. In particular, diets that consist largely or exclusively of maize or millet predispose to this disease. The signs and symptoms of pellagra are often remembered by the mnemonic four Ds: dermatitis, diarrhea, dementia, and death. The classic cutaneous changes are inflammation, hyperpigmentation, and

Figure 13-12

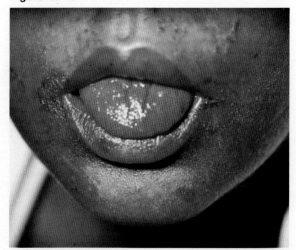

scaling in symmetric distribution and in areas exposed to heat or sunlight. Typical areas of involvement are the hands and forearms, legs and feet, and face and neck. Figure 13-11 shows moderate changes on the feet and legs. Figure 13-12 shows the scaling dermatitis on the face and an angular cheilitis. Edema and inflammation of the tongue are also common features of pellagra. The addition of supplemental niacin to the diet brings a quick resolution to the disease.

Figure 13-13

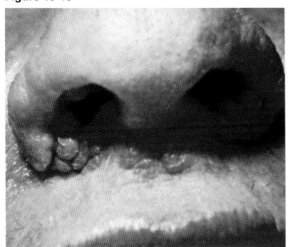

Lipoid proteinosis This is a rare autosomal recessive disease that is caused by the deposition of hyaline material in the skin and mucous membranes. Laryngeal involvement may be present from birth and eventually produces a characteristic hoarseness in every affected individual. Cutaneous disease begins during the first 2 years of life and consists of papules, nodules, and areas of thickening and hyperkeratosis.

Figure 13-14

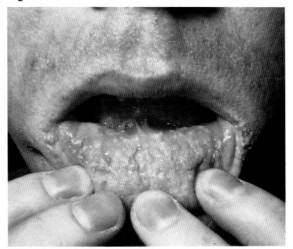

The cutaneous lesions on the alae nasi and in the choanae are shown in Fig. 13-13. In Fig. 13-14, the mucosal surface of the lower lip is extensively involved with the characteristic papules. Not shown here are the numerous small papules that dot the free margins of the eyelids. The disorder is due to a defect in the extracellular matrix protein 1 gene mapped to chromosome 1q21.

Figure 13-15

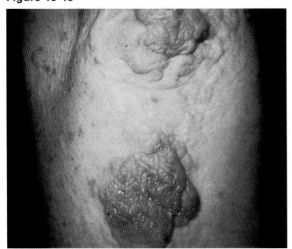

Lipoid proteinosis Pictured in Fig. 13-15 are a plaque and lesions of smaller sizes on and around the elbow. Most children with lipoid proteinosis continue to develop additional lesions during adult life. Lesions in the mouth and oropharynx cause the most serious sequelae. The tongue may become thick and bound down, and dysphagia and respiratory obstruction may result from lesions in the pharynx and larynx. Finally, intracranial calcifications are a common feature of lipoid proteinosis. For most patients, these are asymptomatic but seizure disorders may occur.

Figure 13-16

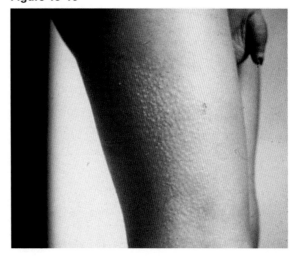

Hurler syndrome This inherited condition results in the accumulation of chondroitin sulfate B in the skin and other organ systems. Dwarfism and an unusual facial appearance are also aspects of the disease. Figure 13-16 is an excellent representation of shagreen skin, an appearance that is also seen in tuberous sclerosis. *Shagreen* refers to a type of leather that is embossed with knobs by processing and then variably stained.

Figure 13-17

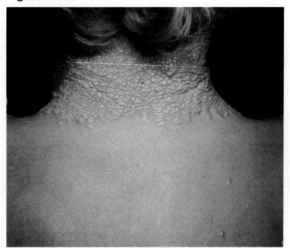

Xanthomatosis Xanthomas are papules or nodules of the skin or mucous membranes that contain lipids. The appearance of xanthomas during childhood should prompt a thorough search for underlying systemic disease. The yellowish papules seen in Fig. 13-17 are a form of planar xanthoma. These may occur on any part of the body and may be an indicator of a hereditary lipoproteinemia, diabetes mellitus, or liver disease. Multiple myeloma and Langerhans cell histiocytosis are less common etiologies. The patient pictured here has biliary cirrhosis.

Figure 13-18

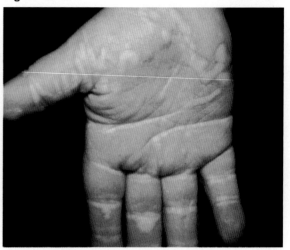

The lesions illustrated in Fig. 13-18 are typical of xanthoma striatum palmare, a form of planar xanthoma. This patient also has biliary cirrhosis. Note how the yellowish papules and plaques follow the creases of the fingers and the palmar folds. The familial hyperlipidemias, particularly types II, III, and V, may present with an identical clinical picture. Patients with these disorders are at high risk for ischemic heart disease.

Figure 13-19

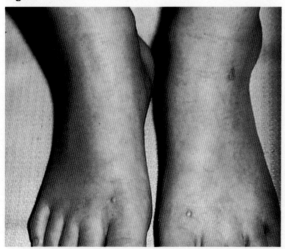

Xanthomatosis These small papules on the dorsa of the feet are also xanthomas. The patient is a 4-year-old child with type II hyperlipoproteinemia. This is an autosomal dominant condition in which there may be massive elevations in serum cholesterol. Individuals with this disease often develop ischemic heart disease during young adulthood. The recognition of the cutaneous lesions is important in identifying children who may require dietary or medical management of their hypercholesterolemia.

Figure 13-20

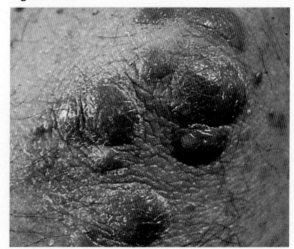

These yellow-red nodules shown in Fig. 13-20, which often occur on the elbows and knees, are termed *tuberous xanthomas*. They may also be found in other areas where ordinary trauma is common, for example, buttocks, knuckles, and heels. Similar lesions that overlie extensor tendons are sometimes called *tendon xanthomas*. Lesions of this sort are almost always caused by a hyperlipoproteinemia and should prompt investigation of serum cholesterol and triglycerides. Types II, IV, and V are those most commonly associated with tuberous and tendon xanthomas.

Figure 13-21

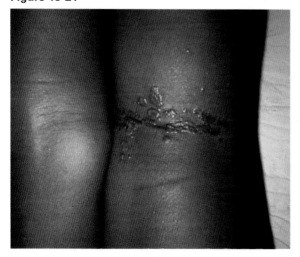

Xanthomatosis Not all xanthomatoses are rooted in abnormalities of cholesterol metabolism or other systemic disease. In Fig. 13-21, xanthomatous papules that developed in a lymphedematous leg are shown. Since serum lipids are normal, local causes stemming from the lymphatic obstruction must account for the lesions. The condition does not have the serious import of those xanthomatoses associated with abnormalities of serum lipids.

Figure 13-22

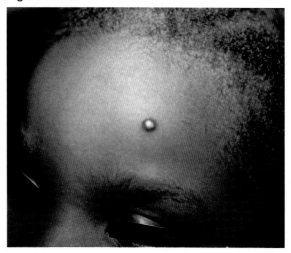

Calcinosis cutis When calcification occurs in the skin, it may represent an isolated local event, or it may be a sign of an underlying systemic disease. The lesion pictured in Fig. 13-22 is a solitary nodular calcification. These sometimes result from local trauma, such as an insect bite, or from the rupture of an epidermal cyst (dystrophic calcinosis cutis). When such nodules occur on the face of an infant, they are usually idiopathic and of no medical significance.

Figure 13-23

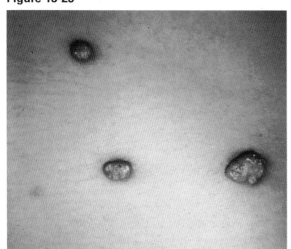

Calcinosis cutis The nodular calcifications pictured in Fig. 13-23 also turned out to be idiopathic. However, grouped calcifications such as these may also be seen in children with CRST syndrome (calcinosis cutis, Raynaud phenomenon, sclerodactyly, telangiectasia) or dermatomyositis. Pseudoxanthoma elasticum and Ehlers-Danlos syndrome are other causes. The so-called metastatic calcinosis cutis, with widespread precipitation of calcium salts, is a sign of abnormal calcium metabolism and may result from parathyroid tumors, chronic renal failure, or vitamin D intoxication.

Figure 13-24

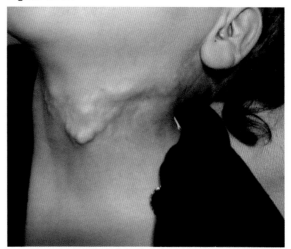

Progressive osseous heteroplasia In this rare disorder, bone forms within skin and muscle tissue. Ectopic bone formation starts in the dermis and subcutaneous fat and gradually extends into other tissues such as tendons and skeletal muscle. Progressive osseous heteroplasia is caused by a mutation in the *GNAS* gene.

Figure 13-25

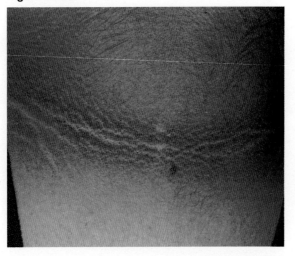

Figure 13-26

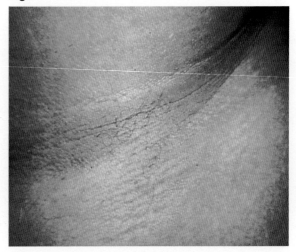

Acanthosis nigricans This common dermatosis is characterized by velvety, brownish-black plaques. The most common area of involvement is the neck, as pictured in Figs. 13-25 and 13-26, and the second most common is the axilla. Lesions also occur on flexural areas of the elbows, knees, and groin, and on the dorsal hands, especially over the fingers.

In children and adolescents, acanthosis nigricans is usually associated with obesity and insulin resistance. It offers a clue to either the diagnosis of type 2 diabetes or for the need for diet and exercise in order to prevent the development of this disease.

Figure 13-27

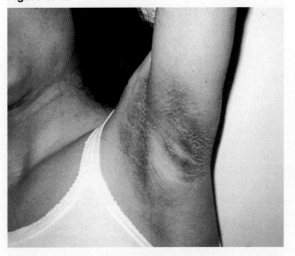

Figure 13-28

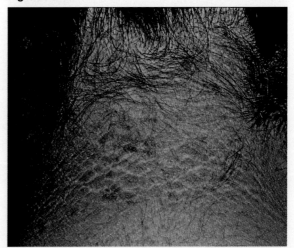

Acanthosis nigricans In some patients, the color and texture of the lesions will improve with the application of topical retinoids. Importantly, the diagnosis of acanthosis nigricans can be seen as an opportunity to counsel overweight and obese patients about diet and physical activity. Patients with hypertension, hypercholesterolemia, hypertriglyceridemia, or elevated fasting glucose may require medical therapy.

Very rarely, acanthosis nigricans develops as a sign of malignancy. It may also occur as a side effect of medications, including niacin, oral contraceptives, and protease inhibitors. Acanthosis nigricans may also be a manifestation of a variety of syndromes, including Costello syndrome and MORFAN syndrome.

Genodermatoses

Figure 14-1

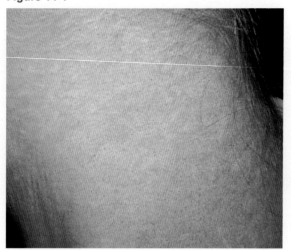

Pseudoxanthoma elasticum This is a generalized condition in which elastic fibers are degenerative. Clinical signs of the phenomenon can be recognized in the skin and eyes. In the skin, patches of yellowish discoloration and general laxness or redundancy develop on the neck ("chicken skin"), in the axillae, and in other places, such as the fossae of limbs and the inguinal folds,

Figure 14-2

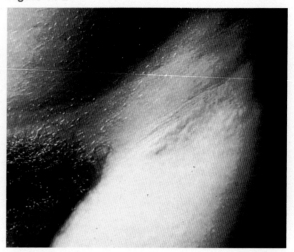

where considerable movement of skin is normal. In the eye, angioid streaks can be seen. They represent the result of faulty elastic fibers in Bruch membrane and generally precede the cutaneous changes. These eye changes frequently result in the loss of central vision and sometimes result in almost complete blindness. Peripheral vision is maintained.

Figure 14-3

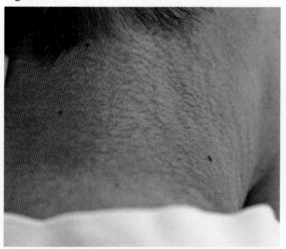

Pseudoxanthoma elasticum Gastrointestinal hemorrhage is the most serious acute consequence, but slower structural damage in various organs may result in hypertension, coronary artery occlusion, diabetes mellitus, thyroid dyscrasia, or ectopic calcinosis. The disease may be inherited in autosomal recessive or autosomal dominant fashion. This entity is caused by mutations in the *ABCC6* gene mapped to chromosome 16p13.1.

Figure 14-4

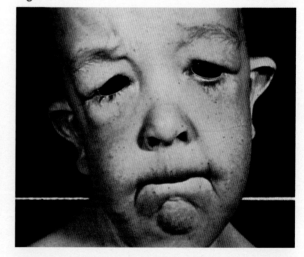

Cutis laxa This disorder may be caused by mutations in genes that are responsible for the formation, assembly, or function of elastic fibers, or may be later in life and related to the destruction of elastic fibers. As seen in this patient, the skin hangs in folds and produces an appearance of premature aging. Because elastic fibers are affected in all organ systems, intestinal and urinary bladder diverticula, rectal prolapse, inguinal hernias, and pulmonary emphysema occur frequently. The last of these is associated with significant mortality.

Figure 14-5

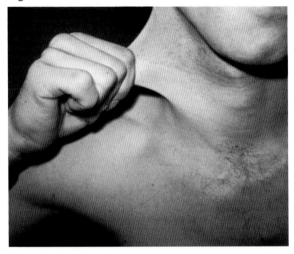

Figure 14-6

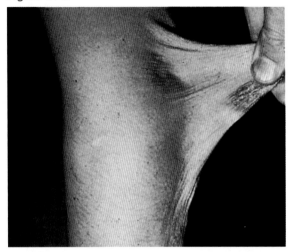

Ehlers-Danlos syndrome This syndrome is actually a collection of six major genetic types with the common features of hyperextensible skin and joints, easy bruising, defective wound healing, and blood vessel fragility. Distinct abnormalities in collagen synthesis have been identified in some of the varieties of Ehlers-Danlos syndrome. The result of the anomaly is extreme stretchability but unimpaired elasticity (ie, the ability to return to normal after stretching). The figures illustrate the phenomenon; Fig. 14-5 shows skin of the neck and Fig. 14-6 shows skin of the elbow extended several times more than normal skin can be pulled out.

Figure 14-7

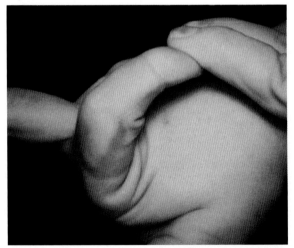

Figure 14-8

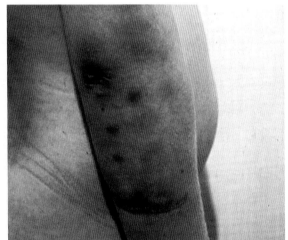

Ehlers-Danlos syndrome In these illustrations, more of the hyperextensible phenomena and the consequences of functional abnormality of elastic fibers and collagen are shown. Figure 14-7 shows hyperextensibility of joints, from which it may be inferred that skin, ligament, tendon, and to some extent bone are also abnormally stretchable. Another way in which softness of muscle and related structures can be appreciated is in the feel of a handshake with a patient who has Ehlers-Danlos syndrome. No matter how hard one presses, there is a feeling that one is not quite through with the handshake. Figures 14-8 illustrates the result of incisions and shearing trauma in the skin of a patient with Ehlers-Danlos syndrome. The result is hemorrhage, failure of healing by primary intention, and finally broad, friable scars.

Figure 14-9

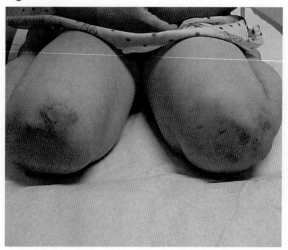

Figure 14-10

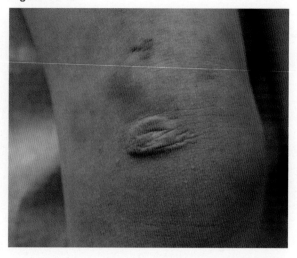

Ehlers-Danlos syndrome Small "pseudotumors" on easily traumatized areas such as the elbows and knees, illustrated in Figs. 14-9 and 14-10, are actually subcutaneous lesions that develop from fibrosis or calcification of hematomas.

Fat-containing cysts that become calcified, known as *spheorids,* are usually found on the forearms and shins. Depending on the type of Ehlers-Danlos, inheritance may be autosomal dominant, autosomal recessive, or X-linked recessive.

Figure 14-11

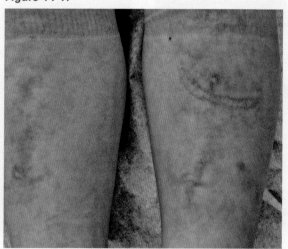

Ehlers-Danlos syndrome Gastrointestinal perforation and rupture of a large artery are the most severe complications of some forms of this syndrome. Premature birth (probably due to fragility of the fetal membranes) is a common event in patients with Ehlers-Danlos syndrome. Figure 14-11 shows another example of the disfiguring scars that are seen in this condition.

Figure 14-12

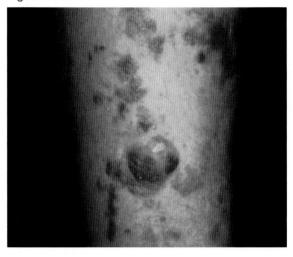

Focal dermal hypoplasia (Goltz syndrome) This syndrome is caused by heterozygous mutation in the *PORCN* gene on chromosome Xp11.23. The syndrome is transmitted in an X-linked dominant fashion. The most common cutaneous lesions are linear or reticulate areas of hypoplasia with telangiectasia, atrophy, and abnormal pigmentation. Figure 14-12 shows some lesions of this type, as well as the nodular fat tumors that are typically present.

Figure 14-13

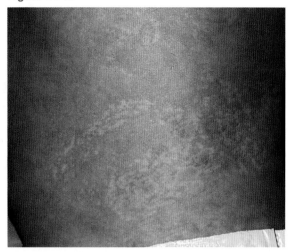

Figure 14-13 shows the whorled nature of the lesions on the trunk following the lines of Blaschko. Ulcers may be present initially in the areas of congenital absence of skin and heal with atrophy. The range of clinical presentation varies from minor involvement on the limbs to extensive distortion of the skin and bony skeleton.

Figure 14-14

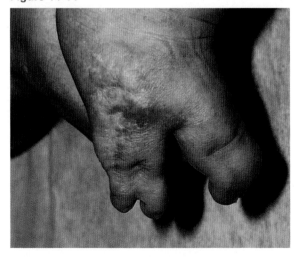

Focal dermal hypoplasia (Goltz syndrome) When bone is involved, syndactyly, polydactyly, oligodactyly with lobster claw deformity (as seen in Fig. 14-14), skeletal asymmetry, and scoliosis may occur. Ocular abnormalities include colobomas, microphthalmia, and strabismus.

Figure 14-15

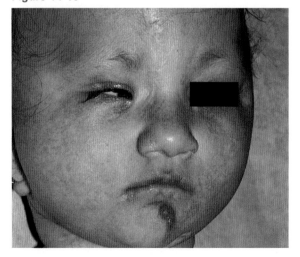

Figure 14-15 shows skin and eye defects that may occur in this syndrome. Note the atrophy on the forehead, the ocular defect in the right eye, and the papillomatous changes on the chin. Papillomas may be present on the lips or in the axillae, periumbilical area, or perineum.

Figure 14-16

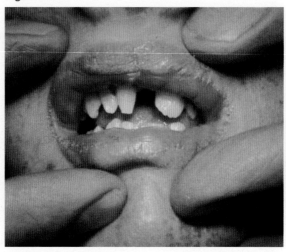

Focal dermal hypoplasia (Goltz syndrome) Figure 14-16 illustrates the frequent involvement of the perioral skin and teeth. Patients may present with hypodontia, oligodontia, or small teeth with dysplastic enamel.

Figure 14-17

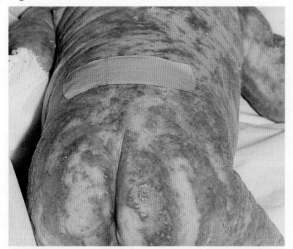

Figure 14-18

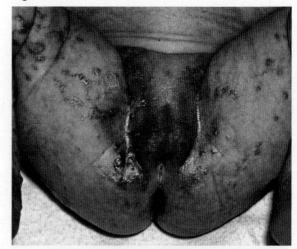

Incontinentia pigmenti This rare condition is characterized by linear and whorled lesions and a wide variety of systemic manifestations. Incontinentia pigmenti is inherited as an X-linked dominant trait linked to the *NEMO* gene and is seen almost exclusively in girls. The cutaneous eruption is usually present at birth and evolves through three stages.

Lesions typical of the first two stages, vesicular and verrucous, are seen in Figs. 14-17 and 14-18. The vesicular phase of incontinentia pigmenti can be quite extensive and lasts for about 2 weeks. Recurrence of vesicular lesions during childhood has also been reported to occur.

Figure 14-19

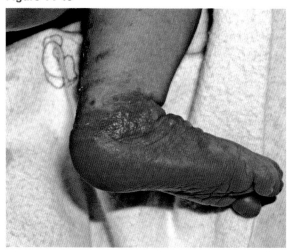

Incontinentia pigmenti The vesicular lesions in this disorder must be differentiated from herpes simplex and other causes of blistering in newborn infants. A skin biopsy often provides definitive evidence of the diagnosis.

Figure 14-20

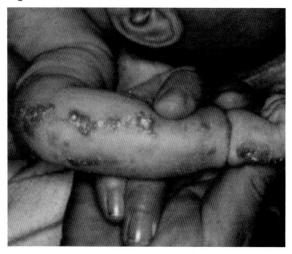

Vesicular and verrucous lesions following the lines of Blaschko are shown in Fig. 14-20. The disorder may also result in scarring alopecia of the scalp, dystrophic nails, and abnormalities of the teeth.

Figure 14-21

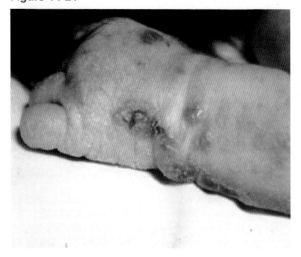

Incontinentia pigmenti A combination of vesicular and verrucous lesions are seen in this newborn girl.

Figure 14-22

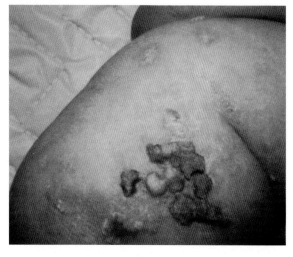

The verrucous phase lasts for about 6 weeks, although it may go on for many months or even for years in rare cases.

Figure 14-23

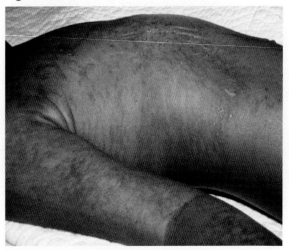

Incontinentia pigmenti Over several months the raised areas flatten, and the patient develops whorled, or "marble-cake," hyperpigmentation, as pictured in Figs. 14-23 to 14-25. In turn, the lesions of this third, hyperpigmented stage fade over a period of several years.

Figure 14-24

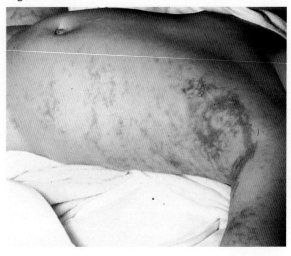

The patients represented in Figs. 14-23 and 14-24 both show details of the marbled hyperpigmentation as well as remnants of the previous papular verrucous stage. A fourth, hypopigmented stage can develop in the second and third decade.

Figure 14-25

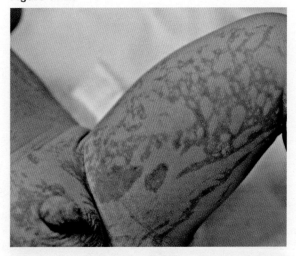

Incontinentia pigmenti This illustration is a good representation of extensive dyschromia. Central nervous system and ocular abnormalities are the most serious aspects of this disease. Some patients will develop seizures, mental retardation, or spastic paralysis. Eye involvement may include the presence of a retrolental mass, retinal detachment, cataracts, and optic atrophy. Skeletal anomalies are sometimes seen.

Figure 14-26

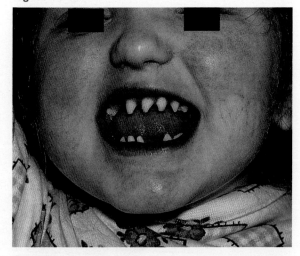

Incontinentia pigmenti The most common extracutaneous abnormality in incontinentia pigmenti involves teeth and occurs in about two-thirds of patients. There may be a marked delay in the eruption of deciduous teeth. Dental defects such as partial or complete absence of teeth as well as conical teeth may be seen.

Figure 14-27

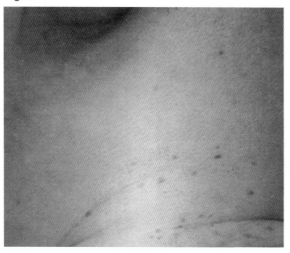

Wiskott-Aldrich syndrome This is another severe immunologic defect with X-linked recessive inheritance. The classic symptoms of this disease, which occurs only in males, are thrombocytopenia, recurrent infection, and a generalized eczematous or exfoliative dermatitis. Children with this disorder have impaired humoral and cell-mediated immunity, with deficient IgM and elevated IgA, and are at risk for sepsis and hemorrhage. Figure 14-27 shows the kind of petechiae that are evidence of the persistent thrombocytopenia.

Figure 14-28

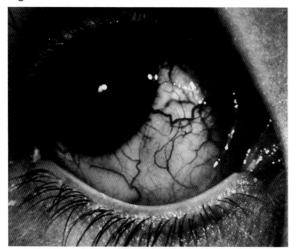

Figure 14-29

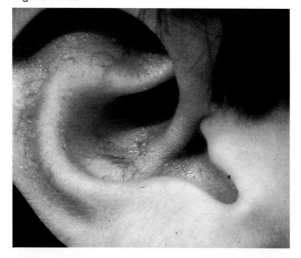

Ataxia telangiectasia This autosomal recessive disorder, caused by a defect in the *ATM* gene, affects the skin and the immunologic and central nervous systems. The onset of the disease, during early childhood, is characterized by the combination of progressive cerebellar ataxia and telangiectasias. The earliest site of telangiectasia is usually the bulbar conjunctiva, as pictured in Fig. 14-28. These vascular lesions also involve the neck, upper chest, face, and, as illustrated in Fig. 14-29, the pinna of the ear.

Later cutaneous changes include blotchy hyper- and hypopigmentation, café-au-lait spots, hirsutism, a generalized eczematous dermatitis, and granulomatous skin lesions. There may be premature graying of the hair. The immunologic abnormalities include decreased levels of IgA and IgE and defective cell-mediated immunity. Children with ataxia telangiectasia suffer from recurrent sinopulmonary infection and may die from bronchiectasis and respiratory failure. Lymphoreticular malignancies are an additional complication.

Figure 14-30

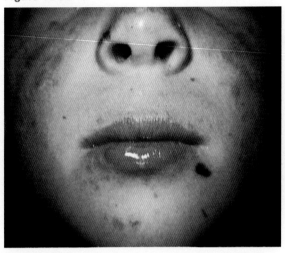

Figure 14-31

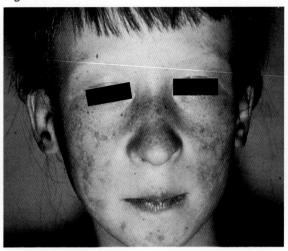

Bloom syndrome The principal cutaneous manifestations of this autosomal recessive syndrome are erythema and telangiectasias of the cheeks and photosensitivity. Café-au-lait spots and acanthosis nigricans may also be present. Children with Bloom syndrome are small at birth and have severe growth retardation throughout life. They also have recurrent respiratory infections and a strong tendency to develop malignancy. This rare disease is due to chromosomal abnormalities and defects in DNA repair. The syndrome is caused by mutation in the gene designated *BLM*, traced to band 15q26.1.

Rothmund-Thomson syndrome (Poikiloderma congenitale) This rare autosomal recessive disorder is attributed to mutations of the *RECQL4* helicase gene on chromosome 8q24. The condition begins during infancy with typically progressive skin changes. Erythema and edema of the facial skin are rapidly followed by the development of atrophy and telangiectasia. The same process occurs on the buttocks and extremities. Cataracts develop in many patients, and these often become apparent during infancy or early childhood. Skeletal deformities and short stature are other occasional features of this disease.

Figure 14-32

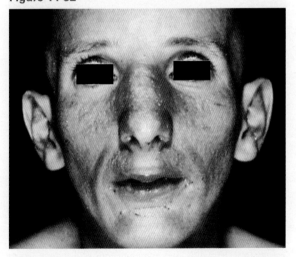

Figure 14-33

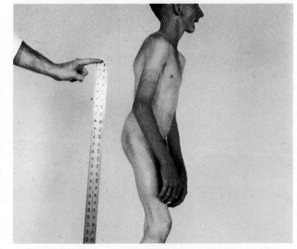

Cockayne syndrome This is another rare autosomal recessive condition characterized by skin changes and dwarfism. During the second year of life, patients develop a scaly photoeruption on the face and upper neck. This resolves with hyperpigmentation. The scaling photodermatitis and typical bird-like facies of this syndrome are illustrated in Fig. 14-32.

In addition to dwarfism (Fig. 14-33), affected individuals may demonstrate sensorineural deafness, microcephaly, and severe mental retardation. Optic atrophy and retinal degeneration may also be present. Characteristic intracranial calcifications are a feature of Cockayne syndrome that may aid in confirmation of the diagnosis. The disorder is due to a defect in DNA repair.

Figure 14-34

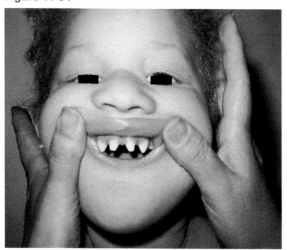

Hypohidrotic ectodermal dysplasia The ectodermal dysplasias are a wide variety of genetic disorders that may affect development of the hair, nails, teeth, and sweat glands. In this most common form, patients lack the ability to sweat and are at risk for developing hyperthermia in warm environmental conditions. There is sparse scalp and body hair and the hair may be, brittle, and slow-growing. Children may have absent teeth or teeth that are small and pointed.

Figure 14-35

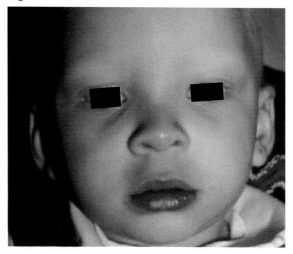

The facial features of hypohidrotic ectodermal dysplasia include thick lips, a prominent forehead, and a flattened nasal bridge. There is often dark and thickened skin around the eyes, and children with this disorder are prone to atopic dermatitis. Most cases are caused by mutations in the *EDA* gene, which is inherited in an X-linked recessive pattern. Other forms are either autosomal dominant or autosomal recessive.

Figure 14-36

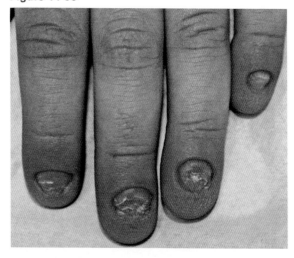

Clouston syndrome This less common form of ectodermal dysplasia is inherited in an autosomal dominant fashion and is due to a mutation in the *GJB6* gene. Abnormal fingernails and toenails are a hallmark of this disorder. The nails are white in early childhood, and later become thick and brittle.

Figure 14-37

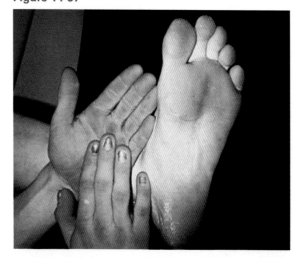

The nail dystrophy may be accompanied by severe hyperkeratosis of the palms and soles, as seen in Fig. 14-37. Topical keratolytics are of some help to affected individuals. Other features of this disorder are hyperpigmentation of the skin over the joints, and clubbing of the nails. Sweating is normal.

Figure 14-38

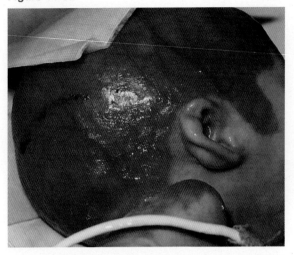

Figure 14-39

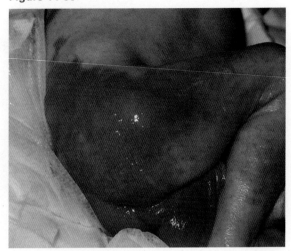

Hay-Well syndrome (AEC) Most infants with this autosomal dominant disorder caused by mutation in the *TP63* gene are born with generalized erythematous and scaly skin. There may be significant erosions as noted on the scalp and buttocks in the infant represented in Figs. 14-38 and 14-39. The erosions can lead to scarring and hair loss.

Skin erosions may occur throughout childhood and at time into adulthood. Other common features include the presence of ankyloblepharon (small strands of skin between the eyelids) at birth, and cleft lip and palate. Limb abnormalities such as syndactyly may be seen.

Figure 14-40

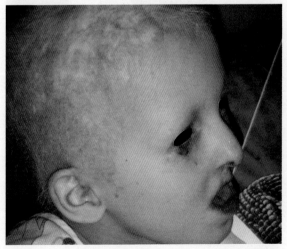

Figure 14-41

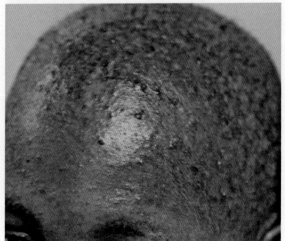

Hay-Well syndrome (AEC) Many patients with this syndrome have persistent problems with an erosive scalp dermatitis, with frequent secondary infection and excessive granulation tissue.

The hair on other parts of the scalp tends to be wiry and coarse. Scarring and hypotrichosis is noted in the patient in Fig. 14-40. In Fig. 14-41 there are pustules scattered throughout the scalp.

Figure 14-42

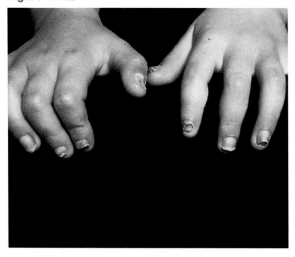

Pachyonychia congenita This condition results from mutations in the genes encoding epidermal keratinocyte keratins, and affects nails, palms and soles, and the mucous membranes of the lips and mouth.

Figure 14-43

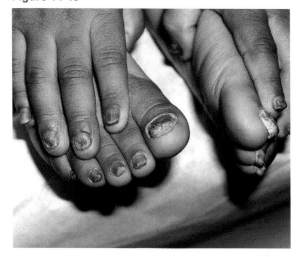

The nail changes are distinctive in their discoloration, hardness, excessive growth, and attachment to hyperkeratotic nail beds. In Fig. 14-43, scleronychia and binding to the nail beds can be appreciated.

Figure 14-44

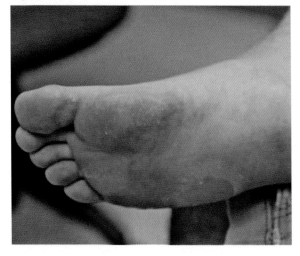

Pachyonychia congenita Figure 14-44 illustrates the severe hyperkeratotic process on the soles of the feet. The palms may also be involved. The plantar involvement can be particularly painful and interfere with normal function.

Figure 14-45

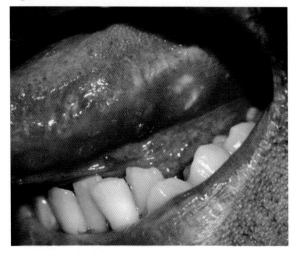

Patients with pachyonychia congenital also develop leukokeratosis of the tongue. Oral lesions occur in approximately 70% of patients, but do not evolve into malignancy.

Figure 14-46

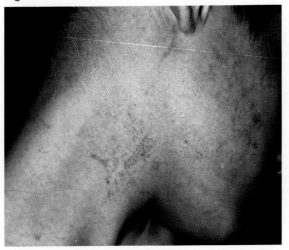

Figure 14-47

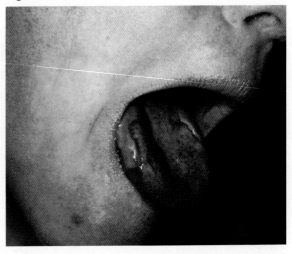

Dyskeratosis congenita This rare congenital condition results from mutations in at least 10 known genes and occurs in X-linked recessive, autosomal dominant, and autosomal recessive subtypes. It is characterized by atrophy and dyschromia of the skin, atrophic dysplasia of nails, and leukoplakia. Figure 14-46 illustrates the typical mottled or retiform poikiloderma. The face, neck, and upper part of the body are characteristically involved.

Mucous membrane involvement is shown in Fig. 14-47. There are two lesions on the tongue that are gray and hypertrophic. The buccal mucosa and the mucosa of the urethra and anus may also be affected. Aside from the cutaneous and mucosal effects, abnormalities such as those seen in Fanconi syndrome may be associated with this condition.

Figure 14-48

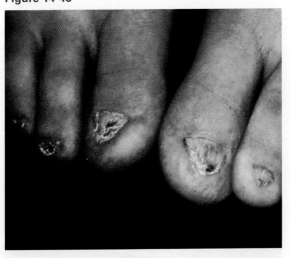

Figure 14-49

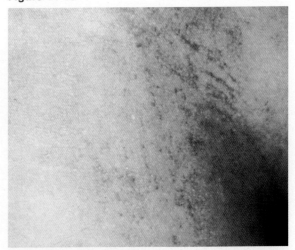

Dyskeratosis congenita Fig. 14-48 shows hypoplastic nail changes that are characteristic. Note how different they are from those of pachyonychia congenita (Figs. 14-42 and 14-43).

Details of the cutaneous changes on glabrous skin in and around the groin, similar to those that occur on the neck and face, are shown in Fig. 14-49. Hyperhidrosis of palms and soles, conjunctivitis, esophageal strictures, intestinal diverticula, mental retardation, and anemia may be part of the syndrome. Malignant degeneration in the leukoplakia of the mucous membranes can occur.

Figure 14-50

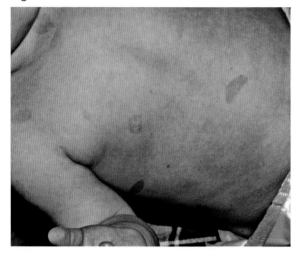

Figure 14-51

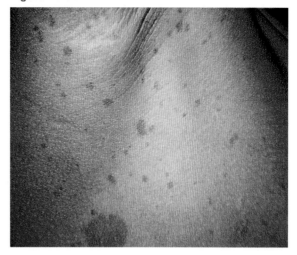

Neurofibromatosis Type I This autosomal dominant disorder includes a number of distinctive cutaneous findings and a wide variety of neurologic manifestations. Figure 14-50 shows multiple café-au-lait macules. Solitary lesions of this type are common in normal individuals; most patients with neurofibromatosis have more than a single macule. The presence of more than six lesions that are larger than 0.5 cm in diameter in prepubescent children and 1.5 cm in diameter in adults is considered one of the major diagnostic criteria for this disease.

In Fig. 14-51, there are numerous macules of hyperpigmentation in the axilla. Axillary freckling, also called *Crowe sign,* is a unique finding in neurofibromatosis. Pigmented hamartomas of the iris, termed *Lisch nodules,* are also present in almost all patients with this condition. Optic gliomas may also be seen. The inheritance of neurofibromatosis is complicated by a highly variable range of expression among those affected. A single family may include some individuals with only cutaneous involvement and others with numerous neurofibromas or severe neurologic disease. Spontaneous mutations are also common.

Figure 14-52

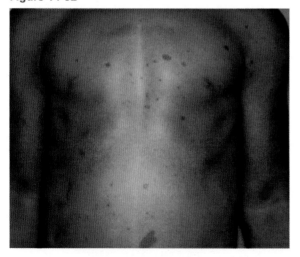

Figure 14-53

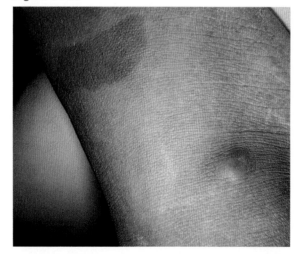

Neurofibromatosis Type I These are more illustrations of the pigmentary anomalies and tumors in the skin of patients with neurofibromatosis. Figure 14-52 shows several café-au-lait spots and small tumors. Figure 14-53 shows a large café-au-lait spot on the left and a tumor on the right. Neurofibromas have variable consistency. The soft lesions can be pushed into the surrounding skin, a process called "buttonholing." Neurofibromas usually begin to develop during puberty and may cause severe

cosmetic disfigurement. Pruritus of the skin that overlies the neurofibroma is a common complaint, and the itching is aggravated by exertion or a warm environment. Malignant degeneration of a benign neurofibroma can occur. In addition, patients with the disease are prone to developing neurofibrosarcomas or malignant schwannomas de novo. Selective surgical removal of neurofibromas, in order to improve either appearance or function, is feasible.

Figure 14-54

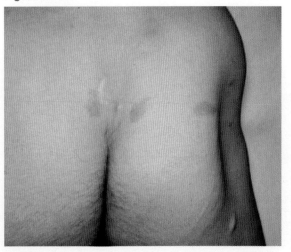

Neurofibromatosis Type I Figure 14-54 shows three café-au-lait spots and a small, soft neurofibroma. Intellectual handicap, and seizures are frequent manifestations of classic, or von Recklinghausen, neurofibromatosis.

Figure 14-55

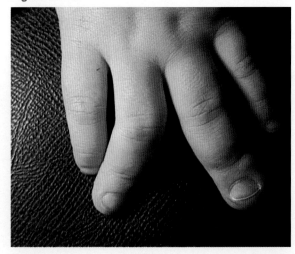

The enlargement in Fig. 14-55 was found to be due to a neurofibroma in the palm and along the length of the digits. Although neurofibromatosis tends to be progressive, it is entirely unpredictable. There is no single aspect of the clinical course that allows the physician to foresee the evolution of other features.

Figure 14-56

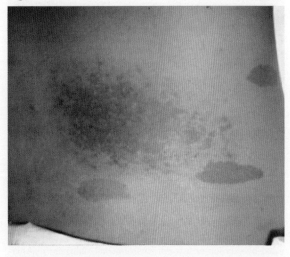

Neurofibromatosis Type I Figure 14-56 illustrates several large café au lait spots, and an area of grayish mottled hyperpigmentation that probably overlies a plexiform neurofibroma. These subcutaneous tumors are pathognomonic for neurofibromatosis type I.

Figure 14-57

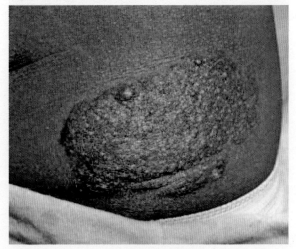

Plexiform neurofibromas may sometimes be subtle, initially presenting only as a patch of hyperpigmentation and/or hypertrichosis. With time, they can grow quite large.

Figure 14-58

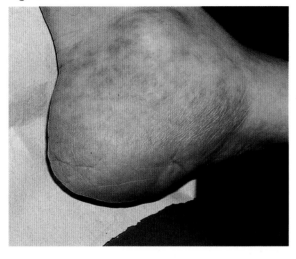

Neurofibromatosis type I Larger plexiform neurofibromas are described as having a "bag of worms" consistency and may be cosmetically disabling.

Figure 14-59

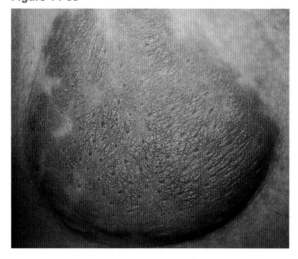

Figure 14-59 shows a large plexiform neurofibroma with overlying darkening and thickening of the skin. Plexiform neurofibromas may also present as firm nodules attached to the nerves. Tumors around nerves may cause pain, muscle weakness, or atrophy.

Figure 14-60

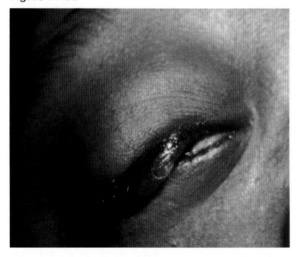

Neurofibromatosis type I Plexiform neurofibromas can invade the orbit or eyelids, obscure the visual axis and cause amgblyopia. In the long term, infiltration of these anatomical structures is potentially vision threatening.

Figure 14-61

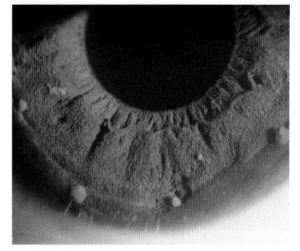

Neurofibromatosis type I (Lisch nodule) Lisch nodules are melanocytic hamartomas occurring on the iris. They can be seen on routine examination of the eye, but a slit lamp is required to distinguish these lesions from nevi. Lisch nodules are brown and dome-shaped and measure up to 2 mm in diameter. The majority of patients with NF1 develop this finding during childhood, and the nodules are present in the vast majority of adolescents and adults with the disorder. The nodules do not cause any ophthalmologic complication.

Figure 14-62

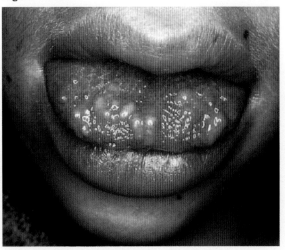

Figure 14-63

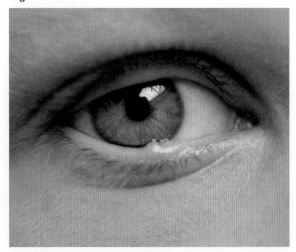

Multiple endocrine neoplasia type 2 The presence of numerous small neuromas of the lips, tongue, and oral mucosa is a marker for a unique autosomal dominant condition. This rare familial syndrome, formerly termed *mucosal neuroma syndrome,* is caused by mutations in the *RET* proto-oncogene, and carries a very high risk for malignancy. Eighty percent of affected individuals will

develop medullary thyroid carcinoma. Pheochromocytoma may also occur. The patient in Fig. 14-62 developed both tumors and had the marfanoid habitus that is frequently seen in patients with the disorder. Note the small lesions in the lower eyelid in Fig. 14-63.

Figure 14-64

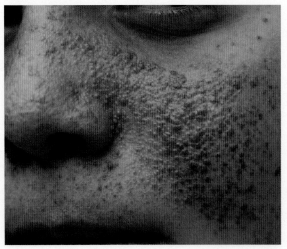

Figure 14-65

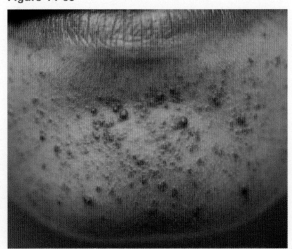

Tuberous sclerosis This autosomal dominant disease with widely variable penetrance has its main effects on the skin, central nervous system, eye, kidney, and heart. Figures 14-64 and 14-65 illustrate angiofibromas, previously named adenoma sebaceum, one of the most common cutaneous manifestations. The pink-to-red dome-shaped papules usually appear between the ages of 2 and 6, and, early in the clinical course, can be confused with acne. The angiofibromas may be symmetrically distributed over the entire face but are usually most concentrated on the cheeks.

In some patients topical sirolimus may be an effective treatment of angiofibromas. The extent of cutaneous involvement is not generally predictive of the severity of the systemic disease. Patients who are severely affected suffer from seizure disorders and mental retardation. Other findings of tuberous sclerosis include retinal and renal hamartomas, cerebral nodules and calcifications, and cardiac rhabdomyomas. This disorder is due to mutations in *TSC1* (hamartin gene) or *TSC2,* (tuberin gene).

Figure 14-66

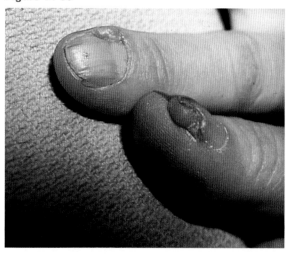

Tuberous sclerosis Figure 14-66 illustrates subungual and periungual fibromas, also known as *Koenen tumors*. These firm lesions arise from the nail beds, usually after puberty. Periungual fibromas may occur in both fingernails and toenails, and can be painful and disfiguring.

Figure 14-67

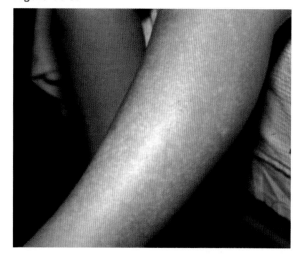

Confetti-like hypopigmented macules may occur on the extremities of children with tuberous sclerosis. This form of hypopigmentation is significantly less common than larger hypopigmented macule (ash leaf spot) illustrated in Fig. 14-68.

Figure 14-68

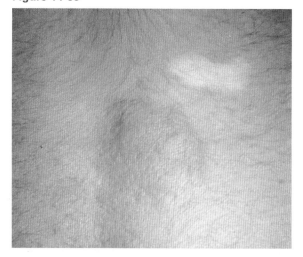

Tuberous sclerosis This figure shows a hypopigmented macule, which sometimes takes the shape of an ash leaf. Hypopigmented macules may occur in healthy infants, but the appearance of several lesions should prompt a search for other manifestations in the patient and family members. These spots are either present at birth or evolve during infancy. Wood light examination may sometimes reveal hypopigmented macules whose presence is otherwise not obvious.

Figure 14-69

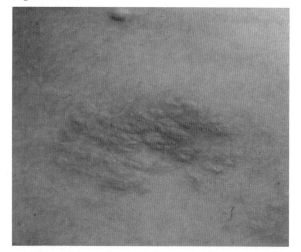

Shown in the center of Fig. 14-68, and in this photo (Fig. 14-69) is the shagreen patch. The lesion, frequently seen in children with tuberous sclerosis, is an area of cutaneous thickening with a pebbled surface. Histologically, this lesion is a form of connective tissue nevus.

Figure 14-70

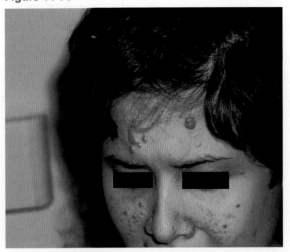

Tuberous sclerosis Another cutaneous finding in tuberous sclerosis is the development of firm fibrous plaques that are located on the forehead, scalp, and cheeks. These lesions, which may be present at birth, are different from angiofibromas in that there is no vascular dilatation associated with the dermal fibrosis.

Figure 14-71

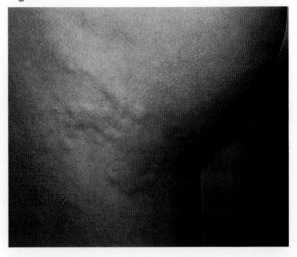

Buschke-Ollendorf syndrome This autosomal dominant syndrome is characterized by the presence of connective tissue nevi of the skin and a radiologic abnormality known as *osteopoikilosis*. The connective tissue nevi are yellowish plaques that tend to appear before puberty and are present on the trunk, buttocks, and arms. Osteopoikilosis is an asymptomatic bony abnormality that presents as round opacities within the carpal and tarsal bones, the phalanges, the epiphyses and metaphyses of the long bones, and the pelvis.

Figure 14-72

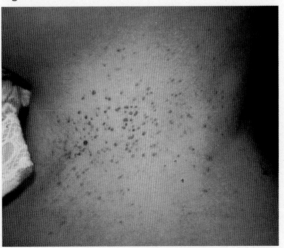

Basal cell nevus syndrome Patients with this autosomal dominant syndrome caused by gene defects in the *PTCH1, PTCH2,* and *SUFU* genes develop multiple basal cell carcinomas and cysts within the mandible. Additional findings include hypertelorism, a variety of other skeletal abnormalities, and calcification of the falx cerebri. Shown in Fig. 14-72 is an example of multiple small basaloid proliferations.

Figure 14-73

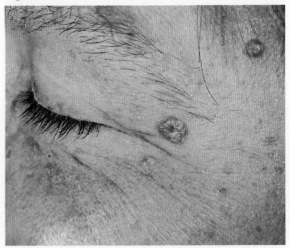

Most patients with basal cell nevus syndrome have more conventional basal cell carcinomas in the form of pearly telangiectatic nodules, sometimes with ulceration, as is shown in Fig. 14-73. Basal cell carcinomas usually develop in these patients after puberty, although they may occur in childhood.

Figure 14-74

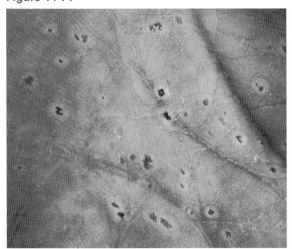

Basal cell nevus syndrome Figure 14-74 shows the palmar pitting that appears during puberty in individuals with this syndrome. Rapidly enlarging basal cell carcinomas must be treated early on with the conventional surgical modalities in order to minimize disfigurement and avoid loss of function. Patients with this syndrome are also at risk for medulloblastoma. This grave complication tends to occur in early childhood.

Figure 14-75

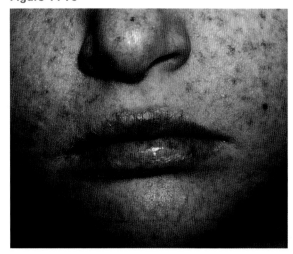

Xeroderma pigmentosum This rare autosomal recessive disease is caused by an inability to repair DNA that has been damaged by ultraviolet light. There are at least eight different molecular defects. Freckling develops on sun-exposed skin at a very early age along with xerosis, scaling, and telangiectasia. Speckled hypo- and hyperpigmentation are also typical.

Figure 14-76

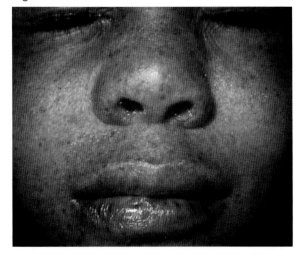

Xeroderma pigmentosum Patients with this disease also tend to develop hyperkeratoses and changes consistent with actinic keratoses. In early childhood, patients with xeroderma pigmentosum begin to develop cutaneous malignancies: basal cell and squamous cell carcinomas and, less commonly, melanomas.

Figure 14-77

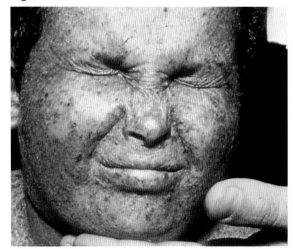

The mortality from this disease is caused by destructive local growth of tumors and by metastases. In addition, patients may suffer from severe neurologic dysfunction, including mental retardation. Although no treatment is available, individuals with this disease benefit from a lifestyle that allows minimal exposure to sunlight.

Ichthyoses and Disorders of Keratinization

Figure 15-1

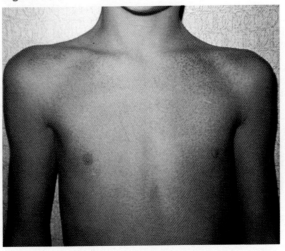

Figure 15-2

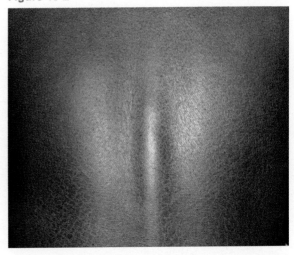

Ichthyosis vulgaris This is the mildest and most common form of ichthyosis, with an incidence in school-aged children as high as 1:250. It is inherited as an autosomal dominant trait and is present in a significant percentage of individuals with atopic dermatitis. It is not present at birth.

The clinical appearance of this ichthyosis varies, depending on location. Figures 15-1 and 15-2 illustrate the fine, bran-like scaling on the upper chest and back. Children with ichthyosis vulgaris are likely to have increased skin markings on the palms and soles and a high incidence of keratosis pilaris (see Figs. 15-61 to 15-64).

Figure 15-3

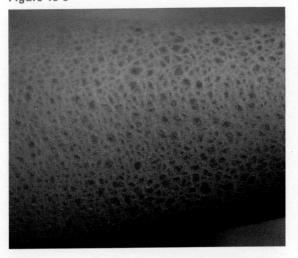

Figure 15-4

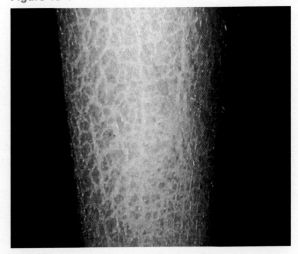

Ichthyosis vulgaris On the anterior lower leg, there are often larger, plate-like scales that resemble the skin of a fish (Figs. 15-3 and 15-4). Facial involvement is usually minimal, and flexural areas are typically spared.

Ichthyosis vulgaris tends to worsen in winter when there is less sweating and lower humidity. Treatment of ichthyosis vulgaris entails the use of emollients and creams and ointments containing urea, lactic acid, and other alpha-hydroxy acids. Excessive bathing and the use of alkaline soaps should be avoided. The exacerbation that frequently occurs in winter months can be lessened if a humidifier is used in the child's room.

Figure 15-5

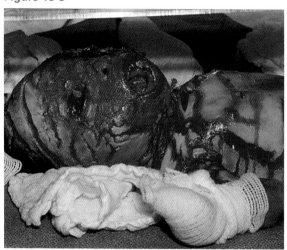

Harlequin–type ichthyosis The newborn infant is covered with thick plates of scale that are often described as resembling a coat of armor. After birth, deep erythematous fissures form between areas of scale. There is also severe facial disfigurement due to eclabium, ectropion, and edema of the conjunctiva. The texture of the skin results in restriction of the respiratory movements of the chest and interferes with normal feeding. This form of ichthyosis is due to a mutation on the *ABCA12* gene.

Figure 15-6

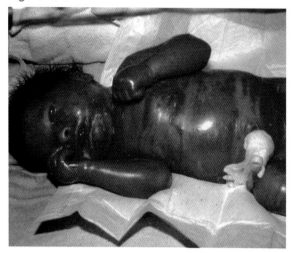

Collodion baby This is a descriptive term for the child who is born encased in a taut, parchment-like membrane, accompanied by ectropion and eclabium. The outcome of this process is unpredictable. When the membrane is completely shed, the infant may go on to develop one of several ichthyosis skin types. Lamellar ichthyosis and congenital ichthyosiform erythroderma (pictured in Fig. 15-6) are the most common. A small percentage of infants go on to have completely normal skin, a phenomenon called "self-healing collodion baby."

Figure 15-7

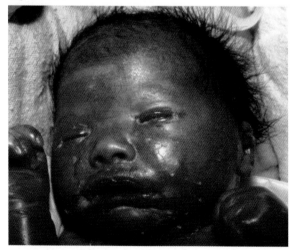

Collodion baby Collodion babies are at risk for complications. These include infection, dehydration, body temperature instability, and pneumonia. Collodion babies should be placed in a high humidity environment, and monitored closely. Gradually, the membrane will come off on its own. The child pictured in Fig. 15-7 also developed congenital ichthyosiform erythroderma.

Figure 15-8

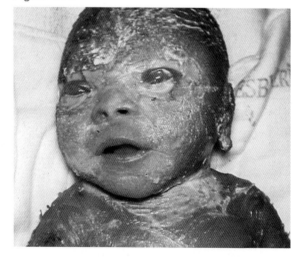

Figure 15-8 is an example of more severe form of collodion baby, with marked ectropion. After spontaneous shedding of the collodion membrane, this child went on to develop lamellar ichthyosis (Figs. 15-9 to 15-16).

Figure 15-9

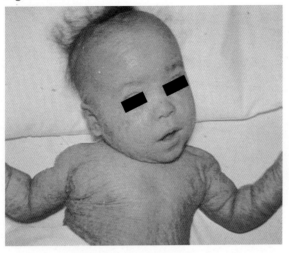

Lamellar ichthyosis Collodion babies, irrespective of the cause, are very often born prematurely. In addition, they are at risk for cutaneous infection, sepsis, pneumonia, and require careful supportive therapy. This infant was formerly a collodion baby and has gradually sloughed his membrane. When the baby was several months of age, he began to develop generalized hyperkeratosis and scaling. This infant has the chronic and severe autosomal recessive disease of lamellar ichthyosis.

Figure 15-10

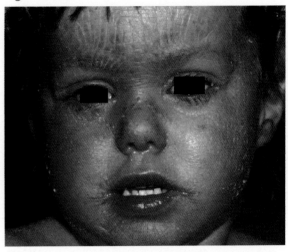

The child in Fig. 15-10 has severe facial involvement. Note the ectropion and tightness of the facial skin as a result of hyperkeratosis. Plate-like scales of the forehead are a particularly common feature.

Figure 15-11

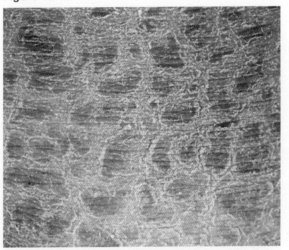

Lamellar ichthyosis Figure 15-11 shows in detail the kind of ichthyosis that gradually becomes established after the disappearance of the collodion membrane. Note the mosaic pattern of the scales and tendency of the edges of the scale to curl away from the surface. The scales are sometimes compared with armored plates. Blister formation does not occur in this condition.

Figure 15-12

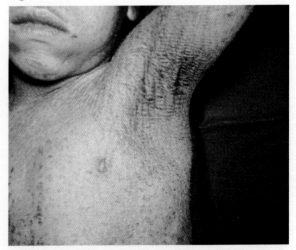

In severe cases, the entire skin surface, including the face, is affected by the hyperkeratotic, scaly, dyschromic dyskeratinization. Involvement tends to be most severe in flexural areas, as in the axilla pictured in Fig. 15-12. Topical therapy with the α-hydroxy acids, such as lactic acid, or with topical N-acetylcysteine is somewhat helpful in reducing the amount of scale and improving the appearance.

Figure 15-13

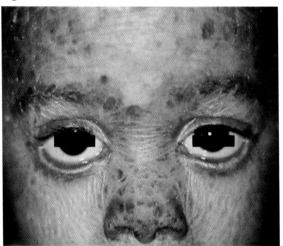

Lamellar icthyosis (cont'd.) In this severe example, there is thick and dark scale involving the entire face, as well as severe ectropion. For many children, eye involvement like this is the most disfiguring aspect of the disease. In addition, scaliness of the scalp may be accompanied by partial hair loss.

Figure 15-14

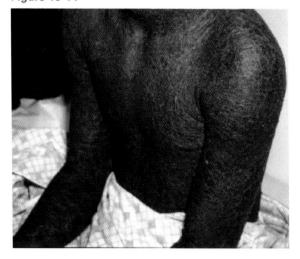

This patient has developed thick scale involving the entire skin surface. One form of lamellar ichthyosis is associated with a deficiency of the enzyme keratinocyte transglutaminase.

Figure 15-15

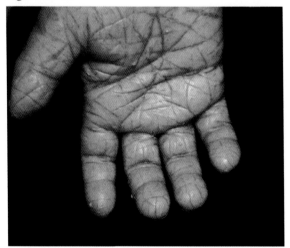

Lamellar ichthyosis Figures 15-15 and 15-16 illustrate involvement of the palms and soles with thick hyperkeratosis and deep grooves.

Figure 15-16

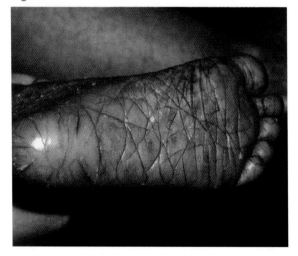

In addition to thickening and fissuring of the palms and soles, the nails may be ridged or thickened, and there may be thick subungual hyperkeratosis.

Figure 15-17

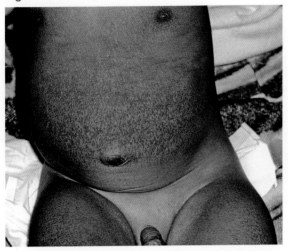

Recessive X-linked ichthyosis This disorder is characterized by ichthyosis that begins at or shortly after birth and persists through adult life. The "dirty" brown and tightly adherent scales are illustrated in Figs. 15-17 to 15-19. The scaling tends to favor the trunk and the extensor surfaces of the extremities. There is relative sparing of the face and flexural areas.

Figure 15-18

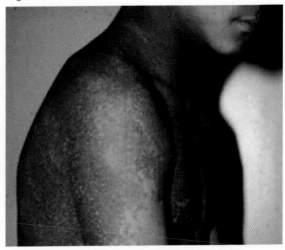

The palms and soles are also spared, and the hair and teeth are normal. Most patients note marked improvement during the summer months, probably related to improved skin hydration. Asymptomatic corneal opacities on the posterior membrane serve as an adult marker for this disease.

Figure 15-19

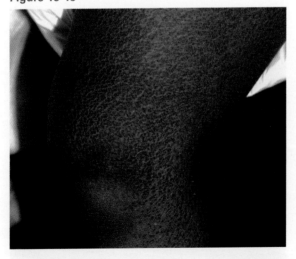

Recessive X-linked ichthyosis In addition, there is a significant incidence of cryptorchidism in individuals with this syndrome. The locus for this rare genodermatosis is now known to affect the STS (steroid sulfatase) gene on the distal short arm of the X chromosome, and the disease is inherited in X-linked recessive fashion. The underlying metabolic disorder is a deficiency in the enzyme steroid sulfatase.

Figure 15-20

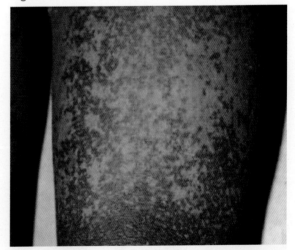

Figure 15-20 gives a closer view of the tightly adherent scales that are seen in this hereditary disorder.

Figure 15-21

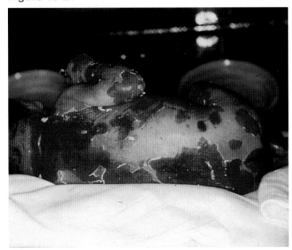

Epidermolytic ichthyosis (formerly epidermolytic hyperkeratosis) The appearance of epidermolytic ichthyosis in a newborn is illustrated in Fig. 15-21. Typically, there are large areas of denuded skin, and sometimes there are intact blisters. The differentiation from epidermolysis bullosa can usually be made by positive family history, the presence of subtle areas of hyperkeratosis, and, most important, the characteristic skin biopsy. Treatment in the newborn period should focus on gentle handling to avoid new blister formation, the maintenance of fluid and electrolyte balance, and the prevention of bacterial superinfection.

Figure 15-22

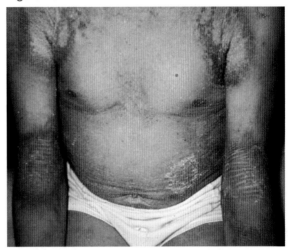

Over time, the generalized blistering resolves, and widespread areas of thick hyperkeratosis and scale develop. In Fig. 15-22, there is a mixed picture; focal erosions are present on the arms and abdomen, and there are areas of thick, discolored, furrowed hyperkeratosis. Note the predilection, which is not seen in ichthyosis vulgaris, for the antecubital fossae and intertriginous spaces.

Figure 15-23

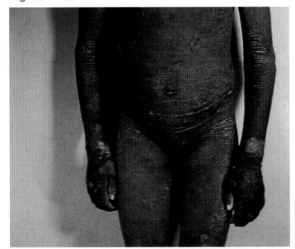

Epidermolytic ichthyosis (formerly epidermolytic hyperkeratosis) This condition was also previously called bullous congenital ichthyosiform erythroderma. It is inherited in an autosomal dominant fashion. The genetic defect lies in mutations in genes encoding keratins 1 and 10. The former is associated with the additional involvement of the palms and soles. Figures 15-23 and 15-24 show bullous ichthyosis in its most severe and generalized form.

Figure 15-24

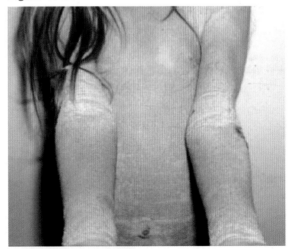

Patients with disease face a very difficult set of problems. Bacterial colonization of this thickened and furrowed skin may result in an extremely unpleasant body odor. The foul smell, along with the disfigurement caused by the disease itself, may interfere enormously with social adaptation. Antibacterial soaps are of some help in reducing odor.

Figure 15-25

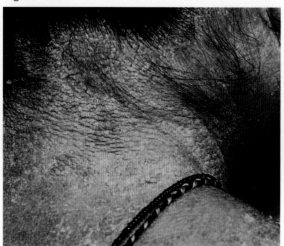

Epidermolytic ichthyosis (formerly epidermolytic hyperker-atosis) Some children remain prone to mechanically induced blisters in areas of friction or trauma. Treatment with kerato-lytics will often induce painful superficial erosions, and the use of oral retinoids, with all of their side effects, has met with little success.

Figure 15-26

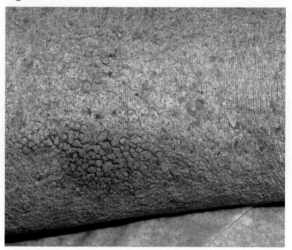

Figure 15-26 illustrates both the darkening and thickening of the skin and the areas of adjacent superficial erosion. Fortunately, in many patients the disease tends to localize to smaller, usually flexural, areas with advancing age.

Figure 15-27

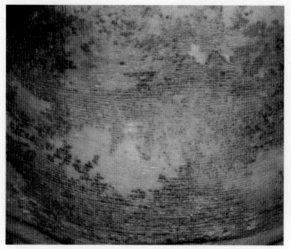

Epidermolytic ichthyosis (formerly epidermolytic hyperker-atosis) Figure 15-27 illustrates the abdomen of a patient with epidermolytic ichthyosis. Note the dark, thickened scale with areas of desquamation that appear to have somewhat more normal skin than the surrounding areas that appear to have a slightly lichenified appearance.

Figure 15-28

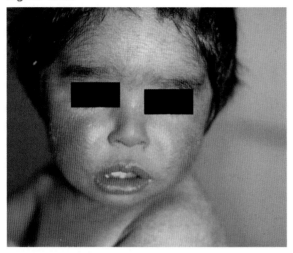

Figure 15-29

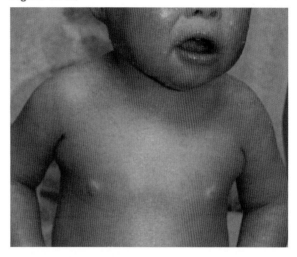

Nonbullous congenital ichthyosiform erythroderma This rare autosomal recessive condition may present with a collodion membrane at birth. The severity of the disease during infancy and later childhood is extremely variable.

The most typical appearance features widespread scaling and moderate to severe erythroderma. The children with most severe involvement may experience difficulty with temperature regulation, and should be followed closely for evidence of secondary infection.

Figure 15-30

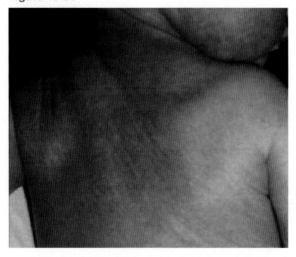

Nonbullous congenital ichthyosiform erythroderma Most cases are caused by mutations in the *ALOXE3*, *ALOX12B*, and *NIPAL4* genes. Improvement sometimes occurs at puberty.

Figure 15-31

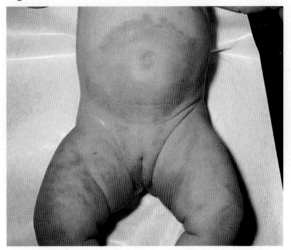

Erythrokeratoderma variabilis This is a rare autosomal dominant condition characterized by migratory areas of erythema and distinct plaques of hyperkeratosis. From an early beginning in infancy, there occur figurate and rapidly (within days) shifting areas of bright erythema on the face, anterior trunk, buttocks, and extensor aspects of the limbs. These may be brought on by changes in environmental temperature. In addition, there are fixed and localized hyperkeratotic plaques.

Figure 15-32

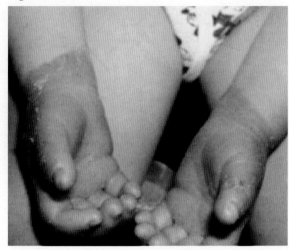

Progressive symmetric erythrokeratoderma This rare disorder develops in early childhood. The lesions are symmetrical large, sharply circumscribed, hyperkeratotic plaques with brownish or orange-red discoloration. The most common locations are the extensor limbs, shoulders, buttocks and fingers. In about half of the patients, palms and soles are involved.

Figure 15-33

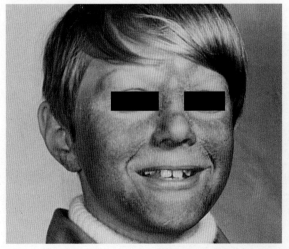

Progressive symmetric erythrokeratoderma As illustrated in Fig. 15-33, facial involvement may also occur. In contrast to patients with erythrokeratoderma variabilis, these lesions are nonmigratory. Therapeutic options are limited and the use of oral retinoids may be considered.

Figure 15-34

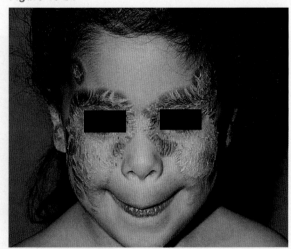

This essentially autosomal dominant disease tends to progress until adolescence, and then may improve spontaneously during adult life.

Figure 15-35

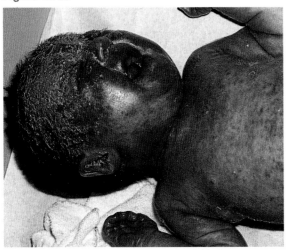

Netherton syndrome This rare autosomal recessive syndrome is associated with mutations in the *SPINK5* gene. It manifests itself in a unique ichthyosis and hair shaft abnormality. At birth, these patients may have a generalized ichthyosiform erythroderma, as seen in Fig. 15-35. Severe hypernatremic dehydration may occur.

Figure 15-36

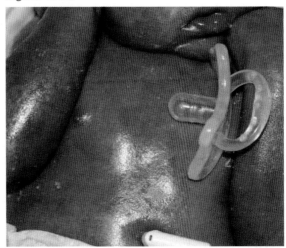

After the newborn period, children with Netherton syndrome may go on to develop a generalized skin rash that is similar in appearance to severe atopic dermatitis. Patients may suffer from itching and frequent superinfection, and are also prone to develop numerous food allergies.

Figure 15-37

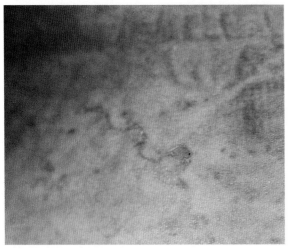

Netherton syndrome The most distinctive cutaneous feature is termed *ichthyosis linearis circumflexa,* a collection of circinate, erythematous, and hyperkeratotic lesions with a very characteristic double-edged scale along the margin (Fig. 15-37 and 15-38).

Figure 15-38

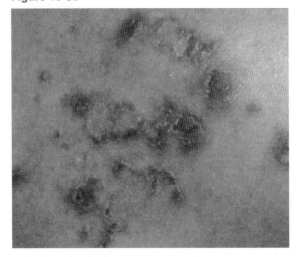

Patients with Netherton syndrome tend to have an atopic diathesis, with some combination of asthma, allergic rhinitis, and eczematous dermatitis. Finally, there is a tendency toward impaired immunity (elevated IgE and immature natural killer cells) and, in some cases, developmental delay.

Figure 15-39

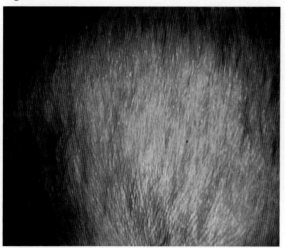

Figure 15-40

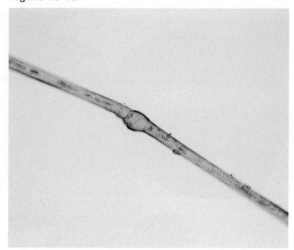

Netherton syndrome The associated hair abnormality is seen in Fig. 15-39. Microscopic examination of these "bamboo hairs" (Fig. 15-40) most often reveals a hair shaft abnormality termed *trichorrhexis invaginata*, a ball-and-socket insertion of the distal hair shaft into the proximal hair.

There may also be pili torti or trichorrhexis nodosa (Figs. 29-34 through Fig 29-37). The hair may be absent at birth and the hair shaft abnormality may sometimes be first found upon examination of eyebrow hair. The hair disorder tends to correct itself with the passage of time.

Figure 15-41

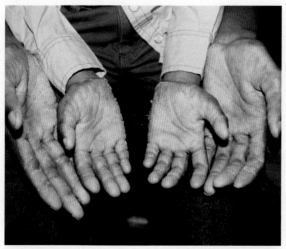

Figure 15-42

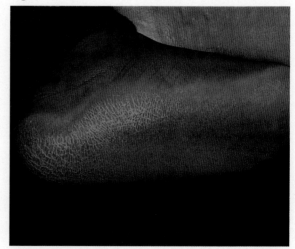

Palmoplantar keratoderma There is a long list of genodermatoses that includes thickening of the palms and soles as either the principal or an associated abnormality. The most common among all of these is Unna-Thost palmoplantar keratoderma, which is caused by mutations in the *KRT1* gene. Well-demarcated hyperkeratosis is noted on the palms and soles with a red band noted at the periphery of the area and is sharply demarcated. The autosomal dominant inheritance of this condition is illustrated by the mother–son involvement in Fig. 15-41 and 15-42. Treatment consists of the use of keratolytic agents and various methods of scraping and paring to remove thickened skin.

Figure 15-43

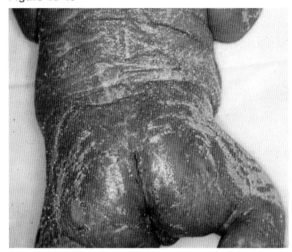

Figure 15-44

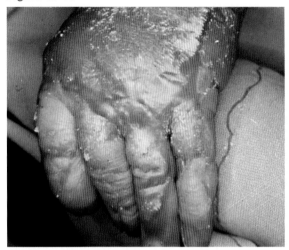

Conradi-Hünermann syndrome This is a rare genetic disorder with multiple systemic effects. Affected infants have generalized redness and scaling (ichthyosiform erythroderma). As illustrated in Figs. 15-43 and 15-44, the lesions occur in a whorled or linear, blotchy pattern. Older children and young adults develop follicular atrophoderma, and sometimes dark and light patches of skin and patchy scarring alopecia.

Conradi-Hünermann syndrome is a form of chondrodysplasia punctata, a group of genetic disorders with shortening of bones, and stippled epiphyses.. This disorder is also associated with cataracts (these may be present at birth or develop after), short stature, and a characteristic facial appearance. Conradi-Hünermann syndrome is caused by mutations of the emopamil-binding protein (*EBP*) gene and is inherited as an X-linked dominant trait. It occurs almost exclusively in girls.

Figure 15-45

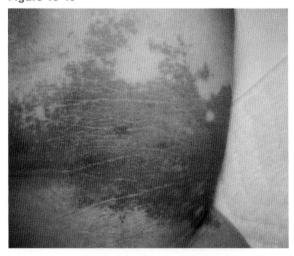

Figure 15-46

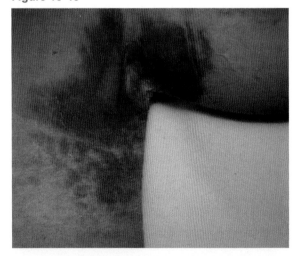

Sjögren-Larsson syndrome This is a rare autosomal recessive genodermatosis that is characterized by spasticity, mental retardation, and congenital ichthyosis. A combination of scaling and erythroderma is seen in the newborn. Over time, the ichthyosis tends to localize to the lower abdomen (Fig. 15-45) and flexural areas (Fig. 15-46). There may be mild involvement of the palms and soles.

The combination of spasticity and psychomotor developmental delay is often quite severe and may be accompanied by a seizure disorder. A specific retinal lesion, the so-called glistening dots, is present in almost all patients with Sjögren-Larsson syndrome after 1 year of age. This syndrome is due to the deficient activity of fatty aldehyde dehydrogenase (FALDH).

Figure 15-47

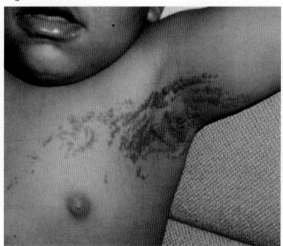

Linear epidermal nevus These lesions consist of verrucous, hyperkeratotic papules that are closely grouped in a linear array. Epidermal nevi are often present at birth but may arise during the first year of life, and occasionally later. They may occur on the head and neck, trunk, or extremities.

Figure 15-48

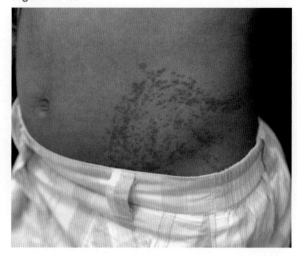

Figure 15-48 illustrates an epidermal nevus on the abdomen. The lesion had been present since birth and there were no associated symptoms. The whorled appearance of the lesion is due to the fact that epidermal nevi characteristically follow the lines of Blaschko.

Figure 15-49

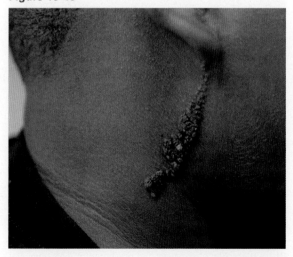

Linear epidermal nevus This linear lesion, present from the time of birth, had gradually become thicker over the course of several years. The benefit of surgical excision must be weighed against the risk of a scar at the site of surgery.

Figure 15-50

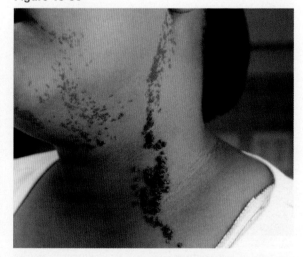

Figure 15-50 shows an extensive epidermal nevus on the face and neck, again following the lines of Blaschko. Epidermal nevi have no malignant potential, except for the extremely rare development of basal cell carcinoma in a preexisting lesion. Surgical treatment is required only when indicated for cosmetic considerations.

Figure 15-51

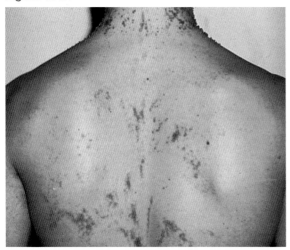

Figure 15-52

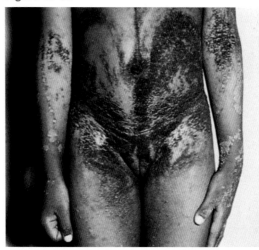

Epidermal nevus syndrome Figures 15-51 and 15-52 show patients with widespread epidermal nevi. Some patients with this phenotype will be diagnosed with epidermal nevus syndrome, which is a group of congenital disorders with a variety of systemic features. Defects in neural crest lead to malformations in skeletal, cardiovascular, ocular, and endocrine systems, and may also result in lipomas. The most frequent malformation in the brain is hemimegalencephaly.

Epidermal nevus syndrome results from genetic mosaicism with a lethal autosomal dominant gene, and a number of specific mutations have been identified. Skeletal abnormalities seen in the epidermal nevus syndrome include limb hypertrophy, bone cysts, and incomplete formation of certain bones. A higher than normal incidence of malignancy, particularly Wilms tumor, has also been associated with this disorder.

Figure 15-53

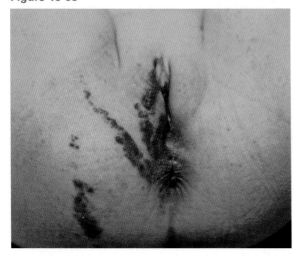

Figure 15-54

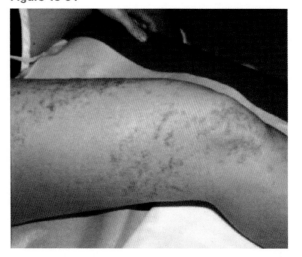

Inflammatory linear verrucous epidermal nevus (ILVEN) This linear array of pruritic papules arises most often during childhood. The lesions are erythematous and scaling and are usually localized to the lower extremities or perineum. Sometimes this entity may be difficult to distinguish from psoriasis.

The persistence of inflammation in one anatomic area and the absence of psoriatic lesions elsewhere favor the diagnosis of ILVEN. Histologically, it may resemble psoriasis or nonspecific chronic dermatitis.

Figure 15-55

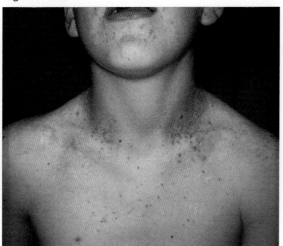

Darier disease (keratosis follicularis) This autosomal dominant disorder usually begins during mid-childhood. It is caused
by a mutation in the gene *ATP2A2*. The primary lesion is a small,
crusted papule; in some areas, these coalesce to form hyperkeratotic, greasy plaques. The lesions tend to favor the so-called
seborrheic areas, and the upper back and chest, as shown in
Figs. 15-55 and 15-56, are the most common locations. Small,
warty papules on the dorsa of the hands are a common finding.

Figure 15-56

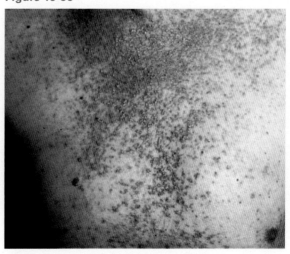

The lesions tend to worsen in the summer; both humidity and
ultraviolet light have a negative effect on the disease process.
Nail involvement is characteristic of Darier disease and may
include red or white longitudinal streaks, thinning or thickening
of the nail plate, and subungual hyperkeratosis.

Figure 15-57

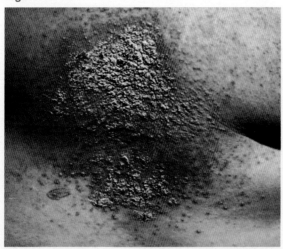

Darier disease (keratosis follicularis) In more severe cases,
there is extensive scalp and facial involvement, and there are
moist, erythematous vegetating plaques in the flexures, as illustrated in Fig. 15-57. The severity of Darier disease varies greatly
among members of the same affected family. The use of synthetic
retinoids in the most severe cases must be balanced against the
problems of long-term toxicity.

Figure 15-58

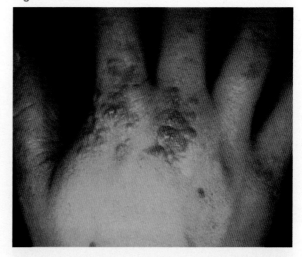

Acrokeratosis verruciformis This autosomal dominant disorder is characterized by numerous flat-topped or verrucous
hyperkeratotic papules that are usually localized to the dorsa of
the hands and feet. They tend to recur after surgical removal.
Histologically, there are distinctive elevations of the epidermis
that resemble church spires. It should be noted that patients with
Darier disease (see Figs. 15-55 to 15-57) may have identical acral
lesions, and this disorder is also associated with defects in the
ATP2A2 gene.

Figure 15-59

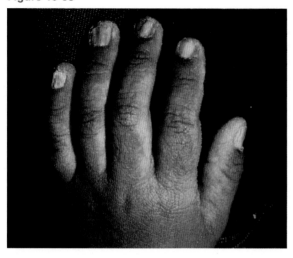

Figure 15-60

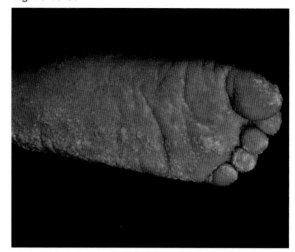

KID syndrome The keratitis-ichthyosis-deafness (KID) syndrome is a multisystem disorder that, in its most severe forms, may be disabling. Cutaneous changes consist of thick keratoderma of the palms and soles, keratotic plaques on the face and extremities, and a diffuse ichthyosis with follicular accentuation. KID syndrome is caused by mutations in the *GJB2* gene, which codes for the protein connexin 26.

Abnormal keratinization may be present at birth. Alopecia, nail dystrophy, and hypoplastic teeth are all part of this disorder. The hearing impairment in this disease is progressive and due to neurosensory deafness. Keratitis begins during childhood and is accompanied by neovascularization. Visual loss may be severe. Recurrent and atypical cutaneous infections may also be seen in KID syndrome.

Figure 15-61

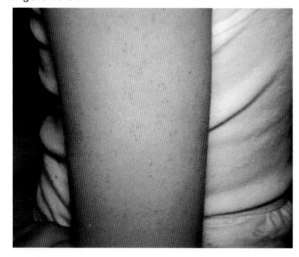

Figure 15-62

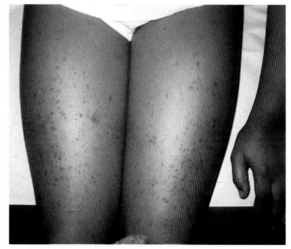

Keratosis pilaris This is an extremely common asymptomatic condition that is often familial and is sometimes associated with atopic dermatitis or ichthyosis vulgaris. Pictured in Figs. 15-61 and 15-62 are typical lesions in the two most common areas of involvement: the lateral aspect of the upper arms and the anterior thighs. The lesions are fine keratotic papules;

each represents a plug in the upper part of a hair follicle. The appearance of the involved areas is often likened to chicken skin or gooseflesh; the sensation on palpation is a grater-like roughness. Keratosis pilaris tends to worsen during the winter months and abates somewhat after puberty. Keratolytics and emollients are somewhat helpful.

Figure 15-63

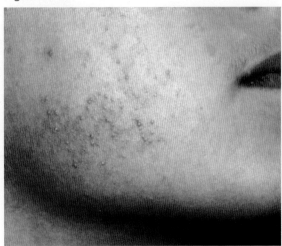

Keratosis pilaris Children with keratosis pilaris sometimes develop the condition's typical follicular papules on the cheeks. When this occurs, there may also be erythema associated with the roughness. This condition is sometimes termed *keratosis pilaris rubra faciei*. Again, mild keratolytics are sometimes helpful.

Figure 15-64

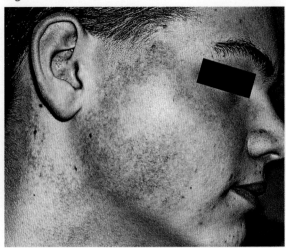

Keratosis pilaris rubra faciei This eruption is sometimes confused with acne, in which comedones are found along with papules, pustules, and sometimes cysts. The prognosis of facial keratosis pilaris is good, although this condition may persist on the extremities.

SECTION

16

Urticarial, Purpuric, and Vascular Reactions

Figure 16-1

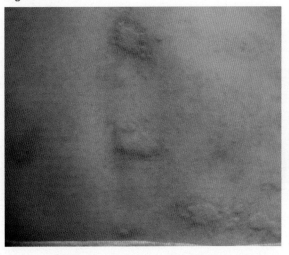

Urticaria A wheal is an edematous papule that may enlarge to form a pink, sharply circumscribed, elevated plaque. The typical lesions of urticaria, pictured in Figs. 16-1 and 16-2, have a suggestion of central clearing.

Figure 16-2

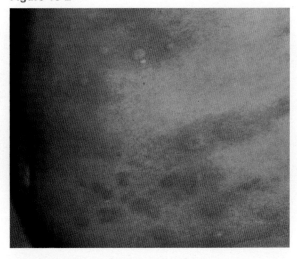

By definition, the individual lesions of urticaria evolve quickly and resolve within 24 to 48 hours. They are usually accompanied by severe pruritus. Urticaria is an extremely common disorder, and the etiology often remains unknown. In most children, the problem resolves spontaneously over time.

Figure 16-3

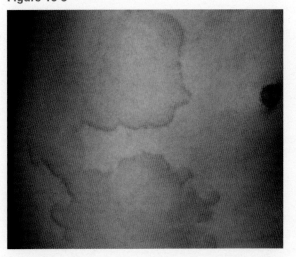

Urticaria Larger, more geographic lesions are pictured in Figs. 16-3 and 16-4. In the cases where a cause is established, the most common etiologies of urticaria are medications, foods (eg, nuts, strawberries, shellfish, and other seafoods), and viral and bacterial infections.

Figure 16-4

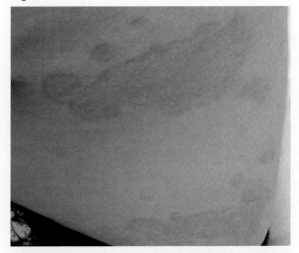

Autoimmune disease, such as autoimmune thyroiditis, and malignancy are extremely rare causes. In the child with chronic urticaria, it is often difficult or impossible to identify a single cause. In these patients, one attempts to control the development of new lesions with a daily schedule of nonsedating antihistamines.

Figure 16-5

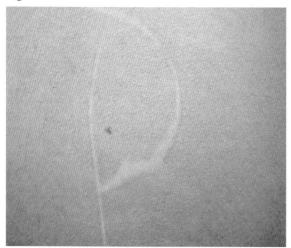

Physical urticarias There are urticarias in which stroking, pressure, cold, heat, or sun exposure are causative. Figure 16-5 shows a wheal produced by stroking the skin with a degree of force that would ordinarily cause nothing more than transient erythema. The phenomenon, called *dermographism,* is present in a small percentage of normal individuals.

Figure 16-6

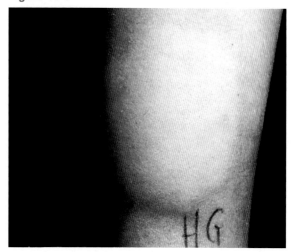

Figure 16-6 shows a large wheal produced by resting an ice cube on the forearm. Cold-induced urticaria may be acquired or inherited. In the most common, acquired form, patients develop lesions shortly after ingesting cold foods or liquids or shortly after exposure to a drop in environmental temperature. Patients with this form of sensitivity are at risk for laryngeal edema or circulatory collapse as a result of significant cold exposure. Antihistamines or doxepin are of some help in preventing attacks. In a very rare syndrome, contact of the skin with water, without respect to its temperature, produces wheals (aquagenic urticaria).

Figure 16-7

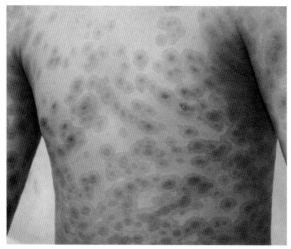

Erythema multiforme This disorder is termed *multiforme* because the morphology of its lesions is so variable. The primary lesion is most often an erythematous macule that evolves into a papule. Early in the course, these lesions may easily be mistaken for urticaria.

Figure 16-8

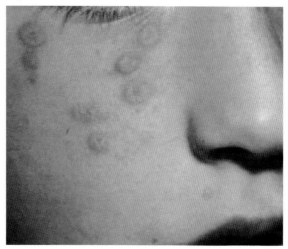

As the lesions enlarge, they form round or irregularly shaped plaques. The central area may blister or become dusky in color; this change represents the necrosis of keratinocytes in areas of active involvement.

Figure 16-9

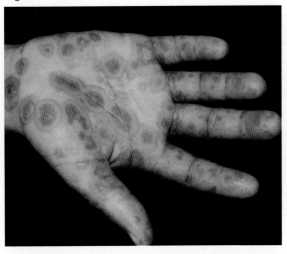

Erythema multiforme Figure 16-9 demonstrates the target-like quality of the variably sized and shaped plaques. Note the redness and edema at the border and the duskier appearance at the center. Mucosal lesions are not uncommon. Erythema multiforme is a self-healing disease, with an average duration of about 2 weeks.

Figure 16-10

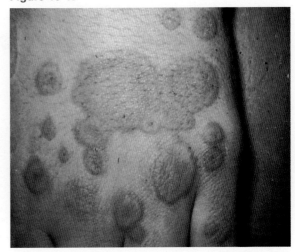

The dorsum of the hand is a particularly common location. Herpes simplex infection is by far the most common etiologic agent. In some patients, frequent recurrences of herpes simplex and erythema multiforme require the use of prophylactic acyclovir or valacyclovir for extended periods of time. A wide variety of drugs, most commonly the sulfonamides, may also cause this syndrome.

Figure 16-11

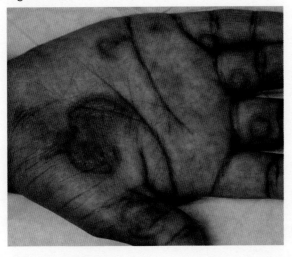

Erythema multiforme Erythema multiforme tends to be acral in distribution. Figure 16-11 illustrates both bulla formation and the crusting of bullae that can occur during the course of the disease.

Figure 16-12

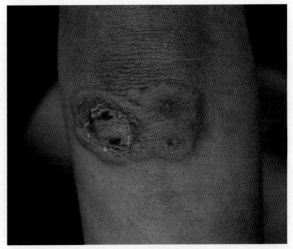

This plaque-like lesion on the elbow illustrates the edematous border and the dusky center, a result of the necrosis of keratinocytes. Erythema multiforme must be distinguished from urticaria multiforme (Figs. 16-21 to 16-23, 21-4,), which has some similar clinical features.

Figure 16-13

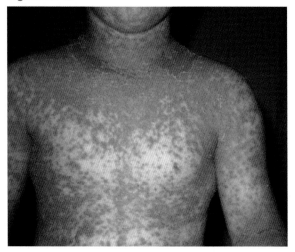

Stevens-Johnson syndrome/toxic epidermal necrolysis Drugs are the major etiologic factor in the development of this severe disorder. The most common agents are sulfonamides, anticonvulsants, and NSAIDs. *Mycoplasma pneumoniae* is the most commonly associated infectious agent. The cutaneous lesions include fixed erythematous macules, target lesions, and bullae.

Figure 16-14

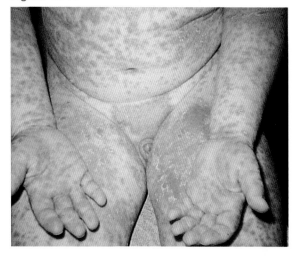

There may be progression to widespread erythema and denudation, leaving underlying erosions. Frozen section processing of a biopsy specimen of toxic epidermal necrolysis allows for rapid diagnosis. In patients with erosions and blisters, one sees necrotic keratinocytes, severe degeneration of the basal layer, and a subepidermal separation.

Figure 16-15

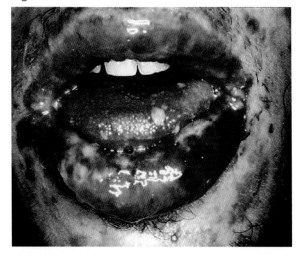

Stevens-Johnson syndrome/toxic epidermal necrolysis The oral cavity is almost always involved, with bullae, ulcerations, and crusting most commonly presenting on the lips, buccal mucosa, and palate. Tracheal and bronchial involvement may result in breathing difficulty. Additionally, patients with Mycoplasma-induced Stevens-Johnson syndrome may have mucositis with minimal or absent skin lesions.

Figure 16-16

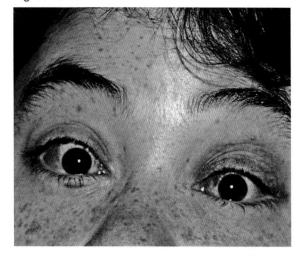

Ocular involvement frequently occurs in this syndrome, significantly affecting the bulbar conjunctiva. Long-term consequences include corneal damage and scarring, which may lead to permanent visual impairment.

Figure 16-17

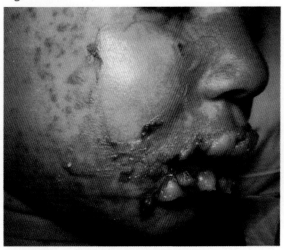

Figure 16-18

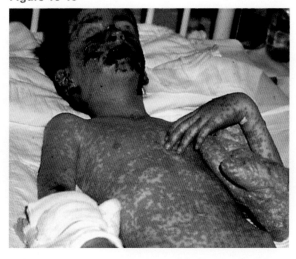

Stevens-Johnson syndrome/toxic epidermal necrolysis Fever, headache, cough, and malaise are frequent features of this disorder. In addition to the lips (pictured in Fig. 16-17) and oral mucous membranes, esophageal involvement may lead to severe dysphagia and difficulty eating and drinking. Involvement of the vulva and vagina in girls, and glans penis in boys may cause dysuria and urinary retention.

In Figs. 16-17 to 16-20, note the extensive involvement with large and small bullous lesions. The mortality rate in this disease is significant; most deaths are related to superinfection and sepsis.

Figure 16-19

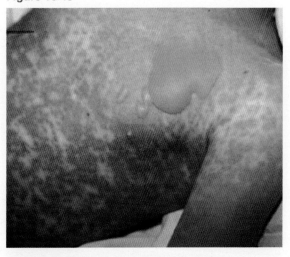

Figure 16-20

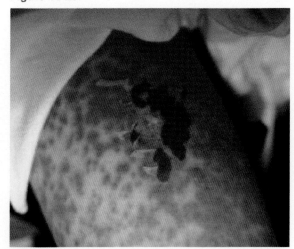

Stevens-Johnson syndrome/toxic epidermal necrolysis Patients with toxic epidermal necrolysis benefit enormously from intensive medical care, in a burn unit when possible. Meticulous attention to the care of blistered and denuded skin and mucous membranes, along with monitoring for electrolyte imbalance, dehydration, and infection significantly improves the possibility of survival.

Both systemic steroids and IVIG have been advocated for the treatment of Stevens-Johnson syndrome/toxic epidermal necrolysis. There is mixed evidence for both of these treatments and their use remains controversial.

Figure 16-21

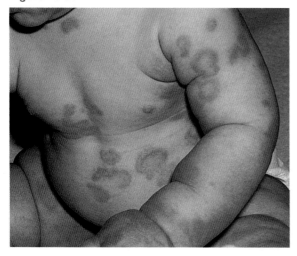

Urticaria multiforme This condition, also known as *acute annular urticaria,* is a benign and fairly common hypersensitivity reaction that presents with urticarial plaques and annular or arcuate urticarial lesions, along with acral edema.

Figure 16-22

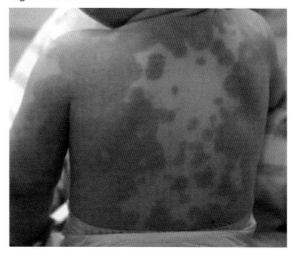

Because the lesions may have an ecchymotic dusky center, this disorder is often misdiagnosed as erythema multiforme. Children with urticaria multiforme may have recently had a viral or bacterial infection.

Figure 16-23

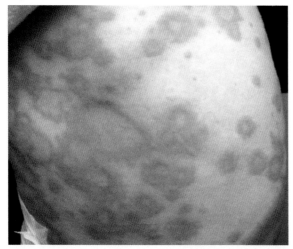

Urticaria multiforme Urticaria multiforme has also been linked to treatment with antibiotics, such as amoxicillin, cephalosporins, and macrolides. Treatment may consist of combination therapy with an H1-antihistamine and an H2-antihistamine.

Figure 16-24

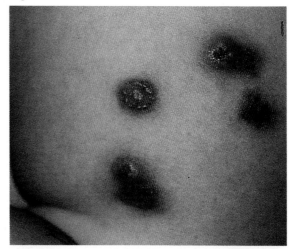

Sweet syndrome (acute febrile neutrophilic dermatosis) This syndrome is characterized by painful, raised, erythematous plaques and nodules. The cutaneous eruption is accompanied by spiking fevers and a neutrophilic leukocytosis. Skin biopsy reveals a widespread infiltrate of polymorphonuclear leukocytes throughout the dermis. Sweet syndrome is often associated with either malignancy or antecedent infection. Systemic corticosteroids are the treatment of choice.

Figure 16-25

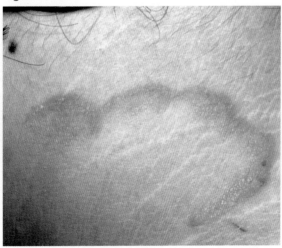

Figure 16-26

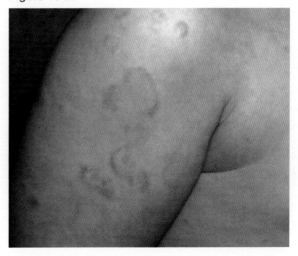

Erythema annulare centrifugum This is an erythematous and edematous lesion that gradually enlarges to form annular, polycyclic, and gyrate shapes. The lesions tend to resolve spontaneously but may reappear. Erythema annulare centrifugum has been attributed to a wide variety of causes.

In some cases, it is temporally related to the development of malignancy and resolves with treatment or removal of the tumor. In other patients, the disease has been related to superficial fungal infections and a wide variety of viral and bacterial diseases.

Figure 16-27

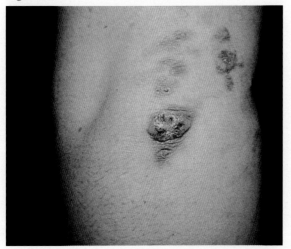

Figure 16-28

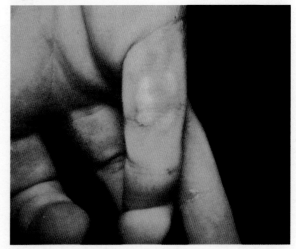

Erythema elevatum diutinum This is a rare skin disease that is characterized by purple or yellowish papules, nodules, and plaques that tend to cluster on the hands, feet, and extensor surfaces of the extremities. The skin overlying joints is a favored location. The distribution is usually symmetrical, and the disease tends to be chronic. Lesions of erythema elevatum diutinum

may be asymptomatic but in some cases are painful. Figure 16-27 shows typical nodules and plaques on the elbow, and yellowish papules on the finger are seen in Fig. 16-28. The etiology of this chronic leukocytoclastic vasculitis remains unknown, but an immune complex etiology has been suggested. Dapsone is one mode of treatment.

Figure 16-29

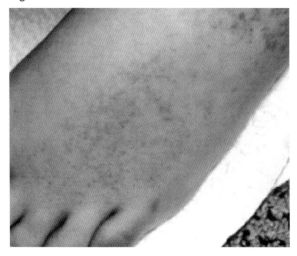

Progressive pigmented purpura (Schamberg disease) This disorder is due to a mild form of capillaritis, leading to extravasation of red cells and the deposition of hemosiderin. Affected children have numerous discrete patches of petechiae.

Figure 16-30

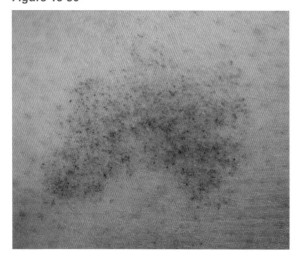

The most common location is the lower extremities. Over time, the individual lesions evolve into typical brown-orange macules containing "cayenne pepper" spots as shown in Fig. 16-30.

Figure 16-31

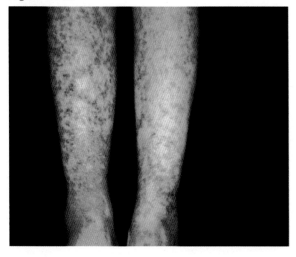

Progressive pigmented purpura (Schamberg disease) Figure 16-31 illustrates a severe case of pigmented purpura, involving both lower extremities. Although less common, pigmented purpura in a segmental distribution on one extremity has been reported to occur.

Figure 16-32

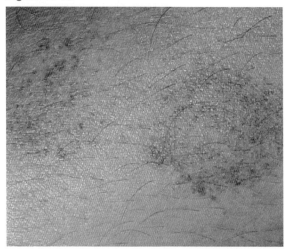

Lichen aureus is a localized form more commonly seen in children and young adults consisting of a solitary or localized group of lesions that is more frequently seen on the leg although any part of the body may be involved. Figure 16-32 shows lesions with a more golden color; only a few petechiae are noted.

Figure 16-33

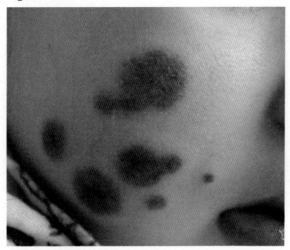

Acute hemorrhagic edema of infancy This striking disorder occurs in infants between 4 months and 2 years of age. The sharply circumscribed lesions favor the extremities and are edematous, ecchymotic, and purpuric. Edema of the ears and eyelids may also be noted.

Figure 16-34

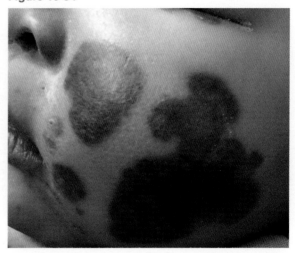

Biopsy of an active lesion reveals an intense leukocytoclastic vasculitis. However, in contrast to Henoch-Schönlein purpura, systemic symptoms are very rare. There may be several outbreaks of new lesions, but the entire process generally resolves in approximately 2 weeks.

Figure 16-35

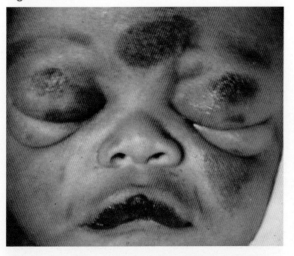

Traumatic purpura Figure 16-35 shows hemorrhage into the skin due to a difficult passage through the birth canal. In this figure, one sees edema and ecchymosis that resulted from molding of the head in a prolonged spontaneous delivery.

Figure 16-36

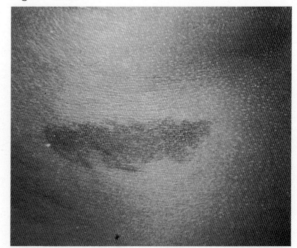

Throughout life, hard knocks in the physical sense are the lot of us all. Rupture of capillaries is thus exceedingly common, and more extensive rupture of arterioles, venules, arteries, or veins is common enough. Petechiae, ecchymoses, vibices, and hematomas are banal, nearly everyday events. The black eye and contusions are of everyone's experience. Illustrated in Fig. 16-36 is a traumatic ecchymosis that may well represent a hickey ("passion purpura"). (*caption by Morris Leider, first edition of Color Atlas of Pediatric Dermatology, 1975*).

Figure 16-37

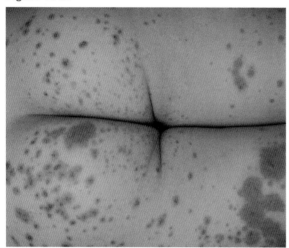

Henoch-Schönlein purpura Palpable purpura is part of a syndrome that is also marked by attacks of arthralgia, abdominal pain, and hematuria. The entire complex of visible cutaneous purpura, arthralgia, and visceral signs and symptoms results from a widespread IgA-related vasculitis. In addition to purpura, the skin may show edematous plaques, vesicles, and even necrosis. The cause of this condition is not known.

Figure 16-38

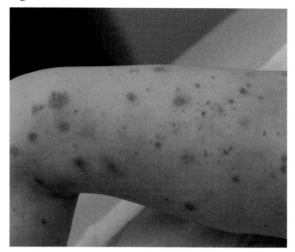

Abdominal pain occurs in up to 65 percent of cases. Usually the pain is colicky, and it can be associated with vomiting and hematemesis. There may also be gross or occult blood in the stools. In unusual cases, there is intussusception, hemorrhage and shock.

Figure 16-39

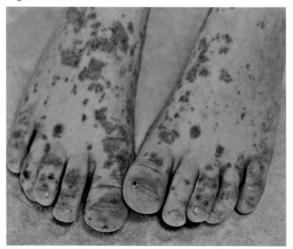

Henoch-Schönlein purpura The most serious consequence of this disease is renal disease. Patients who develop kidney involvement may do so months after the onset of cutaneous purpura. The most common manifestation of renal disease is hematuria. Proteinuria and hematuria may rarely progress to renal insufficiency.

Figure 16-40

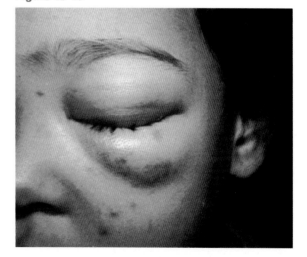

Figure 16-40 is a good representation of both the purpuric elements and the edema that may appear in the Henoch-Schönlein syndrome. Rare manifestations of this disorder are pulmonary hemorrhage and central nervous system involvement with seizures and behavioral changes. Scrotal swelling and testicular torsion has also been reported.

Figure 16-41

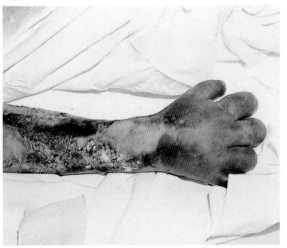

Purpura fulminans This condition is a rare and exceedingly serious consequence of certain acute infectious diseases. Scarlet fever of bygone days, meningococcal meningitis, severe varicella, and congenital protein C deficiency have been known to be complicated by fulminating purpura that went on to gangrene, extreme toxicity, shock, and death.

Figure 16-42

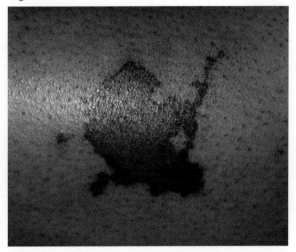

This is an additional example of purpura fulminans due to meningococcemia. The cause of the condition is a necrotizing vasculitis associated with defects of clotting (disseminated intravascular coagulation).

Figure 16-43

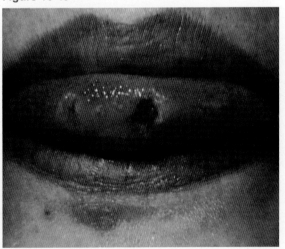

Aphthous stomatitis This very common condition is characterized by recurrent episodes of painful ulceration on the lip, tongue, or buccal surfaces. The individual lesions quickly evolve from erythematous macules to papules and then to yellowish ulcerations with a surrounding pink or red halo.

Figure 16-44

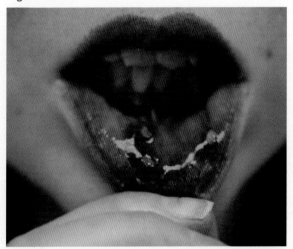

The etiology is not known, and the ulcers heal in 7 to 10 days without scarring. Whereas a solitary lesion is the cause of only temporary, minor discomfort, there are some individuals who develop deeper and larger ulcers or numerous erosions. For them, aphthous stomatitis can be a severe problem.

Figure 16-45

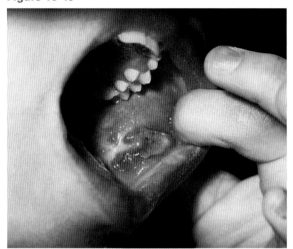

Figure 16-46

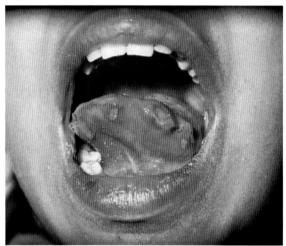

Behçet syndrome This rare disease is characterized by a classic triad of recurrent ulcerations of the oral mucosa, genital ulcers, and eye involvement. The oral ulcers, pictured in Figs. 16-45 and 16-46, tend to be larger, more numerous, and more frequently recurrent than those of simple aphthous stomatitis. Genital lesions occur on the penis and scrotum in males, and on the vulva in females. These frequently recurrent ulcers tend to heal with scarring. The various forms of eye involvement include uveitis and keratoconjunctivitis and may eventuate in blindness.

Other cutaneous lesions may be widespread and include papules, vesicles, abscesses, and lesions of erythema nodosum. In addition to the eyes and skin, a number of other organ systems may become involved. Severe chronic arthritis and thrombophlebitis are common occurrences. Gastrointestinal disease ranges from mild abdominal discomfort to chronic diarrhea and an ulcerative colitis-like illness.

Figure 16-47

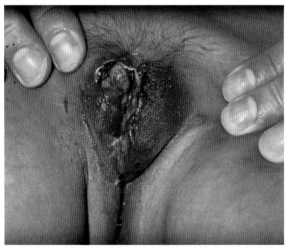

Behçet syndrome Typical vaginal lesions are pictured in Fig. 16-47. Neurologic manifestations, including recurrent meningoencephalitis and brain stem lesions, are often the most serious and can be life threatening. Diagnosis of Behçet syndrome is based on the presence of the typical clinical findings. The disease is difficult to treat, but colchicine, immunosuppressive drugs, and corticosteroids are the most frequently used therapies. Tumor necrosis factor inhibitors also have a varying degree of success.

Figure 16-48

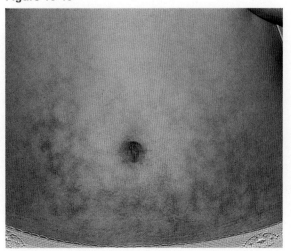

Figure 16-49

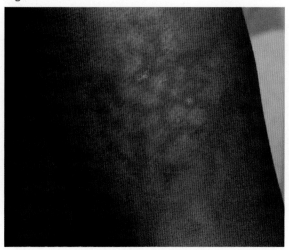

Erythema ab igne This disorder results from prolonged and repeated exposure to infrared radiation. Historically, and before the advent of central heating, erythema ab igne was seen on the legs of individuals who sat or stood in front of heating devices. In this era, more common causes are hot water bottles and heating pads. The patient in Fig. 16-48 used a heating pad for relief from menstrual cramps; the patient in Fig. 16-49 applied heat to his thigh after an injury.

Erythema ab igne on the anterior thighs may be caused by the warmth from a laptop computer. Typical lesions are characterized by reticular erythema and brownish pigmentation. Epidermal atrophy and subepidermal blisters may also occur.

Bullous, Pustular, and Ulcerating Diseases

Figure 17-1

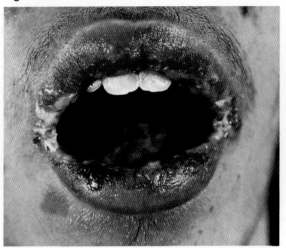

Pemphigus vulgaris Pemphigus vulgaris is a rare autoimmune, bullous disease that occasionally occurs during childhood. The disease affects both the skin and mucous membranes and can be life threatening. The typical lesions of pemphigus vulgaris are pictured in Fig. 17-1. Erosions of the lips, gums, tongue, and palate, as pictured here, are a common presenting symptom and may be misdiagnosed early in the course of the disease. The difficulty in chewing and swallowing that may occur can become a significant complication.

Figure 17-2

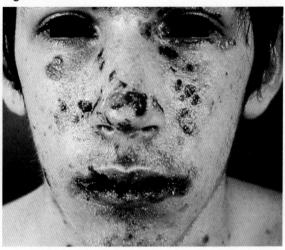

Cutaneous lesions consist of flaccid weeping blisters that quickly erode to leave large denuded areas of skin. Nikolsky sign, the extension of blistering by lateral finger pressure, is seen in the presence of widespread disease. Figure 17-2 shows the kind of crusting that develops as the blisters open. Antibodies to desmoglein 1 are associated with skin lesions and antibodies to desmoglein 3 are associated with oral lesions.

Figure 17-3

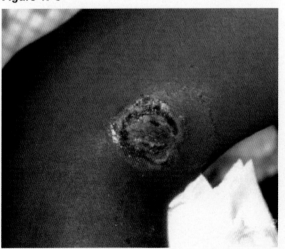

Pemphigus vulgaris The blisters of pemphigus vulgaris may arise on an erythematous base, or on normal-appearing skin, as pictured in Fig. 17-3. A variety of modalities have been employed in the treatment of this disease. The patient who is seriously ill requires hospitalization.

Figure 17-4

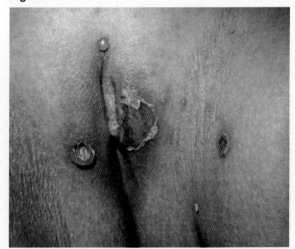

Figure 17-4 illustrates both intact blisters and superficial erosions. For most patients, the most rapidly effective treatment remains high-dose systemic steroids. Patients undergoing this form of therapy are at risk for infection and must be followed with extreme care. Rituximab, a monoclonal antibody against the B cell surface protein CD20, is the most promising new treatment for this disease. Immunosuppressive agents such as azathioprine, mycophenolate mofetil, intravenous immunoglobulin, and plasmapheresis are useful therapies.

Figure 17-5

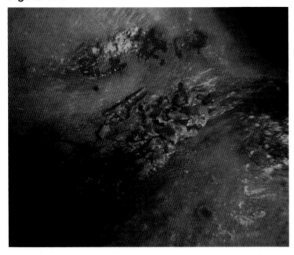

Pemphigus vegetans When the cutaneous changes of pemphigus take place in intertriginous spaces, clear blistering is not evident. Rather, one sees boggy inflammation. The essential histologic process is again epidermal acantholysis, but blister roofs part almost at once and secondary infection is inevitable. This figure is a good representation of the kind of clinical appearance that develops in pemphigus vegetans. Lesions on other parts of the body take the form of pemphigus vulgaris.

Figure 17-6

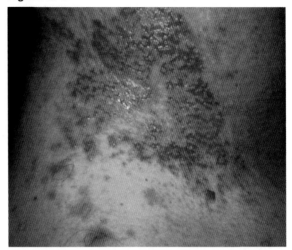

Familial benign chronic pemphigus (Hailey-Hailey disease) This blistering disease is inherited in autosomal dominant fashion. Onset tends to occur during late adolescence. Patients with this disorder have a pruritic vesicular eruption in intertriginous areas that is worse during the summer months. Intact bullae may be absent, and often there is only an erosive and crusted intertrigo in the axillae, in the groin, and on the neck. Control of this condition is best achieved by the avoidance of the causative factor, such as heat or friction, and the treatment of superinfection when it occurs.

Figure 17-7

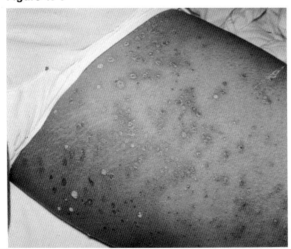

Subcorneal pustulosis (Sneddon-Wilkinson disease) This condition is most common during adulthood, but it does occur in children. Characteristically, crops of vesicles and pustules spring up and evolve into areas of superficial crusts and scales. As the lesions coalesce, they form the type of arcuate plaque that is illustrated in Fig. 17-7. The most common locations are the axillae, groin, and flexures of the upper and lower extremities. The lesions are often pruritic, and, especially in childhood, there may be fever and an elevated white blood count.

Figure 17-8

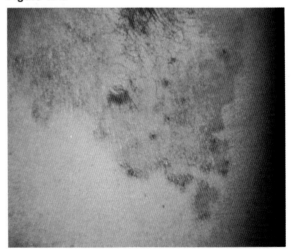

The etiology of this condition is completely unknown. Diagnosis is best confirmed by classic histologic appearance, which consists of collections of neutrophils just beneath the stratum corneum. The disease process is essentially benign, but dapsone is an effective therapy for the patient with frequent or severe recurrences.

Figure 17-9

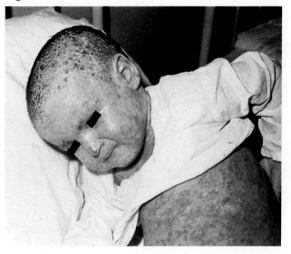

Pemphigus foliaceus This form of pemphigus is less severe than pemphigus vulgaris because blister formation occurs higher in the epidermis. As a result, there is less compromise of vital cutaneous functions. In most areas of the world, pemphigus foliaceus is extremely unusual in children. In rural areas of Brazil, there is an endemic form of pemphigus foliaceus, termed *fogo selvagem*, which affects individuals of all ages.

Figure 17-10

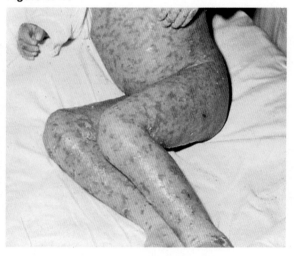

Pictured in Figs. 17-9 and 17-10 are the typical lesions of pemphigus foliaceus. The disease often begins in the scalp with areas of erythema and scaling. As it progresses to involve the trunk and extremities, there evolve numerous crusting and erythematous plaques. Severe scaling is common, but usually there is no blister formation and no involvement of the oral cavity. Treatment consists of topical or systemic steroids, depending on the severity of the disease.

Figure 17-11

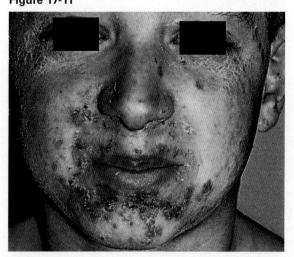

Pemphigus foliaceus Lesions in the perioral area, as seen in Fig. 17-11, are quite common. Oral mucosal involvement is less common, in contrast to pemphigus vulgaris. Often, patients with pemphigus foliaceus are initially thought to have recurrent impetigo, although the infection does not totally clear with appropriate antibiotics. It is important to realize that secondary infection often occurs in these patients, and this should be considered when patients have flare-ups or the disease is difficult to control.

Figure 17-12

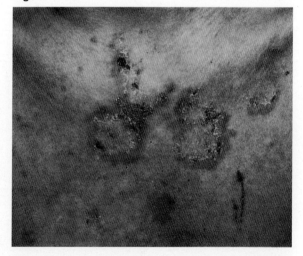

Figure 17-12 shows annular lesions that are seen in childhood forms of pemphigus foliaceus. Direct immunofluorescence is important in making the diagnosis. In addition, antibodies to desmoglein, an epidermal desmosomal component, are found.

Figure 17-13

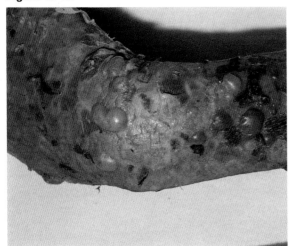

Figure 17-14

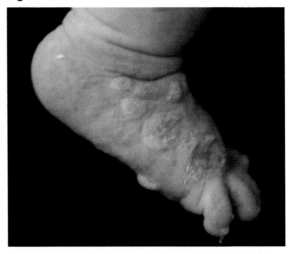

Bullous pemphigoid This autoimmune blistering disorder is due to antibodies to various components of the basement membrane. It is extremely rare during childhood. Tense blisters can arise on either erythematous or normal skin and may be pruritic. Lesions tend to cluster and may be preceded by the development of urticarial plaques. Sites of predilection include the face, groin, and inner thighs.

Palm and sole involvement is sometimes seen in children, and mouth lesions are extremely unusual. Blisters generally heal without scarring but may leave temporary hyper- or hypopigmentation. The prognosis is generally good, and initial treatment consists of topical and/or systemic corticosteroids.

Figure 17-15

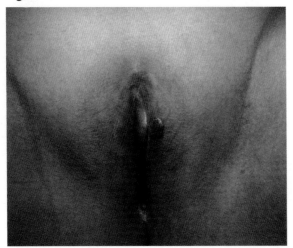

Vulvar pemphigoid Patients with bullous pemphigoid may develop both genital and oral lesions. Rarely, in young girls, pemphigoid is limited to the vulva and may result in scarring. Localized vulvar pemphigoid must be distinguished from lichen sclerosus et atrophicus (Figs. 20-12 and 20-13), which can also result in chronic blistering and pain in this anatomic location.

Figure 17-16

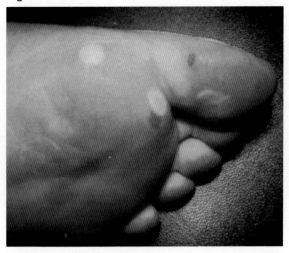

Epidermolysis bullosa simplex (EBS) The most common types of epidermolysis bullosa simplex (EBS) are autosomal dominant and the lesions are localized. Other subtypes of EBS, including autosomal recessive forms, have now been characterized. The blisters in EBS are in the epidermis, and can be either suprabasal or basal. Multiple genetic mutations have been identified; most forms of EBS are associated with mutations in genes coding for keratins 5 and 14.

Figure 17-17

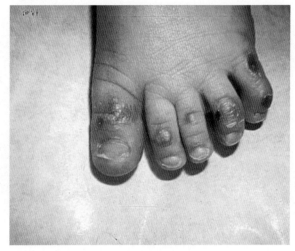

Epidermolysis bullosa simplex begins at birth or in early infancy, and throughout life the site of blistering corresponds to areas of friction or other trauma. The localized form of EBS, previously known as the Weber-Cockayne type (Fig. 17-17), is associated with onset in early childhood and with blisters forming on the hands and feet. Milia and scarring are rarely associated with this form, and hyperkeratosis of the palms and soles may develop in adulthood.

Figure 17-18

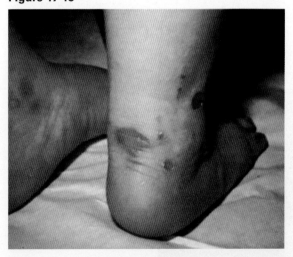

Epidermolysis bullosa simplex (EBS) During infancy, blisters occur on the neck, lower extremities, and hands and feet. In the child who is old enough to wear shoes, the dorsa of the toes are a common site of bulla formation. In this condition, cleavage occurs through the basal cell layer of the epidermis, and the dermoepidermal junction is otherwise undisturbed. The lesions are superficial, but sometimes are painful and cause difficulty in walking. In children with this disorder, mucous membrane involvement is minimal and usually does not produce serious difficulty. There may be some nail dystrophy, but this also heals with the cutaneous process.

Figure 17-19

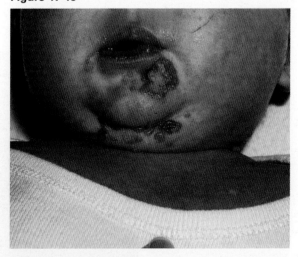

Epidermolysis bullosa simplex (Dowling-Meara) This disorder is characterized by grouped, herpetiform blistering that generally occurs on the trunk but is also seen on the face and extremities. Blistering in infancy is often severe and extensive, and can be fatal. After a few months, infants develop frequent blistering of the palms and soles, along with periungual lesions. The blistering can lead to milia, scarring, dystrophic nails, and a diffuse palmoplantar keratoderma. Blistering tends to improve with age.

Figure 17-20

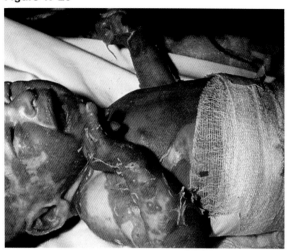

Epidermolysis bullosa, junctional type (JEB) JEB may be generalized or localized, with some uncommon forms associated with pyloric atresia or respiratory or renal involvement. Blisters in this form of epidermolysis bullosa develop within the lamina lucida of the skin basement membrane zone. The infant in Fig. 17-20 has severe, generalized JEB, formerly known as the Herlitz type. Blisters and erosions were present at birth. Patients with the severe, generalized form of JEB develop scarring, have dystrophic or absent nails, and develop exuberant granulation tissue.

Figure 17-21

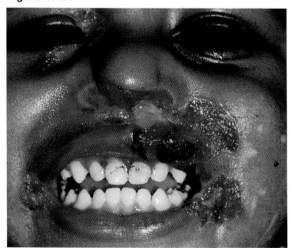

Epidermolysis bullosa, junctional type (JEB) Chronic, non-healing erosions associated with granulation tissue tends to be most severe around the nose and mouth, and it is not unusual for granulation tissue to cause obstruction of the nares. Mucosal involvement of the both, the oral cavity and the gastrointestinal tract, lead to poor feeding, malnutrition, anemia, and growth retardation.

Figure 17-22

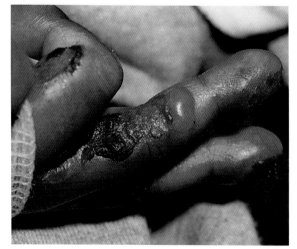

There is blister formation surrounding a nonhealing erosion in Fig. 17-22. Scalp erosions and chronic paronychia with nail loss are common. The prognosis varies according to disease severity, but in the severe JEB type there is a high rate of mortality during early childhood. In the generalized intermediate type, formerly known as the non-Herlitz type, there is absent to rare development of granulation tissue.

Figure 17-23

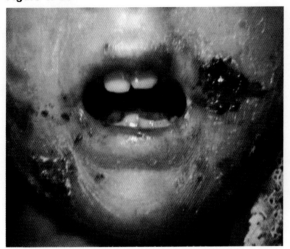

Figure 17-24

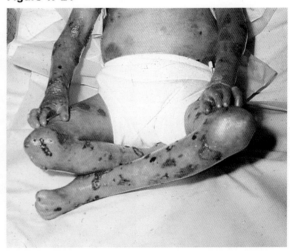

Epidermolysis bullosa recessive dystrophic type (RDEB) The dystrophic forms of epidermolysis bullosa are characterized by blister formation in the sublamina densa of the dermis, associated with defects on collagen VII. There are recessive and dominant dystrophic forms. Epidermolysis bullosa recessive dystrophic type (RDEB) may be generalized of localized. The generalized form of RDEB is a multisystem disease characterized by chronic and recurrent blistering that leads to scarring as well as the development of chronic, nonhealing wounds.

The disorder often leads to severe disability, interfering with normal growth and development. Blister formation begins at or shortly after birth, and intraoral involvement may lead to early feeding difficulties. Normal handling of the infant with this disease results in the formation of bullae that quickly evolve into ulcerations. The typical blisters, crusts, and erosions of RDEB are seen in Figs. 17-23 and 17-24.

Figure 17-25

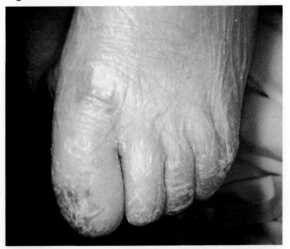

Figure 17-26

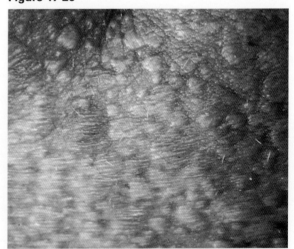

Epidermolysis bullosa recessive dystrophic type (RDEB) Figure 17-25 shows a foot with complete destruction of the toenails, induced syndactyly of the fourth and fifth toes, and typical wrinkled scarring of the skin surface. Appropriate care for the child with epidermolysis bullosa must begin in the nursery and involves the use of topical dressings to protect eroded skin and the careful handling of the infant to avoid new blister formation. Subsequent management includes efforts to minimize skin trauma, good dental and ophthalmic care, and careful attention to diet and nutrition.

Epidermolysis bullosa dominant dystrophic type, generalized (DDEB) Figure 17-26 shows a specific form of DDEB which was previously known as albopapuloid or Pasini type. This form of epidermolysis bullosa presents with generalized blistering at birth. During puberty, patients may develop distinctive ivory-white follicular papules on the chest and lower back. The prognosis tends to be good.

Figure 17-27

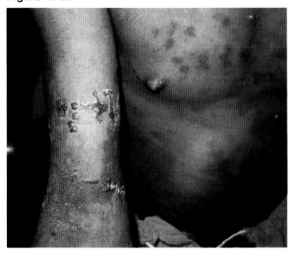

Dystrophic epidermolysis bullosa, dominant type (DDEB)
Figure 17-27 illustrates another patient with a dominant form of scarring epidermolysis bullosa. Previously known as the Cockayne-Touraine type, this form tends to begin during infancy and is associated with widespread blistering and milia formation. Shown here are a number of tense bullae on the flexor surface of the arm. Mouth involvement and nail dystrophy may also occur.

Figure 17-28

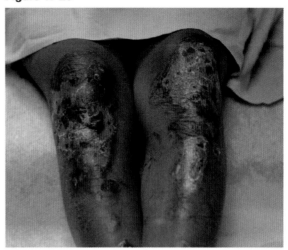

Some forms of DDEB have blistering limited to the elbows, hands, knees, and feet. The blisters heal with scarring. Figure 17-28 reveals atrophic scarring, scaling, and hemorrhagic bullae on the knees and pretibial area.

Figure 17-29

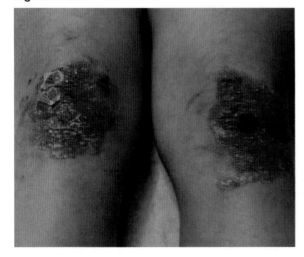

Dystrophic epidermolysis bullosa, dominant type (DDEB)
Figure 17-29 illustrates atrophic scarring on the knees. Patients with localized forms of DDEB also develop a nail dystrophy secondary to the blistering, at times leading to loss of the fingernails and toenails.

Figure 17-30

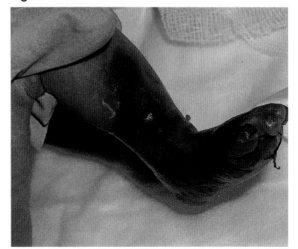

Epidermolysis bullosa with congenital absence of skin There are patients born with well-defined areas of absence of skin limited to the legs and feet. In some cases, this occurrence is familial. This condition may represent a localized type of aplasia cutis congenita or of dominant dystrophic epidemolysis bullosa. Atrophic scarring is associated with this presentation.

Figure 17-31

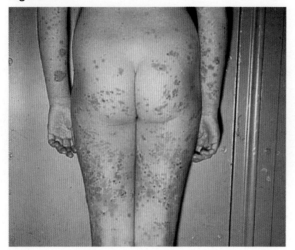

Figure 17-32

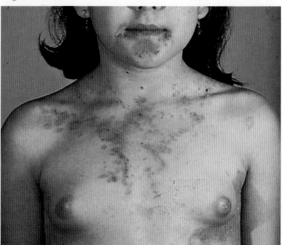

Dermatitis herpetiformis This intensely pruritic papulovesicular eruption is fairly unusual during childhood. Figure 17-31 shows the symmetrical distribution of the grouped, excoriated lesions on the extensor extremities and buttocks. Additional papules and vesicles on the upper chest and face are seen in Fig. 17-32. Dermatitis herpetiformis affects both the skin and the gastrointestinal tract. The majority of children with this disorder have a gluten-sensitive enteropathy.

This may lead to diarrhea and malabsorption, or it may be evidenced only by villous atrophy on jejunal biopsy. The approaches to treatment of this disease include sulfapyridine or dapsone and a gluten-free diet. As mentioned above, children treated with dapsone or sulfapyridine must be carefully monitored for the development of hemolytic anemia. Adherence to a diet that contains no gluten is difficult but, if accomplished, will often lead to prolonged remission.

Figure 17-33

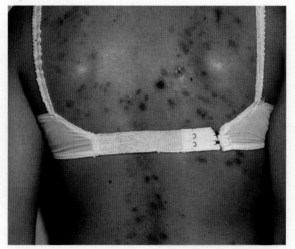

Dermatitis herpetiformis Figure 17-33 shows highly characteristic distribution of lesions of dermatitis herpetiformis on the back. Because of the intense pruritus, excoriations tend to outnumber the primary papulovesicles. Direct immunofluorescence of perilesional skin is an effective means of confirming the diagnosis of dermatitis herpetiformis. Typically, there are granular deposits of IgA at the tips of the dermal papillae.

Figure 17-34

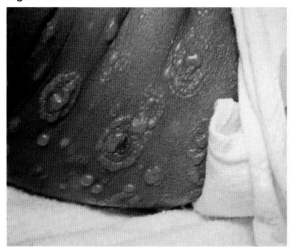

Figure 17-35

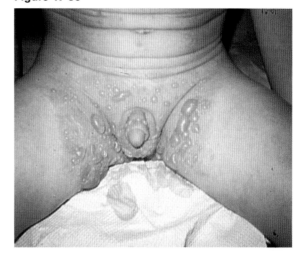

Linear Ig A dermatosis (chronic bullous dermatosis of childhood) This is a distinct blistering disease that occurs exclusively during childhood, most commonly during the first 5 years of life. The disorder is characterized by large, tense bullae that tend to occur in the genital area, lower abdomen and back, and lower extremities. The degree of pruritus is variable. Figure 17-34 illustrates the particular fashion in which the blisters tend to cluster. Note the circular or oval configuration of blisters.

As an early lesion heals with crusting and hyperpigmentation, new lesions arise in a string-of-pearls or rosette-like pattern along the periphery. The blisters themselves may be elongated or sausage-shaped. Figure 17-35 shows the clustering of tense blisters on the inner thighs. This is probably the most common location for linear IgA dermatosis.

Figure 17-36

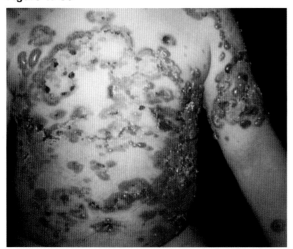

Figure 17-37

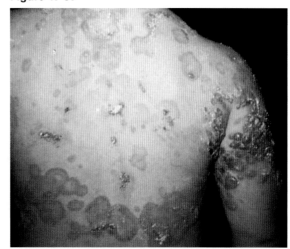

Linear IgA dermatosis (chronic bullous dermatosis of childhood) Figures 17-36 and 17-37 show the annular and polycyclic clustering of blisters that is so typical of this disorder. Biopsy of a lesion reveals a subepidermal blister with an infiltrate of neutrophils and/or eosinophils. Immunofluorescence is more distinctive and usually shows a linear deposit of IgA along the basement membrane (in the lamina lucida). In most patients, there are also circulating IgA antibodies directed against the basement membrane.

For most affected children this is a self-limited disease and it resolves spontaneously over a period of several years. Sulfapyridine and dapsone are the most effective therapies. These drugs have hemolytic activity, and the patients must be monitored for induced anemia and methemoglobinemia. A test for glucose-6-phosphate dehydrogenase should be done before initiation of therapy, and hemoglobin determinations should be made subsequently until stabilization occurs.

Cutaneous Manifestations of HIV Disease

Figure 18-1

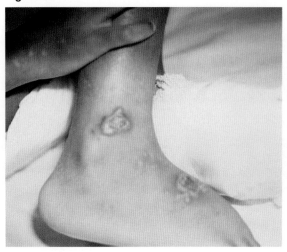

Cutaneous manifestations of HIV infection (chronic varicella zoster infection) Figure 18-1 illustrates a form of infection with varicella zoster virus that is unique to patients with immune suppression from HIV. The 6-year-old child pictured here developed recurrent vesicular and ulcerative lesions of the trunk and extremities following an episode of chickenpox. The lesions contain numerous multinucleated giant cells and are culture-positive for varicella zoster virus.

Figure 18-2

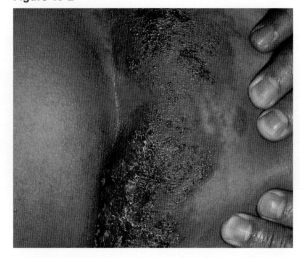

Cutaneous manifestations of HIV infection (herpes zoster infection) In addition to chronic infections with varicella zoster, many patients develop unusual forms of herpes zoster infection. These patients also develop prolonged episodes of shingles that do not respond quickly to appropriate antiviral agents; they may also develop generalized varicella zoster infections.

Figure 18-3

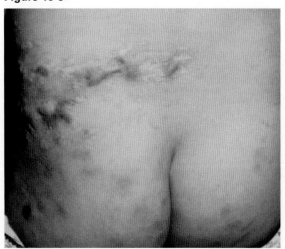

Cutaneous manifestations of HIV infection (scarring from herpes zoster) Figure 18-3 shows a 3-year-old girl developed herpes zoster as an early manifestation of her immune deficiency. Despite therapy with intravenous acyclovir, severe scarring resulted. Herpes zoster generally occurs more frequently in children who have had chickenpox very early in life. Although herpes zoster is certainly seen in the healthy child, its occurrence in a child who is at risk for HIV infection should signal concern.

Figure 18-4

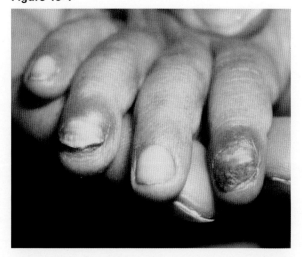

Cutaneous manifestations of HIV infection (candidal paronychias and nail dystrophy) Candidiasis is the most common mucocutaneous manifestation of pediatric HIV infection. Children with AIDS or lesser forms of HIV-related disease frequently develop oral thrush, which recurs or persists despite topical antifungal therapy. Recalcitrant infections of the diaper area and neck folds are also common. Illustrated in Fig. 18-4 are chronic paronychias with a resultant nail dystrophy.

Figure 18-5

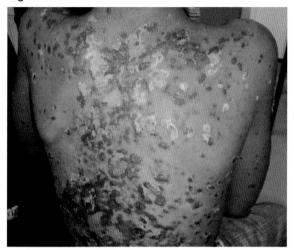

Cutaneous manifestations of HIV infection (drug eruption)
Drug eruptions, usually due to therapy with trimethoprim-
sulfamethoxazole, are particularly common among children
with HIV infection. This child shown in Fig. 18-5 developed
Steven-Johnson syndrome, which is a fairly frequent occurrence
among children infected with HIV. The frequency of drug eruptions in children with AIDS illustrates the complex effect of HIV
on the immune system.

Figure 18-6

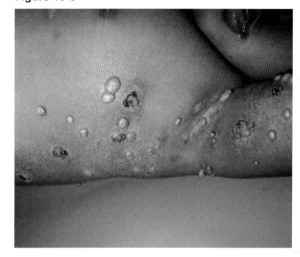

**Cutaneous manifestations of HIV infection (molluscum
contagiosum)** Children in general are prone to infection with
the virus causing molluscum contagiosum. Children infected
with the HIV are more likely to develop persistent, widespread
eruptions due to molluscum contagiosum, and are more likely
to develop the numerous giant lesions that are pictured in
Fig. 18-6.

Figure 18-7

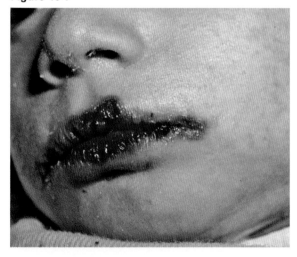

**Cutaneous manifestations of HIV infection (chronic herpetic
gingivostomatitis)** Children with AIDS frequently suffer from
persistent herpetic infections of the mucous membranes or skin.
The gingivostomatitis shown in Fig. 18-7 would be typical of primary infection in a healthy child. One would then expect recurrences to be considerably milder. By contrast, the child with HIV
infection may have recurrent episodes of gingivostomatitis or
may develop infection that does not respond at all to acyclovir
or related drugs.

Figure 18-8

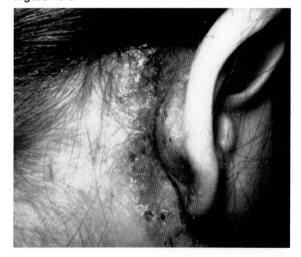

**Cutaneous manifestations of HIV infection (seborrheic
dermatitis)** Seborrheic dermatitis occurs with particular severity in individuals who are infected with HIV. The infantile form
consists of severe scaling and erythema of the scalp and flexural areas and sometimes of the entire skin surface. Illustrated in
Fig. 18-8 is an older child with recalcitrant inflammation behind
the ears. She also had crusting and scaling of the entire scalp.

Figure 18-9

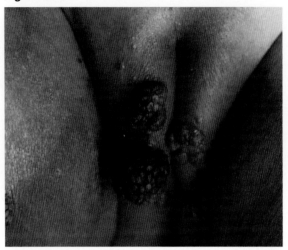

Figure 18-10

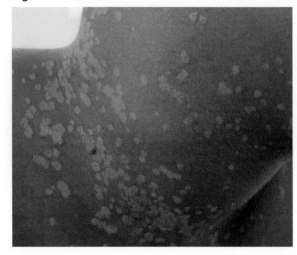

Cutaneous manifestations of HIV infection (condylomata acuminata) Children who are infected with the HIV are prone to a wide variety of cutaneous viral infections. Lesions caused by human papillomavirus (HPV) may be unusually widespread and persistent. A case of condylomata acuminata in a 1-year-old girl is illustrated in Fig. 18-9.

Cutaneous manifestations of HIV infection (widespread flat warts) These coalescent shiny gray macules and slightly elevated plaques are typical of a distinctive clinical manifestation of HPV infection in children with HIV/AIDS. There is a strong tendency for the lesions to Koebnerize (develop in a linear array) where the skin has been scratched. Unlike other cutaneous manifestations of HIV infection, these warts tend not to resolve during successful antiretroviral therapy.

Figure 18-11

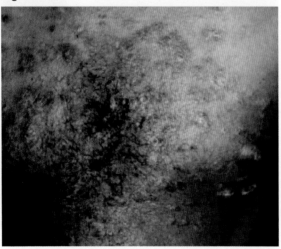

Figure 18-12

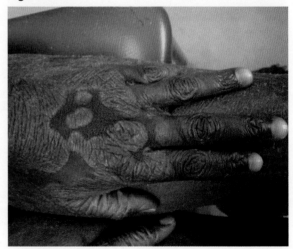

Cutaneous manifestations of HIV infection (psoriasis) Psoriasis is significantly more common among children and adolescents with HIV infection, and often occurs in the absence of a family history. The two patients shown in Figs. 18-11 and 18-12 have severe and generalized plaque psoriasis.

Eryrthrodermic and inverse psoriasis are also seen in the context of HIV infection, and some patients simultaneously develop several morphologic types. Most patients with HIV-related psoriasis improve with successful antiretroviral therapy.

Cutaneous Manifestations of Systemic Disease

Figure 19-1

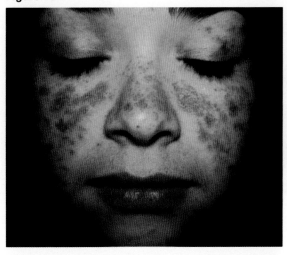

Figure 19-2

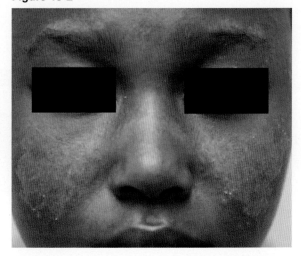

Systemic lupus erythematosus Figures 19-1 and 19-2 illustrate cutaneous involvement of systemic lupus erythematosus (SLE) in the classic butterfly pattern on the face. This macular and intensely erythematous eruption is frequently aggravated by sun exposure and may flare with other symptoms of systemic disease.

This autoimmune disease of unknown etiology affects almost every organ system. The most common findings in the child with SLE are fever, arthralgias, and arthritis. In addition, pleuritis, pericarditis, and central nervous system involvement are frequently seen in children with SLE. Lupus nephritis develops in the vast majority of affected children and may eventually cause renal failure.

Figure 19-3

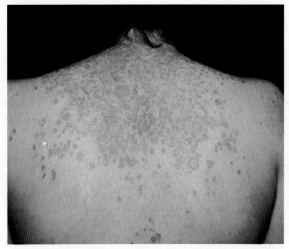

Figure 19-4

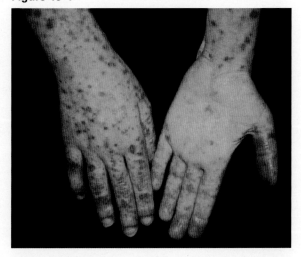

Systemic lupus erythematosus These figures illustrate additional cutaneous features of SLE. The lesions on the back (Fig. 19-3) and the hands (Fig. 19-4) are intensely erythematous macules and slightly edematous papules and plaques. Childhood SLE occurs most frequently during adolescence and is more common among African-Americans and among girls.

Clinical criteria include rash (either malar or discoid), photosensitivity, oral ulcers, and disease of the joints, lungs, kidneys, and central nervous system.

Figure 19-5

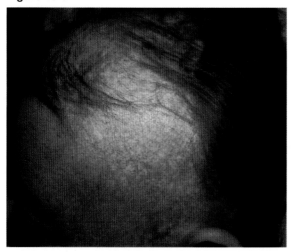

Figure 19-6

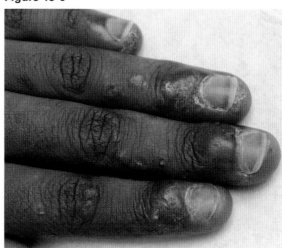

Systemic lupus erythematosus Figure 19-5 shows the temporary alopecia that is also a hallmark of SLE. The single most reliable laboratory test for SLE is antinuclear antibody which will be positive in almost every case of childhood SLE. Other laboratory criteria include leukopenia, thrombocytopenia, and the presence of antinative DNA antibodies.

Involvement of the distal fingers is a common occurrence in children with SLE. Findings include telangiectasia of the nail folds, splinter hemorrhages, and digital infarcts as shown in Fig. 19-6.

Figure 19-7

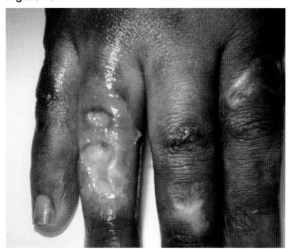

Systemic lupus erythematosus vasculitis Cutaneous vasculitis occurs commonly in patients with SLE. The vasculitis may lead to ulceration as shown in Fig. 19-7.

Figure 19-8

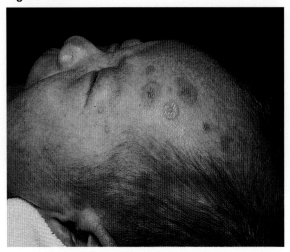

Neonatal lupus erythematosus This condition is primarily due to the transplacental passage mainly of anti-Ro (anti-SS-A) antibodies from mother to infant. Maternal anti-La (anti-SS-B) and anti-RNP antibodies may be implicated. The mother may herself suffer from a form of connective tissue disease or may be completely asymptomatic.

Figure 19-9

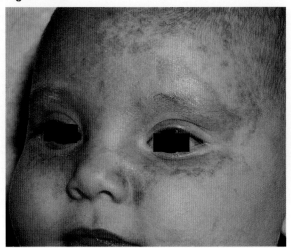

The infants pictured in Figs. 19-8 and 19-9 were born with these atrophic and telangiectatic plaques on the face. Symmetrical involvement of the skin around the eyes is one common pattern. The skin lesions, which are slightly more common in girls, tend to resolve without scarring. Nonfluorinated topical steroids and avoidance of the sun are the only treatments that may be required.

Figure 19-10

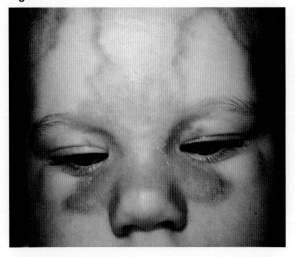

Neonatal lupus erythematosus Figure 19-11 shows the atrophic telangiectatic changes that are most often seen on the temple and scalp, and which may lead to permanent alopecia.

Figure 19-11

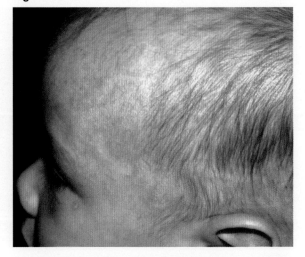

A frequent complication of neonatal lupus is congenital heart block, which may be found in utero. This situation is potentially life threatening and may sometimes require implantation of a pacemaker. Although neonatal lupus is self-limited, there are reports of affected infants going on to develop connective tissue disease during adolescence.

Figure 19-12

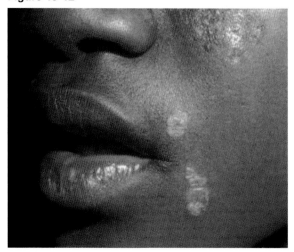

Figure 19-13

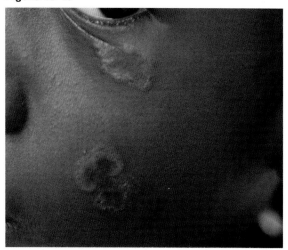

Discoid lupus erythematosus Figures 19-12 and 19-13 show the characteristic plaques of discoid lupus erythematosus. There is a violaceous hue at the border and central atrophy with scarring. Similar involvement in the scalp can cause permanent alopecia.

The majority of children with discoid lupus erythematosus do not go on to develop systemic disease. However, discoid lesions may be a cutaneous manifestation of SLE and children with this disorder should be monitored for the development of systemic disease.

Figure 19-14

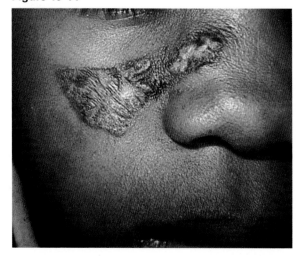

Figure 19-15

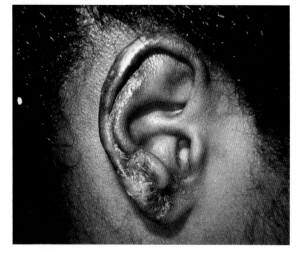

Discoid lupus erythematosus Treatment consists of avoidance of the sun or the use of sunscreens, antimalarial agents, and topical or intralesional corticosteroids.

Illustrated in Fig. 19-15 is a plaque of discoid lupus erythematosus involving the pinna of the ear. Lesions are commonly found in this location, and also within the conchal bowl of the ear.

Figure 19-16

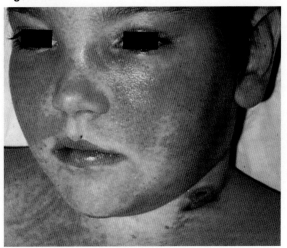

Dermatomyositis This collagen vascular disease is characterized by a combination of symmetrical proximal upper and lower extremity muscle weakness and cutaneous disease. Early symptoms of muscle involvement include general malaise, difficulty in playing or climbing stairs, myalgias, and muscle tenderness.

Figure 19-17

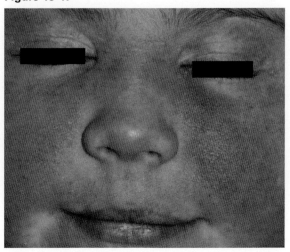

Figures 19-16 and 19-17 show symmetrical, intense erythema and edema of the face. The violaceous color of the periorbital rash is sometimes described as heliotrope in hue; the edema is so intense that it makes the face look puffy.

Figure 19-18

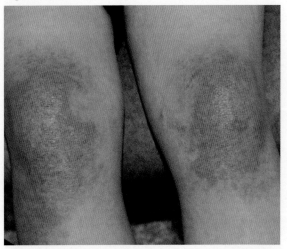

Dermatomyositis Erythematous and edematous papules and plaques may also be present on the elbows and knees. Scaling may also be present, as illustrated in Fig. 19-18, and this manifestation of dermatomyositis may be confused with psoriasis. Psoriasiform scalp involvement may also be a presenting feature.

Figure 19-19

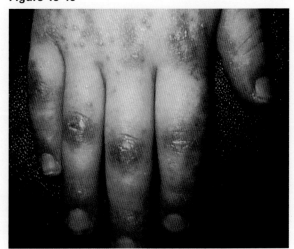

Figure 19-19 illustrates typical papules and plaques located on the dorsum of the hand.

Figure 19-20

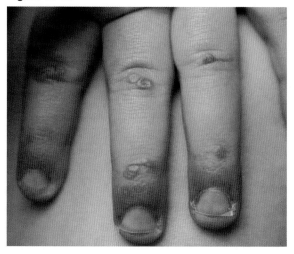

Dermatomyositis Figures 19-20 through 19-22 illustrate involvement of the dorsal hands. Gottron's papules are classically situated over the knuckle joints, and unlike other dermatoses involving the hands, conspicuously spare the skin between those joints.

Figure 19-21

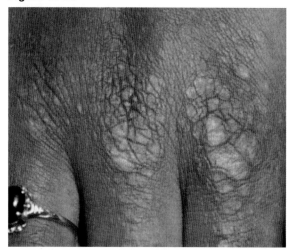

In skin of color, the papules are significantly less erythematous, but show the same characteristic morphology and distribution.

Figure 19-22

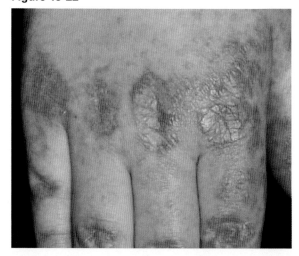

Dermatomyositis The diagnosis of dermatomyositis is usually made on the basis of elevated muscle enzymes (especially creatinine phosphokinase and aldolase), magnetic resonance imaging (MRI), and muscle biopsy if necessary. Skin biopsy tends not to be helpful in differentiating dermatomyositis from other collagen vascular disease. Some patients may develop typical Gottron's papules in the absence of muscle disease (dermatomyositis sine myositis).

Figure 19-23

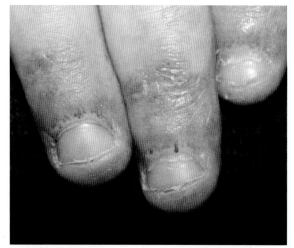

Figure 19-23 shows erythema and telangiectasia in the proximal nail fold. Early and aggressive therapy is vital in the treatment of the muscle disease and in the prevention of calcinosis. In contrast to the adult form of the disease, childhood dermatomyositis is not associated with malignancy.

Figure 19-24

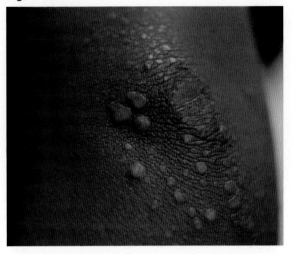

Figure 19-25

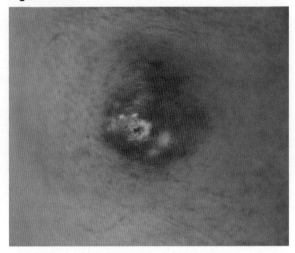

Dermatomyositis Although Gottron's papules are most commonly seen on the dorsal hands, they also may occur on the bilateral elbows. In that case, they should be distinguished from erythema elevatum diutinum (figures 16-27 and 16-28) frictional lichenoid dermatitis (figures 9-20 and 9-21) and an id reaction to nickel.

An additional cutaneous finding, which is particularly characteristic of childhood dermatomyositis, is calcinosis cutis. This may present as firm, superficial nodules or plaques or as painful deposits of calcium in muscle or fascia. Treatment for this troubling disorder is challenging.

Figure 19-26

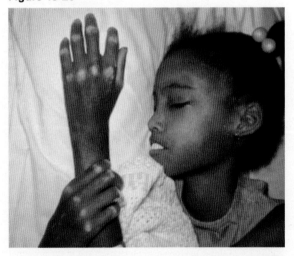

Figure 19-27

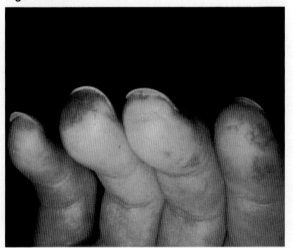

Scleroderma (progressive systemic sclerosis) This is a multisystem connective tissue disease that is relatively rare in childhood. Patients may suffer from arthritis and muscle weakness and from the results of pulmonary, esophageal, cardiac, and renal involvement. The induration of the skin on the face and hands is shown in Fig. 19-26. The pallor of the knuckles gives a sense of the inflexibility of the fingers.

Figure 19-27 shows the pallor of Raynaud phenomenon and telangiectasia. The patient also has scleroderma of the hands, forearms, and face. If calcinosis cutis were also present, this type of case would be designated as the CREST syndrome, characterized by calcinosis, Raynaud phenomenon, esophageal dysmotility, sclerodactyly, and telangiectasia. Such a combination is the most severe of the cutaneous possibilities of scleroderma.

Figure 19-28

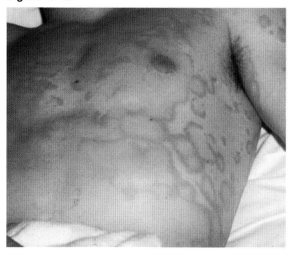

Cutaneous expression of rheumatic fever *Erythema marginatum* is a specific cutaneous expression of rheumatic fever. The lesions, transient and recurrent over days and weeks, may precede cardiac or joint symptoms or signs.

Figure 19-29

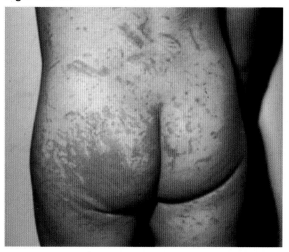

Cutaneous expression of rheumatoid arthritis Patients with rheumatoid arthritis may develop dermographism or edematous erythema provoked by scratching. These lesions are most evident during a febrile period of the illness. Figure 19-29 shows persistent and transient stripes of erythema and edema on the back and buttocks.

Figure 19-30

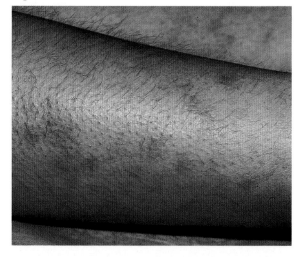

Cutaneous expressions of polyarteritis nodosa This multisystem disease is a form of necrotizing vasculitis that affects small and medium-sized arteries. Frequent areas of systemic involvement are the gastrointestinal tract and kidneys. Palpable purpura is the most common cutaneous manifestation of this disease. In addition, there may be necrotic ulcers and distal gangrene.

Figure 19-31

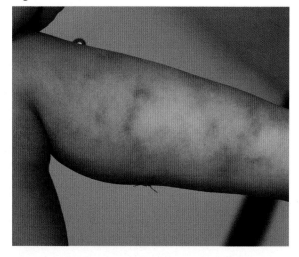

Tender cutaneous nodules, which may be transient, are occasionally seen (Fig. 19-30), but these are more characteristic of benign cutaneous periarteritis nodosa, which has no systemic manifestations. A livedo reticularis pattern is often seen in this condition (Fig. 19-31).

Figure 19-32

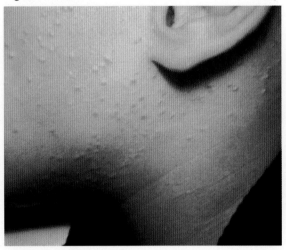

Figure 19-33

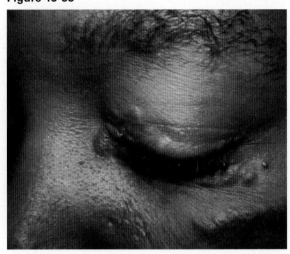

Sarcoidosis This is a disease of unknown etiology that is characterized by the formation of noncaseating granulomas in many different organ systems. It is unusual in children but it does occur. During childhood, the most common presenting signs and symptoms are lymphadenopathy, uveitis, and cutaneous disease. In very young children, arthritis, eye disease, and skin disease tend to predominate. Figure 19-32 illustrates the erythematous and flesh-colored papules that may be the sole cutaneous manifestation of sarcoidosis.

Sarcoidosis is more common among African-Americans. Children and adolescents with sarcoidosis may also have weight loss, fever, and respiratory involvement. Disorders of calcium metabolism are evidenced by hypercalcemia and hypercalciuria. Systemic steroids remain the treatment of choice in this disease. Illustrated here are highly characteristic papules of sarcoidosis on and around the eyelids. Similar lesions are common around the nose and mouth. Investigation for systemic disease should include X-rays of the lungs and pulmonary function tests. The eyes should be examined for uveitis and lacrimal gland enlargement.

Figure 19-34

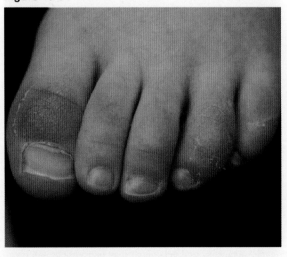

Figure 19-35

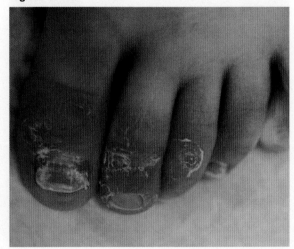

Pernio Children with pernio develop recurrent painful or pruritic, erythematous or violaceous nodules or plaques on the distal fingers or toes. The development of lesions is usually related to cold exposure, and episodes last 2 to 3 weeks.

In the majority of patients, pernio is an isolated benign finding However, less commonly, it is a symptom of cryoglobulinemia, antiphospholipid antibody syndrome, connective tissue disease, or hematologic malignancy. The best treatment is prevention: keeping fingers and toes warm in cold weather.

Figure 19-36

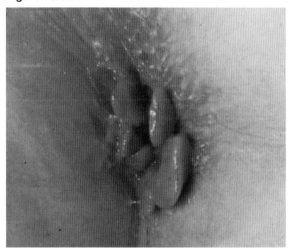

Figure 19-37

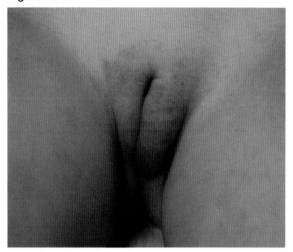

Cutaneous manifestations of Crohn disease This chronic inflammatory bowel disease has several cutaneous manifestations. Most common are perianal fissures, fistulas, and granulomatous nodules. The exophytic lesions shown in Fig. 19-36 could easily be confused with condylomata acuminata. Metastatic Crohn disease may present with ulcerations in intertriginous folds. Children with Crohn disease may also suffer from erythema nodosum and aphthous ulcers.

Crohn disease may also present with erythema and edema of the labia majora, which can progresses to extensive ulcer formation. This form of skin involvement, which may be unilateral or bilateral, may develop before or after the gastrointestinal symptoms.

Figure 19-38

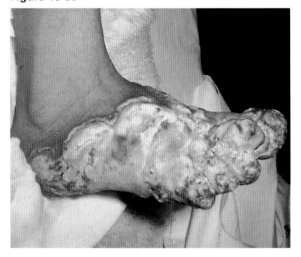

Figure 19-39

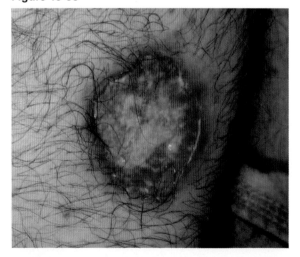

Pyoderma gangrenosum This form of gradually enlarging necrotic ulceration usually involves the distal lower extremity. Typical characteristics include a purulent base and a purplish undermined border. Etiologies include inflammatory bowel disease, chronic active hepatitis, and Behçet syndrome. Arthritis may be an associated finding.

Treatment consists of bed rest, local care, and may include injection of intralesional steroids along the border of the lesion. Oral corticosteroids, cyclosporin A, dapsone, mycophenolate mofetil, and azathioprine are additional therapies, and the anti-TNF agents may also be useful.

Figure 19-40

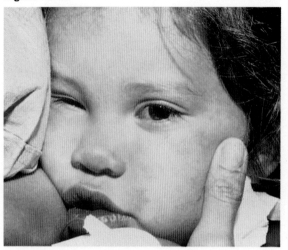

Kawasaki disease This childhood disease of unknown etiology is officially diagnosed by the presence of high fever lasting for 5 or more days, and four of the following criteria: conjunctival injection (Fig. 19-40), mucous membrane changes (Figs. 19-41 and 19-42), erythema or edema of the palms and soles, rash (Fig. 19-43), and cervical lymphadenopathy.

Figure 19-41

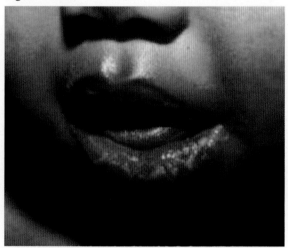

The clinical features of Kawasaki disease are often evanescent, and, frequently the diagnosis is only considered during the second week of illness. For this reason, careful attention to the recent history of oral and cutaneous findings is extremely important.

Figure 19-42

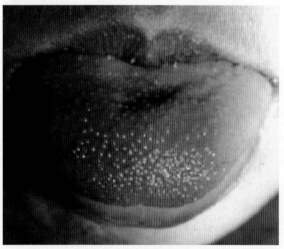

Kawasaki disease Pictured in Fig. 19-42 is a child with straw-berry tongue, a finding also seen in scarlet fever and toxic shock syndrome. Systemic aspects of Kawasaki disease include arthritis, aseptic meningitis, and hydrops of the gallbladder.

Figure 19-43

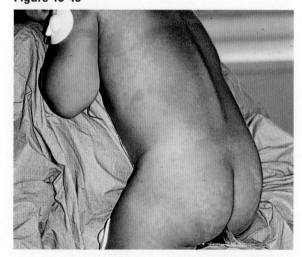

Coronary artery aneurysms develop in 20 percent of patients who are not treated, and some children go on to develop myocardial infarction. Current therapy, consisting of aspirin and intravenous gamma globulin, reduces the incidence of cardiac disease.

Figure 19-44

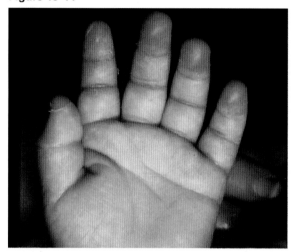

Kawasaki disease A common cutaneous finding during the second week of the illness is desquamation of the palms and soles beginning around the distal portion of the digits and then extending upward.

Figure 19-45

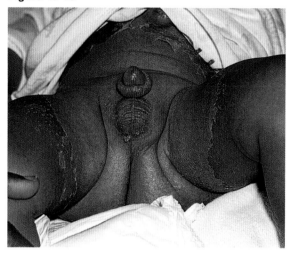

Figure 19-45 illustrates the desquamation of the diaper area that frequently occurs in Kawasaki disease. All children with a history of Kawasaki disease should be followed with serial two-dimensional echocardiography to monitor for the progression of cardiac involvement.

Figure 19-46

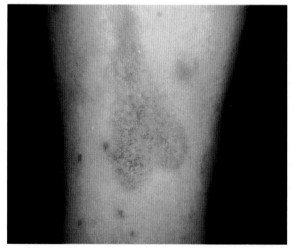

Necrobiosis lipoidica This condition usually occurs in patients with diabetes but is also rarely associated with rheumatoid arthritis. The most common location is on the shins, and the condition is often bilateral. The lesions are usually asymptomatic, but may also be tender. The lesion may be erythematous at first, but eventually evolves into an indurated plaque with a yellowish or brown tint.

Figure 19-47

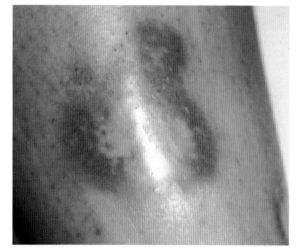

This condition has some histologic and clinical resemblance to granuloma annulare (Figs. 20-24 to 20-29), but the two conditions are distinct. The lesions of necrobiosis lipoidica are generally much larger than those of granuloma annulare and patients with necrobiosis lipoidica can develop atrophy and scarring, as illustrated in Fig. 19-47.

Disorders of the Dermis (Infiltrates, Atrophies, and Nodules)

Figure 20-1

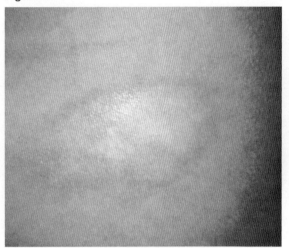

Figure 20-2

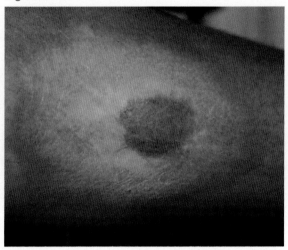

Morphea This condition is characterized by discrete areas of hardened and discolored skin. The areas vary in size and shape, and may be single or multiple. Morphea is also sometimes referred to as *localized scleroderma,* but this condition must not be confused with scleroderma, a generalized disease with organ involvement. Families must be cautioned of this important difference so that their internet searches do not lead to unnecessary worry.

The solitary or individual lesion is a circle or oval of firm skin that is whitish, slightly depressed, and sometimes surrounded by a different color—lilac or purple. A lesion with a prominent purple vascular border is illustrated in Fig. 20-2. There may be only one such lesion, or multiple smaller and larger lesions covering large parts of the skin surface. The course of the condition is variable. Spontaneous recovery in children is common, but a wide variety of topical and systemic therapies have been recommended for lesions that cause significant problems with respect to appearance and function.

Figure 20-3

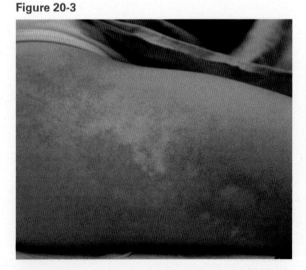

Figure 20-4

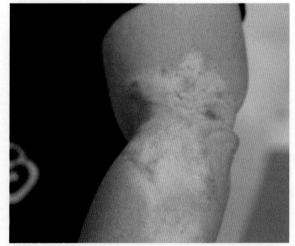

Morphea (linear) Figure 20-3 shows a type of morphea that is linear in shape and situated on the lateral surface of the leg. Again the affected skin is hard, slightly depressed, and dyschromic. Extensive areas of linear morphea are the most difficult to treat. There is a tendency toward permanent deformity. In this case, linear morphea appears to follow the lines of Blaschko, and suggests the possibility of mosaicism.

When the lesions cross over a joint, the rapid development of atrophy or contractures may occur. In those cases, systemic therapy, usually with pulsed intravenous steroids and methotrexate, is required.

Figure 20-5

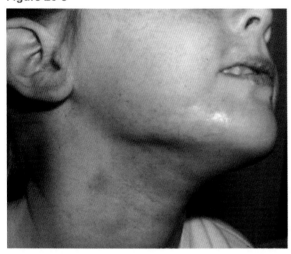

Morphea (linear) This is an example of linear morphea involving the lip, chin, and neck. The skin is hard to the touch, and shiny with prominent vasculature. Rarely, linear morphea occurring in this location may lead to involvement of the gums and tongue.

Figure 20-6

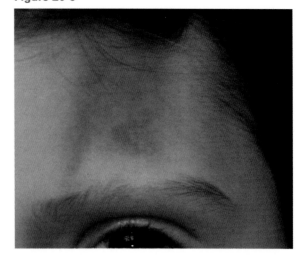

Morphea (linear, en coup de sabre) This term refers to linear morphea occurring on the forehead and scalp. Rarely, the central nervous system is affected. Neurologic manifestations include seizures, focal neurologic deficits, and movement disorders. MRI in affected children shows some areas of T2 hyperintensity and evidence of focal tissue atrophy in the brain.

Figure 20-7

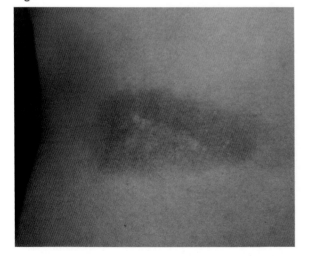

Morphea Illustrated in Fig. 20-7 is a lesion of morphea that is resolving. The first sign of improvement is softening in the area of involvement. In this patient, the lesion is becoming softer, and turning brown. In the center there is still an area of sclerosis.

Figure 20-8

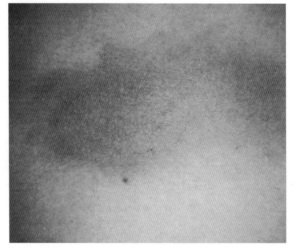

Figure 20-8 shows a lesion that is reddish-brown and is now level with the surrounding skin. It will eventually completely resolve or leave minor dyschromia. The cause of morphea is unknown.

Figure 20-9

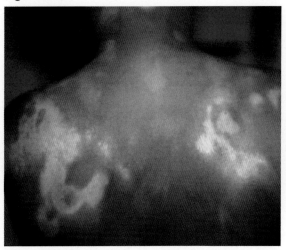

Figure 20-10

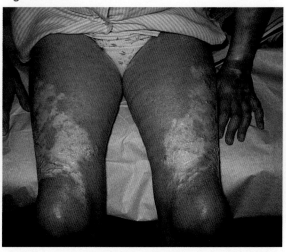

Generalized morphea Sometimes morphea can be more extensive and involve large areas of the skin surface. The lesions begin as erythematous to violaceous plaques and become sclerotic with a central ivory color. Sometimes only hyperpigmentation can be discerned.

These lesions may enlarge peripherally, becoming quite extensive. When involvement occurs on the extremities, contractures and atrophy may result. Scarring may result in disability, but these patients do not have the internal organ involvement that is seen in scleroderma (systemic sclerosis).

Figure 20-11

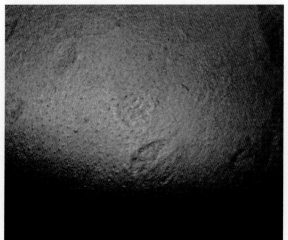

Atrophoderma (Pasini-Pierini) This condition is most common in adolescent girls, and its etiology is completely unknown. Characteristically, there develop single or multiple well-circumscribed, slightly hyperpigmented areas of cutaneous atrophy, with a sharp "cliff-drop" border. The lesions tend to enlarge slowly and then persist. Some believe that this form of atrophoderma represents a variant of morphea, in which atrophy is more evident than is sclerosis.

Figure 20-12

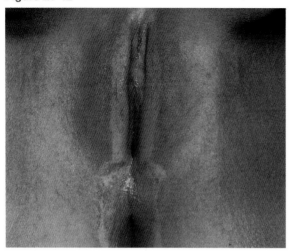

Figure 20-13

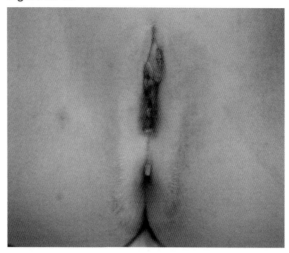

Lichen sclerosus et atrophicus Figures 20-12 and 20-13 illustrate lichen sclerosus et atrophicus in its most typical location. This cutaneous disorder is more common in girls and is usually confined to the skin surrounding the anogenital region. The onset of the disease may be accompanied by pruritus, burning, constipation, or vaginal discharge, or it may be completely asymptomatic. Porcelain-colored or slightly erythematous macules gradually coalesce to form plaques.

The end result is an area of shiny atrophy in an hourglass shape around the rectum and vagina. Childhood lichen sclerosus et atrophicus tends to be a self-limited disease, with improvement occurring at the time of puberty. It may persist into adulthood. The use of topical corticosteroids provides symptomatic relief and may hasten the resolution of the process.

Figure 20-14

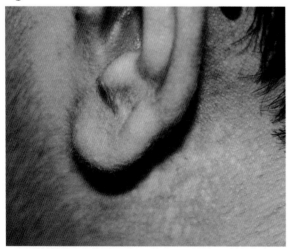

Figure 20-15

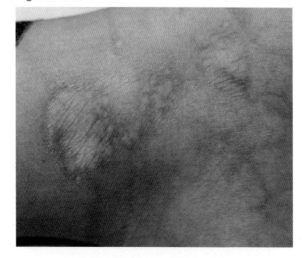

Lichen sclerosus et atrophicus Figure 20-14 shows the discrete and confluent ivory-colored macules that are typical of extragenital lichen sclerosus et atrophicus. Involvement as shown here, on the skin behind the ear is unusual. Extragenital lesions tend to be asymptomatic.

Figure 20-15 illustrates lichen sclerosus et atrophicus involving the ankle, which is not an unusual location. The classic lesion contains numerous white round and oval-shaped macules that, in some cases, form areas of confluence. Rarely, extragenital lichen sclerosus is widespread and disfiguring.

Figure 20-16

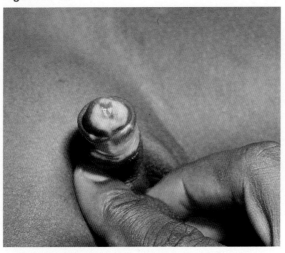

Figure 20-17

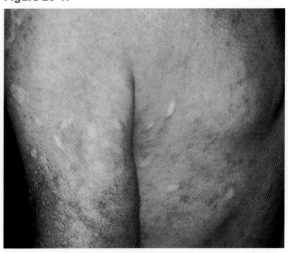

Lichen sclerosus et atrophicus (Balanitis xerotica obliterans) This is a form of lichen sclerosus et atrophicus affecting the penis. It usually presents as recurrent balanitis, associated with redness, tightening, and fissuring of the foreskin. Eventually, the disease process may result in phimosis and difficulty in urination. In many cases, circumcision is either very helpful or curative. However, involvement of the glans penis may persist after surgery. Although this disorder is generally rare, it is not an unusual finding among young boys who present with phimosis.

Anetoderma (macular atrophy) The term *anetoderma*, meaning slack skin, is used to describe a form of cutaneous atrophy. The classic lesion is a macule of atrophic and wrinkled skin. The lesions of anteoderma may be preceded by inflammation, or may occur de novo on normal skin. Anetoderma may arise without a known cause, or it may be a sequelae of syphilis, or lupus erythematosus.

Figure 20-18

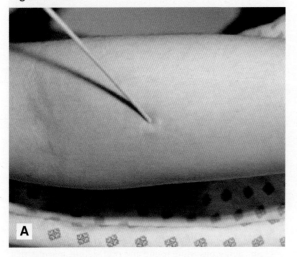

A

Figure 20-18

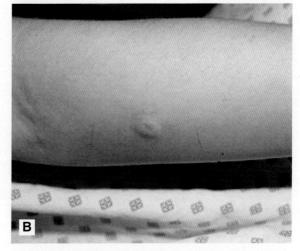

B

Anetoderma Illustrated in Fig. 20-18 is a lesion of anetoderma on the arm of a teenage girl. Direct pressure with a wooden

applicator causes an inpouching of the involved skin.

Figure 20-19

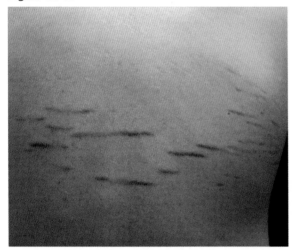

Figure 20-20

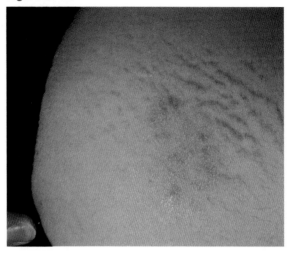

Striae distensae Stretch marks are parallel streaks of glossy and erythematous skin, that gradually become hypopigmented and scar-like in appearance. The stretch marks often have a different texture from normal skin and may be slightly depressed. Striae are commonly seen in healthy adolescents and may be found on the back, around the breasts, upper arms, hips, inner thighs, and around the popliteal fossae.

Other causes of striae include pregnancy and rapid weight gain. Striae may also be seen in children with Cushing syndrome. Athletes, particularly weight lifters, sometimes develop striae distensae. In Fig. 20-19, one sees striae on the back that may well be of a weight lifter. Figure 20-20 shows striae and telangiectasia as a side effect of topical corticosteroids, which is most frequent in older children and adolescents.

Figure 20-21

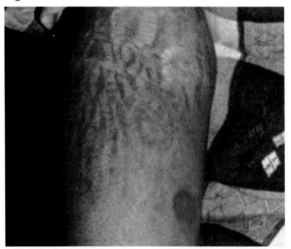

Striae distensae This is an example of striae resulting from the use of topical corticosteroids in the antecubetal fossa, a typical area of involvement of atopic dermatitis. Older children and teenagers must be made particularly aware of this potential side effect, and should be cautioned against using stronger topical steroids on the inner thighs and axillae.

Figure 20-22

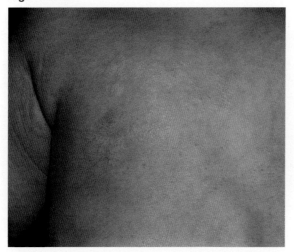

Figure 20-23

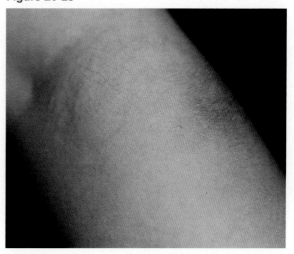

Connective tissue nevus This group of hamartomas may be composed of various elements of the extracellular connective tissue: collagen, elastic fibers, and glycosaminoglycans. One example of the collagen variety is the shagreen patch, a cutaneous manifestation of tuberous sclerosis (Fig 14-69). These yellow or orange plaques of coalescent papules are often seen in the lumbosacral area. Other varieties of connective tissue nevus are not associated with tuberous sclerosis and may be seen elsewhere on the body.

Particularly, collagenomas may be seen in solitary (Figs. 20-22 and 20-23), eruptive, and multiple forms. The last of these is a familial disorder. Elastic fibers are found in isolated elastomas and in the small yellowish papules of the autosomal dominant Buschke-Ollendorf syndrome (Fig 14-71). The latter is also characterized by asymptomatic sclerotic densities of the bones.

Figure 20-24

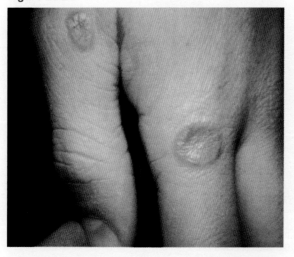

Figure 20-25

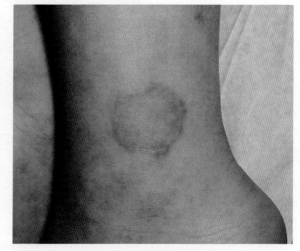

Granuloma annulare This benign condition is characterized by one or more circular plaques consisting of rings of papules around a depressed center. The hands and feet are the most common location for granuloma annulare. The majority of patients have only one or several lesions, but occasionally, eruptive and widespread lesions occur.

Granuloma annulare, when it occurs in children, is not associated with any other disease, nor is there any known cause. The condition is symptomless. Lesions may persist for months or years before response to therapy or spontaneous resolution.

Figure 20-26

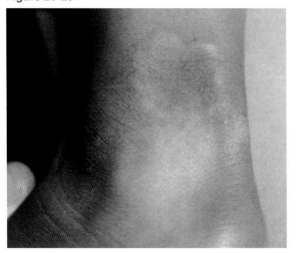

Granuloma annulare Figure 20-26 illustrates a very typical lesion of granuloma annulare in a common location. Because of the circular appearance with central clearing, granuloma annulare is often mistaken for a fungal infection. However, the indurated nature of the periphery and the absence of scale make the diagnosis obvious in most cases.

Figure 20-27

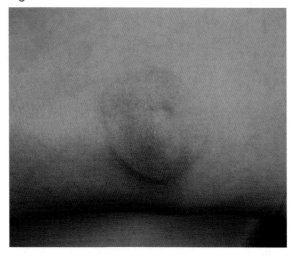

Subcutaneous granuloma annulare This form of granuloma annulare presents with deep nodules. In some cases, as illustrated in Fig. 20-27, a more typical annular lesion may surround the nodule. These lesions are most frequently localized to the digits, scalp, dorsa of the feet, or anterior tibial region.

Figure 20-28

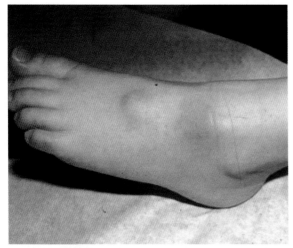

Subcutaneous granuloma annulare This patient in Fig. 20-28 developed a subcutaneous nodule on the dorsum of the foot. The lesion is not painful or tender, and has a rubbery consistency. In some cases, the diagnosis of subcutaneous granluloma annulare can be confirmed by the presence of typical annular lesions in other locations.

Figure 20-29

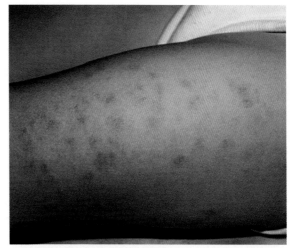

Eruptive granuloma annulare This generalized form of the disease is more unusual. It presents with numerous flesh-colored or pink-red papules. In some cases, they coalesce into round or reticulate clusters. A subtle annularity, especially noted on palpation of a lesion, may be the clue to diagnosis. In most children, eruptive granuloma annulare favors the trunk, but it is occasionally seen in a photodistribution. In children, this disorder does not appear to be associated with any systemic illness.

Figure 20-30

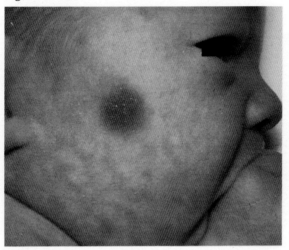

Figure 20-31

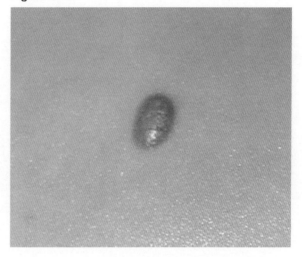

Juvenile xanthogranuloma This is a common and completely benign cutaneous nodule. Typically, a juvenile xanthogranuloma is firm and dome-shaped. At first, the lesion is reddish as in Fig. 20-30, but develops a fairly typical orange-brown hue over time (Figs. 20-31 to 20-33).

The bright orange color seen in this lesion is virtually pathognomonic for juvenile xanthogranuloma. Most juvenile xanthogranulomas are located on the head or neck, but the lesions sometimes occur on the trunk or extremities. They may be present at birth, but most develop during the first year of life.

Figure 20-32

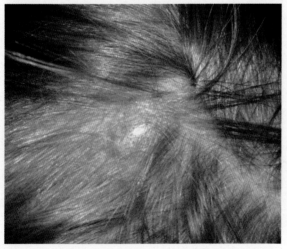

Figure 20-33

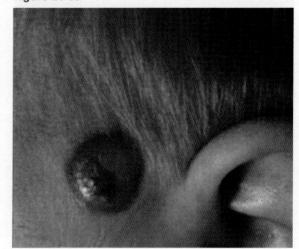

Juvenile xanthogranuloma Juvenile xanthogranuloma is not associated with abnormalities in serum cholesterol or triglycerides, and the individual lesions undergo spontaneous involution, usually over a period of 1 to 2 years.

A diagnostic biopsy analysis is sometimes needed; surgical intervention is possible, but certainly not required. Larger lesions may resolve with an area of atrophic skin or a hyperpigmented or hypopigmented macule.

Figure 20-34

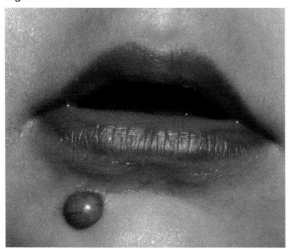

Juvenile xanthogranuloma Pictured in Fig. 20-34 is a solitary nodular facial lesion. Multiple juvenile xanthogranulomas on the skin may be accompanied by intraocular lesions. For this reason, the physician must pay careful attention to the examination of the eyes and consider an ophthalmologic referral for the child with multiple lesions. Certainly, an abnormality in the color of the iris or an enlargement of the globe should trigger a prompt referral.

Figure 20-35

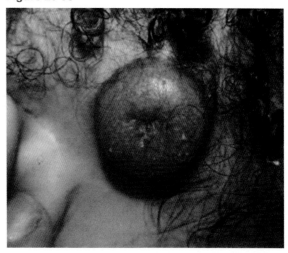

Rarely, as illustrated in Fig. 20-35, a juvenile xanthogranuloma can grow very large. In this case, surgical excision may well be desirable approach.

Figure 20-36

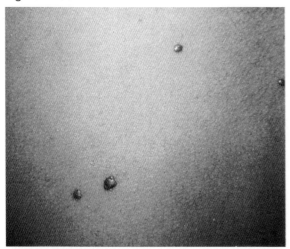

Juvenile xanthogranuloma Figure 20-36 shows four lesions. It is somewhat more common to see multiple juvenile xanthogranulomas than a solitary lesion. Rarely, they may number in the hundreds. As mentioned, juvenile xanthogranuloma of the eye is the most common complication of this generally benign and self-limited condition.

Figure 20-37

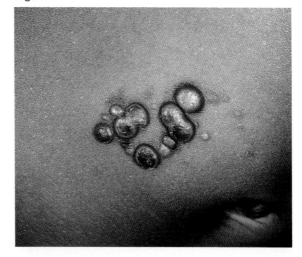

When multiple small juvenile xanthogranulomas are seen in children with neurofibromatosis, these patients have an additional tendency toward the development of juvenile chronic myelocytic leukemia. Rarely, as illustrated in Fig. 20-37, juvenile xanthogranulomas may become agminated and appear as a plaque.

Figure 20-38

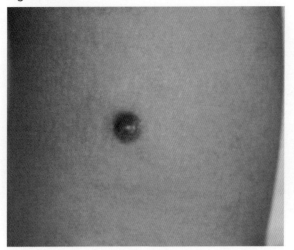

Figure 20-39

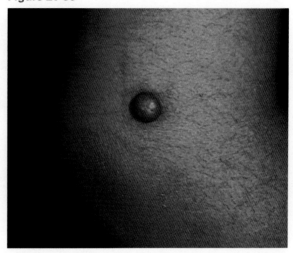

Dermatofibroma These are benign dermal nodules that represent a focal proliferation of fibroblasts; the overlying epidermis is slightly thickened. Their occurrence is not unusual in children and adolescents. Dermatofibromas are firm and may be black, red, brown, or flesh-colored. Their diameter generally ranges from 0.5 to 1.5 cm, although they may occasionally be larger. Dermatofibromas may be solitary or multiple, and they develop either spontaneously or after minor trauma to the skin, such as an insect bite.

Most are asymptomatic but sometimes dermatofibromas may be painful on palpation. A very useful diagnostic maneuver is executed by exerting lateral pressure on the lesion. The skin overlying a dermatofibroma will frequently dimple. Dermatofibromas require surgical treatment only when they are of cosmetic concern to the patient. However, biopsy is occasionally required in order to confirm the diagnosis and to differentiate it from more serious disorders.

Figure 20-40

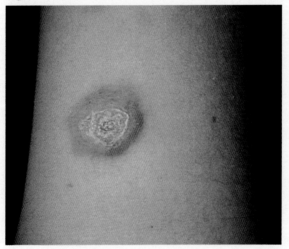

Figure 20-41

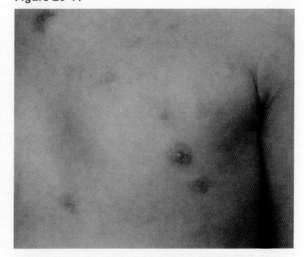

Granular cell tumor These are unusual nodular lesions that vary from 0.5 to 3.0 cm in diameter. They may be single (Fig. 20-40) or multiple (Fig. 20-41) and are firm, elevated, and circumscribed. The tongue is a common site. The lesions pictured in both figures are fairly typical of the cutaneous variety.

The original name *granular cell myoblastoma* derived from an early theory that these tumors arise from immature striated muscle cells. In fact, granular cell tumors are of neural derivation.

Figure 20-42

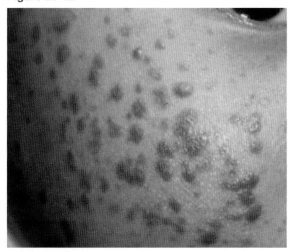

Figure 20-43

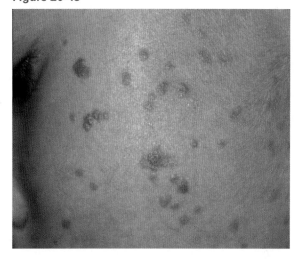

Benign cephalic histiocytosis This very distinctive eruption consists of numerous brownish-yellow macules and papules involving the head and neck. The mucous membranes are spared. Benign cephalic histiocytosis usually begins during the first 3 years of life, and the lesions continue to evolve for several years. The condition then resolves spontaneously during childhood but may leave small atrophic or pigmented scars.

Children with benign cephalic histiocytosis do not develop systemic disease and are not at risk for Langerhans cell disease. This disorder can be diagnosed by skin biopsy with appropriate immunostains.

Figure 20-44

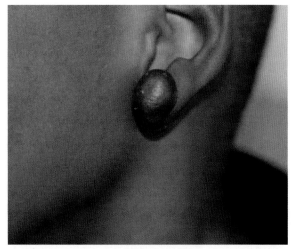

Figure 20-45

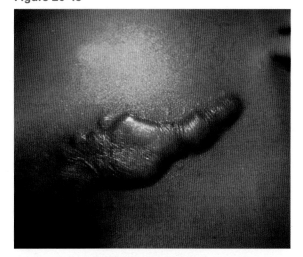

Keloids The lesions pictured in Fig. 20-44 are typical of the disfiguring changes that sometimes occur after trauma to the skin. In children, a laceration, a surgical procedure, or a bout of chicken pox may be the inciting event for keloid formation. This figure shows a keloid that was caused by ear piercing. Keloid formation is more common in African-American children, is very rare in infants, and becomes somewhat more frequent with increasing age. Keloids begin as firm, telangiectatic plaques confined to the site of the initial wound. Over time, they become less erythematous and extend beyond the site of injury.

Pruritus, burning, and hyperesthesia are frequent complaints. In contrast to hypertrophic scars, keloids extend beyond the limits of the original scar and do not resolve spontaneously. In fact, they may continue to grow over a period of years. The intralesional injection of corticosteroids is currently the preferred treatment for most keloids. Surgical excision will almost always result in recurrence but is somewhat more successful when accompanied by the injection of corticosteroids during the process of healing.

Figure 20-46

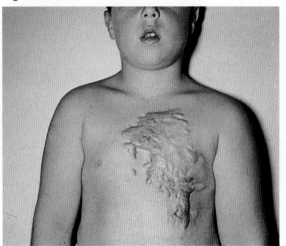

Keloids The keloid pictured in Fig. 20-46 is a common variety that develops after a thermal burn. The irregular contour and crab-like projections are characteristic and illustrate the root of the word *keloid:* from the Greek word *chele,* meaning crab's claw. The size and thickness of lesions of this type make treatment difficult. The chest and back are also common sites for keloids of another cause, namely, inflammatory acne. In that situation, repeated injections of intralesional corticosteroids are often of cosmetic benefit.

Figure 20-47

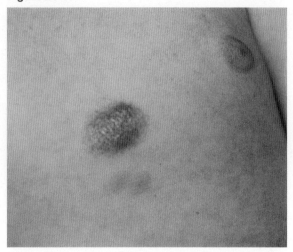

Fibrous hamartoma of infancy This benign growth may be present at birth, or develop during the first 2 years of life. The solitary subcutaneous nodule ranges from 2 to 5 cm in diameter and is sometimes lumpy on palpation. In most cases, the lesion occurs on the axilla, shoulder, upper arm, and chest wall. Other possible sites are the inguinal region and the buttocks. Diagnosis depends on histopathological examination, and the treatment of choice is excision.

Figure 20-48

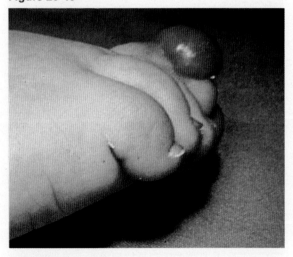

Digital fibrous tumor of childhood This is a rare fibromatosis that starts in infants either as a single nodule or, less commonly, as several nodules. Parents may be alarmed by the rapid growth of the lesions. Digital fibrous tumors usually occur on the dorsal and sometimes on the lateral aspects of the distal phalanges of fingers and toes.

Figure 20-49

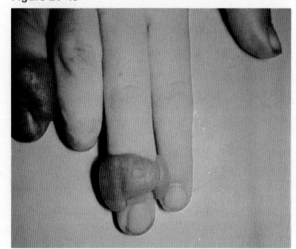

They may be globular, red, and smooth as illustrated in Fig. 20-48, or reddish-brown and convoluted, especially when they wrap around digits, as illustrated in Fig. 20-49. Deformity of the adjacent nail plate may occur. The lesions are benign and have never been known to become malignant or metastasize.

Figure 20-50

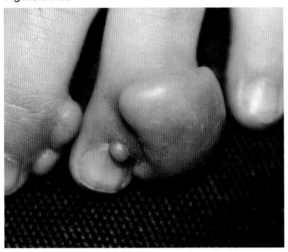

Digital fibrous tumor of childhood Recurrence is a common event after surgical excision, but many such tumors will involute without treatment over a period of several years. In most cases, the best treatment is simple observation

Figure 20-51

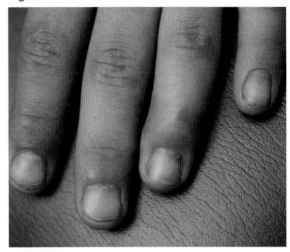

Figures 20-50 and 20-51 are of the same patient, and illustrate the process of spontaneous involution over several years.

Figure 20-52

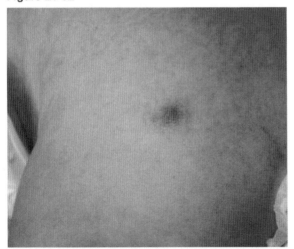

Infantile myofibromatosis The majority of lesions present at birth or shortly thereafter. They may be superficial or may involve the subcutaneous tissue and muscle. The typical lesion of infantile myofibromatosis is a rubbery or firm nodule (Fig. 20-52), sometimes measuring up to 7 cm in diameter (Fig. 20-53). Solitary lesions tend to occur on the head and neck, and resolve spontaneously, sometimes leaving areas of atrophy or pigmentary alteration.

Figure 20-53

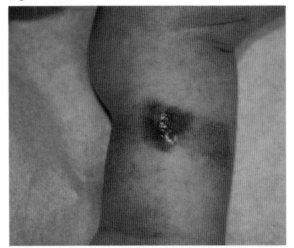

Children with multiple lesions (the generalized form) are particularly at risk for visceral and bone involvement. While the skin and bone lesions in these children also tend to disappear spontaneously, the visceral lesions (lungs, heart, and gastrointestinal tract) are a significant cause of morbidity and mortality.

Figure 20-54

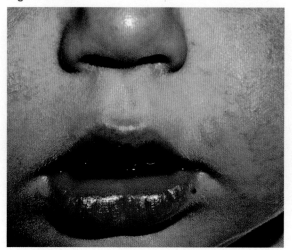

Mastocytoma This is one of a group of disorders that are characterized by the accumulation of mast cells in the skin and sometimes in other organs. The plaque shown in Fig. 20-54 represents a solitary mastocytoma, which occurs almost exclusively during infancy. This is most often a reddish-brown or orange nodule or plaque that is rubbery in consistency. There is occasionally a history of repeated swelling or even blister formation on the surface.

Figure 20-55

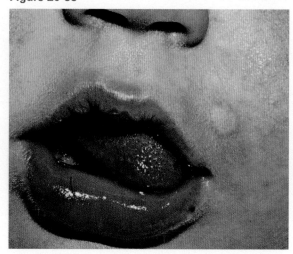

Pictured in Fig. 20-55 is the same patient as in the previous photo. When a solitary mastocytoma or a lesion of mastocytosis is firmly rubbed, the area will turn red, swell, and occasionally blister. This diagnostic test is termed *Darier's sign* and it is virtually diagnostic of mast cell disease. Mechanical trauma is thought to degranulate mast cells and cause a local release of histamine. Dermographism in uninvolved skin is not uncommon.

Figure 20-56

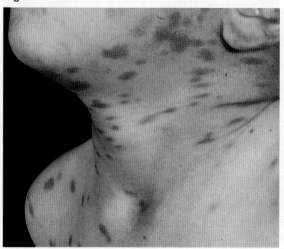

Mastocytosis Figure 20-56 shows the numerous macules and papules of reddish or brownish hue that are typical of urticaria pigmentosa. This generalized form is the most common type of mastocytosis, and it also usually develops during early childhood.

Figure 20-57

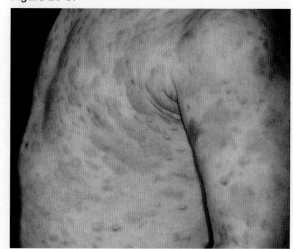

Figure 20-57 illustrates the typical lesions of generalized mastocytosis (urticaria pigmentosa). Numerous brown and orange papules are coalescing to form plaques.

Figure 20-58

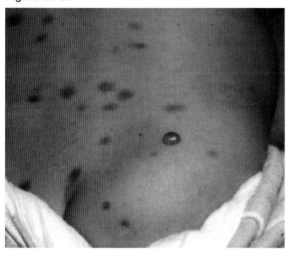

Mastocytosis (cont.) Patients who develop urticaria pigmentosa during early childhood tend to have only cutaneous involvement, and their disease will almost always involute over a period of years. Figure 20-58 illustrates a child with widespread lesions; one has spontaneously blistered due to the release of histamines.

Figure 20-59

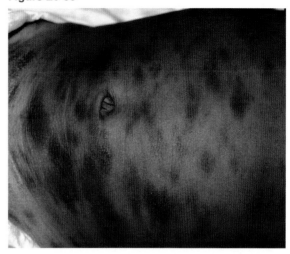

Figure 20-59 shows the same process in child with skin of color. In general, no treatment is necessary, but it is important to provide the parents with a list of medications that might cause the sudden and potentially life-threatening release of histamine. These include aspirin, codeine, morphine, polymyxin B, aminoglycosides, and NSAIDs. Immersion in a very hot bath may have the same effect.

Figure 20-60

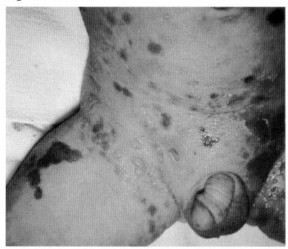

Bullous mastocytosis (Diffuse cutaneous mastocytosis) This disease form is much less common than urticaria pigmentosa and much more serious. The disease may be present at birth, or begin during infancy. The skin tends to be leathery and thickened as a result of widespread infiltration of mast cells in the dermis. Children suffer from severe recurrent episodes of urticaria and blistering.

Figure 20-61

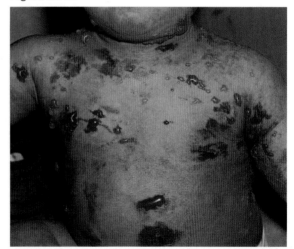

As illustrated in Fig. 20-61, the blisters vary in size and may be hemorrhagic. The occurrence of bullae may be accompanied by wheezing, diarrhea, hypotension, and shock-like symptoms. In such patients, management of the disease may present a significant challenge. In the newborn, diffuse cutaneous mastocytosis must be differentiated from other blistering disorders, including staphylococcal scalded skin syndrome (Figs. 3-7 through 3-11), and a skin biopsy is mandatory. Familial occurrence of bullous mastocytosis has been reported.

Figure 20-62

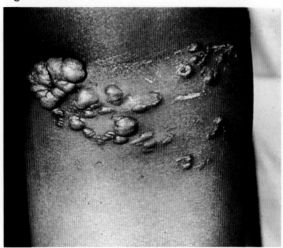

Nevus lipomatosus superficialis This is a hamartoma composed of fat tissue situated in dermis. The lesions are papillomatosis and have a yellowish hue. Nevus lipomatosus is not associated with any syndromes or underlying disorders, and can be excised if disfiguring.

Figure 20-63

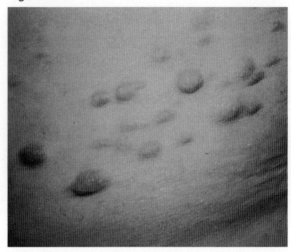

Leiomyoma The lesions are fleshy papules or nodules. In some case, they are associated with intense pain. They have no malignant potential. Surgical removal is curative for solitary lesions but may be more complicated for numerous and widely spaced lesions such as those illustrated in Fig. 20-63.

Figure 20-64

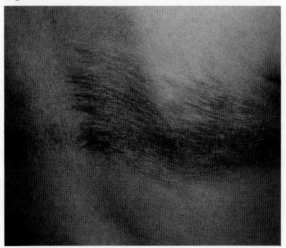

Smooth muscle and pilar hamartoma This lesion typically presents as a solitary firm plaque, most often located on the trunk or proximal extremities and noted at birth or within the first few weeks of life. The lesions are flesh-colored to slightly erythematous initially, but eventually tend to develop a light brown color. There is usually increased hair growth within the lesion.

Figure 20-65

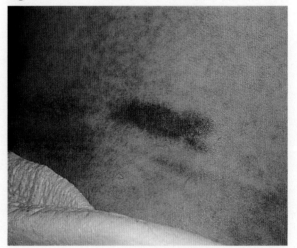

Histologically, the lesion is characterized by the presence of well-defined bundles of smooth muscle. Firm stroking may elicit fasciculations, a phenomenon noted in the lesion pictured in Fig. 20-65). This is termed *pseudo-Darier's sign*. The term is based on a similarity to Darier sign: the swelling of a lesion of mastocytosis elicited also by stroking (Fig 20-55).

Figure 20-66

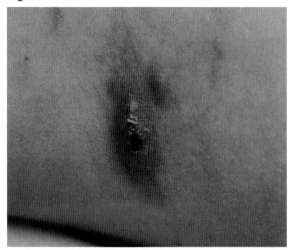

Figure 20-67

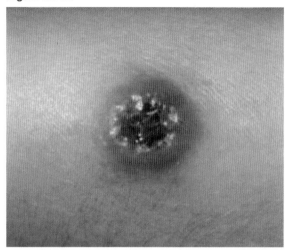

Lymphomatoid papulosis This uncommon skin disorder is characterized by recurrent episodes of red to brown papules and nodules. Most common locations are the trunk and extremities, and the face is usually spared. The crops of lesions may last for several weeks, but larger nodules may be more persistent.

Ulceration is not uncommon, as illustrated in Figs. 20-67 and 20-68, and lesions may heal with hyperpigmentation, hypopigmentation, or true scarring.

Figure 20-68

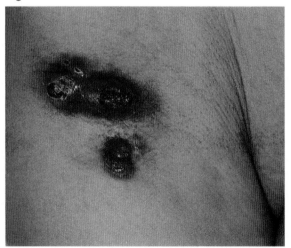

Lymphomatoid papulosis The prognosis of lymphomatoid papulosis is variable. In some patients, there is complete resolution after a single episode, and, in others, recurrences occur for a period of years. In adult patients, there is a significant risk of developing some form of malignant lymphoma. In children, the risk appears to be less, but there are reported cases of lymphomatoid papulosis developing into non-Hodgkin lymphoma.

SECTION

21

Drug Eruptions

Figure 21-1

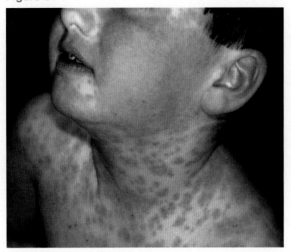

Drug eruptions Diagnosing drug eruptions has become a common experience to practitioners in all branches of modern medicine. The profusion of drugs now available, the continuous influx of new drugs, and the capability of drugs to cause actions different from or in addition to their pharmacologically desirable actions make adverse cutaneous reactions an inevitable fact of modern medical practice. The kinds of cutaneous reactions are varied. Illustrated in Fig. 21-1 is a reaction to amoxicillin. Eruptions from amoxicillin are more frequently seen in children with infectious mononucleosis.

Figure 21-2

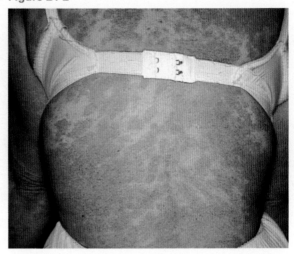

Morbiliform rashes are the most common form of drug eruption. Illustrated in Fig. 21-2 is a reaction to chloroquine (Plaquenil). Other common causes are amoxicillin, cephalosporins, semisynthetic penicillins, and barbiturates. Constitutional symptoms of low-grade fever and malaise may be associated with such drug eruptions.

Figure 21-3

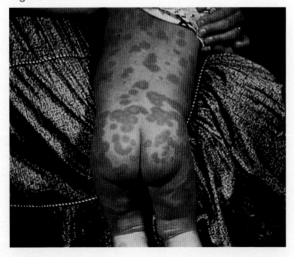

Drug eruptions Drug eruptions may be uncomfortably pruritic, but they are rarely serious and usually subside fairly quickly upon elimination of the causative drug. Illustrated in Fig. 21-3 is reaction to a sulfonamide.

Figure 21-4

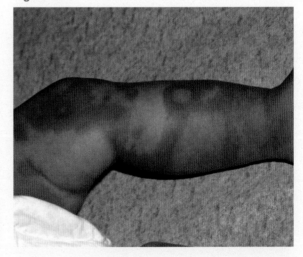

Urticaria multiforme (also Figs. 16-21 to 16-23) This condition, also known as acute annular urticaria, is a benign and fairly common hypersensitivity reaction that presents with urticarial plaques and annular or arcuate urticarial lesions, along with acral edema. When the cause is a medication, the most likely culprits are amoxicillin, cephalosporins, and macrolides.

Figure 21-5

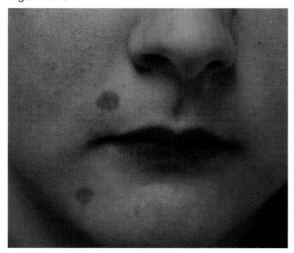

Fixed drug eruption Another common type of adverse reaction to drugs is the so-called fixed drug eruption. The term *fixed* is intended to suggest that the cutaneous change, occurring for the first time in given sites (anywhere), recurs in those same sites upon subsequent and repeated administration. Upon subsequent provocation, new reactions in new sites may occur, but original sites always flare again.

Figure 21-6

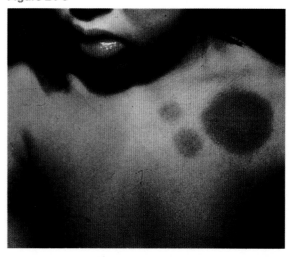

There are a number of drugs that are well known for their propensity to cause fixed drug eruptions. The most common are the tetracyclines, sulfonamides, and, NSAIDs, Other causes are aspirin, dapsone, and a variety of sedatives. The clinical morphology of a fixed drug eruption is usually a roundish plaque that is palpably edematous and purplish as shown in Fig. 21-6. Sometimes fixed drug eruptions are bullous.

Figure 21-7

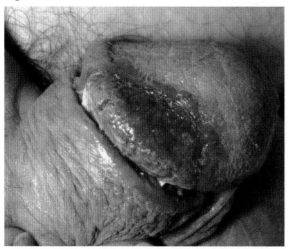

Fixed drug eruption Figure 21-7 illustrates fixed drug eruption in a particularly common location. Proof of a drug as cause of an eruption is sometimes certain, on the basis of repeated experience, but often conjectural or circumstantial, especially in the case of newly introduced drugs.

Figure 21-8

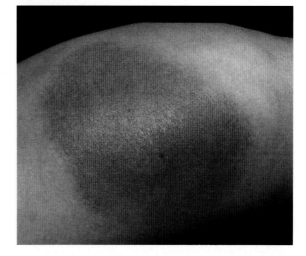

Figure 21-8 illustrates a larger lesion. The erythema of acute inflammation and the residual pigmentary change from a previous episode are seen simultaneously. The area of dark skin does not always completely fade between episodes.

Figure 21-9

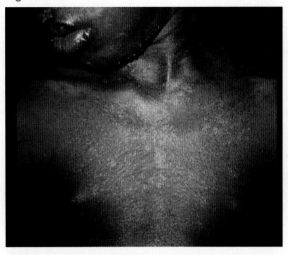

Hypersensitivity syndrome Each of the anticonvulsant medications phenytoin (Dilantin), phenobarbital, and carbamazepine (Tegretol), as well as numerous other medications have been reported to cause this severe form of drug reaction. The mucocutaneous manifestations are strawberry tongue and a generalized scarlatiniform eruption that is followed by desquamation. The rash may also be purpuric. The presence of high fever, lymphadenopathy, and hepatosplenomegaly may give the false impression of an infectious disease. Elevations in blood urea nitrogen, liver enzymes, and peripheral eosinophil count may also be present.

Figure 21-10

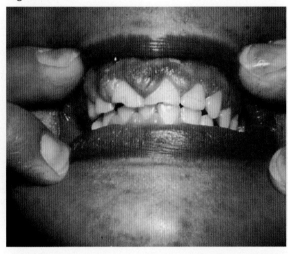

Drug-induced gingival overgrowth Drug-induced gingival overgrowth can be caused by phenytoin, cyclosporine, and a number of calcium channel blockers. There is evidence that genetic predisposition, length of treatment with the above medications, and poor dental hygiene all contribute to the evolution of this disorder.

Figure 21-11

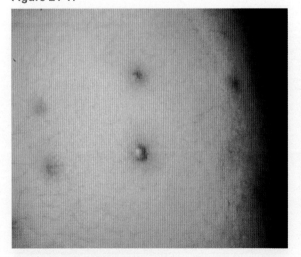

Iododerma and bromoderma Iodides and bromides are drugs that can cause severe adverse cutaneous reactions. These can be acneiform, furuncular, carbuncular, chancriform, pyodermatous, or granulomatous. Iodides and bromides are widely distributed, not only in foods and in the environment, but also in proprietary and formally prescribed medications.

Figure 21-12

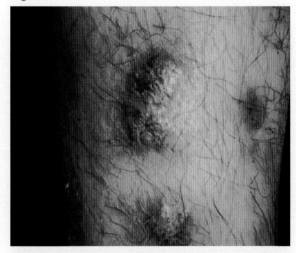

Figures 21-11 and 21-12 show adverse reactions from the two halides. Lesions like those of acne or folliculitis caused by an iodide are shown in Fig. 21-11. Figure 21-12 shows a granulomatous reaction caused by a bromide.

Figure 21-13

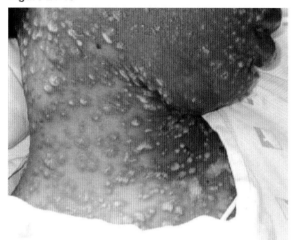

Figure 21-14

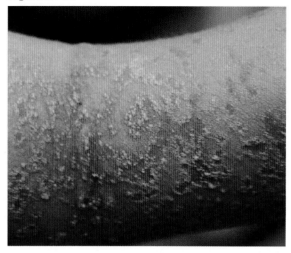

Acute generalized exanthematous pustulosis (AGEP) This severe form of drug eruption begins with high fever. Patients develop a generalized redness and edema, followed by numerous pustules that are sterile and do not necessarily arise from hair follicles. The entire process resolves with generalized desquamation.

Treatment consists of withdrawal of the causative medication (often a beta-lactam or macrolide antibiotic), and, sometimes, systemic corticosteroids. Rarely, AGEP may be the result of an antecedent infection and not a reaction to a drug.

Panniculopathies

Figure 22-1

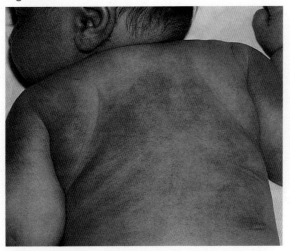

Subcutaneous fat necrosis of the newborn This is a self-resolving and benign condition that is seen in healthy newborns. The etiology of this disorder is probably ischemic injury to subcutaneous fat. Lesions often develop at sites of pressure.

Figure 22-2

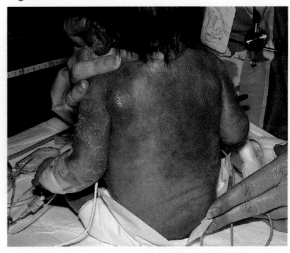

The infants develop single or multiple firm red-purple nodules or plaques that are asymptomatic. Cheeks, back, buttocks, and thighs are the most common locations. It is difficult to capture the quality of panniculitis in the figure, but a sense of it can be appreciated on the back of the patient pictured in Fig. 22-2.

Figure 22-3

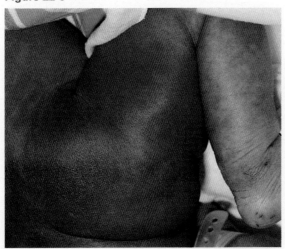

Subcutaneous fat necrosis Lesions may be present at birth, or they may develop during the first month of life. Most lesions resolve spontaneously over a period of 2 to 4 weeks, but some last significantly longer. There is usually no residual atrophy or scarring. Subcutaneous fat necrosis is occasionally associated with hypercalcemia, as was the case in this patient.

Figure 22-4

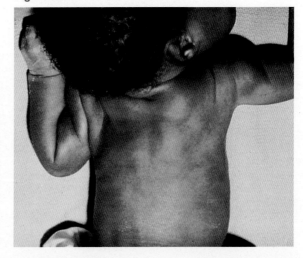

Sclerema neonatorum Unlike the condition just described, sclerema neonatorum presents itself as symmetrical areas of induration on cheeks, shoulders, buttocks, and calves. The skin over involved subcutaneous fat is uniformly board-like, cold, and livid in color, as though frozen. Infants so affected appear rigid because mobility is interfered with by the sclerema and they are severely ill. Mortality is high. The condition is more common in premature infants and in those with severe underlying disease, such as sepsis or dehydration.

Figure 22-5

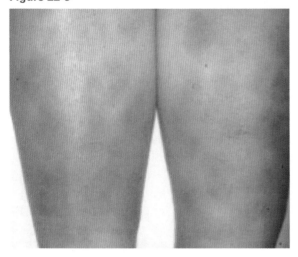

Figure 22-6

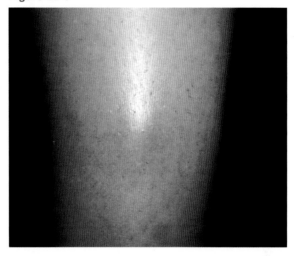

Erythema nodosum This condition, characterized by red, tender, subcutaneous nodules on the extensor aspects of the legs between knees and ankles has numerous causes. The most important conditions are streptococcal upper-respiratory infections, ulcerative colitis, histoplasmosis, coccidioidomycosis, tuberculosis, syphilis, and leprosy.

Another condition that is sometimes revealed by investigation of erythema nodosum is sarcoidosis. Drugs, including oral contraceptives, appear to be the cause of particular cases of erythema nodosum. In many cases, however, no clear etiology can be found.

Figure 22-7

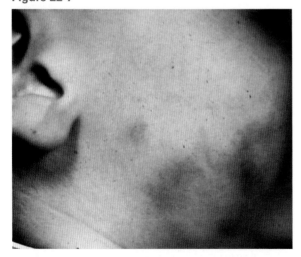

Figure 22-8

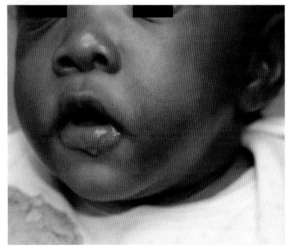

Panniculitis from cold Local exposure to cold leads to the formation of ice crystals within cells. Injury to cell contents occurs during both cooling and thawing. Cold panniculitis may occur in a child whose glove or boot has filled with snow. The patient shown in Fig. 22-7 was out in freezing weather with a strap holding her hat.

Cold panniculitis can also occur in a youngster who has been sucking on a frozen dessert product. So-called "popsicle panniculitis" is illustrated in Fig. 22-8. This condition is self-limited and requires only symptomatic relief.

Figure 22-9

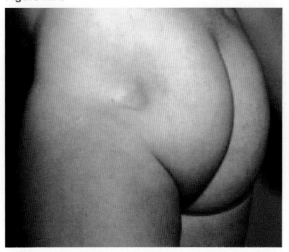

Lipoatrophy (localized) A localized area of fat atrophy may result from the injection of insulin or corticosteroids. In most cases, the change in the subcutaneous tissue is temporary. In this patient, as sometimes occurs, there was no antecedent injection and the etiology was unknown.

Figure 22-10

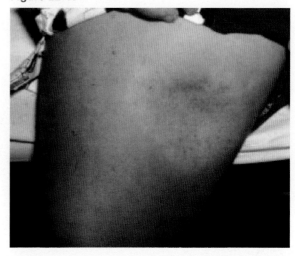

Lipoatrophy secondary to reticular hemangioma A rare form of hemangioma of infancy presents as a macular lesion with numerous fine telangiectasias. This lesion, now referred to as *reticular hemangioma*, has also been termed *abortive or minimal-growth hemangioma*. Hemangiomas of this type may be associated with a focal area of cutaneous depression, as pictured in Fig. 22-10, or a larger band-like or segmental area of lipoatrophy.

Figure 22-11

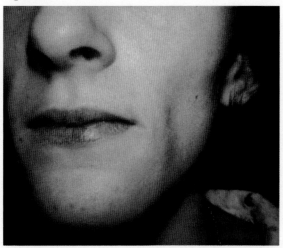

Progressive partial lipodystrophy This disorder is characterized by the loss of all adipose tissues in the upper portion of the body. Patients characteristically have the emaciated "sunken cheek" appearance that is seen in Fig. 22-11. A frequent complication of progressive lipoatrophy is membranoproliferative glomerulonephritis, associated with decreased levels of the third component of complement. The majority of patients are female.

Figure 22-12

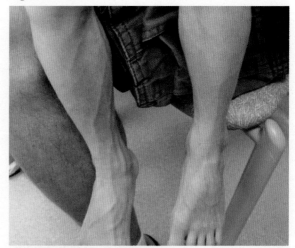

Acquired generalized lipodystrophy This rare disorder develops during childhood and adolescence and is characterized by loss of subcutaneous fat involving the face, trunk, abdomen, and extremities. Figure 22-12 illustrates the prominence of veins and muscles in a child lacking subcutaneous fat. Patients may develop diabetes, elevated serum triglycerides, and autoimmune thyroid disease.

Hemangiomas and Vascular and Lymphatic Disorders

Figure 23-1

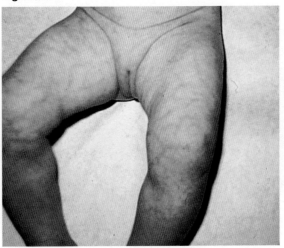

Cutis marmorata This term means "marbled skin" and is intended to describe the appearance of the skin in which the terminal vessels are so superficial and dilated that they are constantly visible in patterns that vaguely suggest veined marble. This condition is physiologic in the newborn and represents a vasomotor response to lowering of the environmental temperature. Persistent cutis marmorata is seen in Down syndrome and in trisomy 18.

Figure 23-2

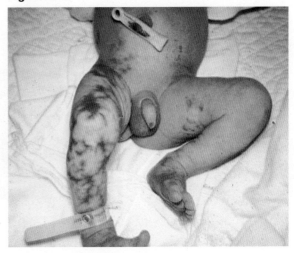

Cutis marmorata telangiectatica congenita This condition is present at birth and consists of accentuated vascular markings (cutis marmorata), along with areas of telangiectasia, and occasionally ulceration, and atrophy. The lesions may be localized, usually to a lower extremity or generalized.

Figure 23-3

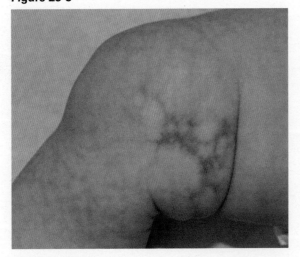

Cutis marmorata telangiectatica congenita A small minority of children with this condition have other abnormalities, including hemiatrophy or hemihypertrophy. The mottling resolves gradually with age in most patients.

Figure 23-4

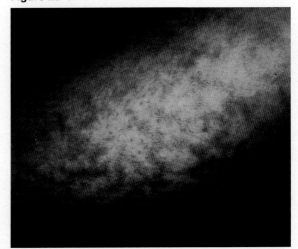

Livedo reticularis *Livedo* means a slate-gray blueness. *Reticularis* means "like a net." The term describes a network of *gray-blueness* that is generally seen on the lower extremities. The idiopathic form of this disorder, most common in young women, carries a good prognosis. However, livedo reticularis is also seen in association with polyarteritis nodosa, SLE, and cryoglobulinemia.

Figure 23-5

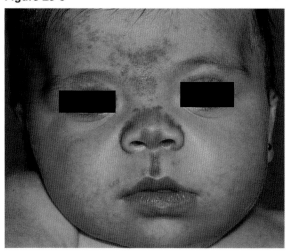

Nevus simplex (salmon patch) Nevus simplex is by far the most common vascular lesion in the newborn. This midline or symmetrical pink macular lesion is most commonly seen on the eyelids, the nape of the neck, and the glabella. The last two are commonly described as "stork bite" and "angel's kiss," respectively. The glabellar lesion in Fig. 23-5 can be expected to resolve spontaneously, as do lesions on the eyelids. Rarely, a nevus simplex on the neck may persist into adult life.

Figure 23-6

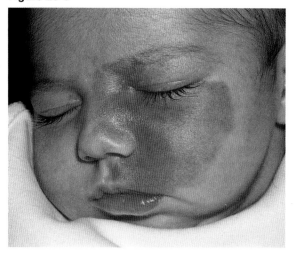

Port-wine stain This unilateral vascular malformation has a markedly different histology, significance, and natural history from that of the nevus simplex. The port-wine stain is made up of capillary ectasias that may be present throughout the dermis and that gradually increase with age. The color may change from pink to purple as the patient grows, and the lesions may become nodular during adult life. Because port-wine stains show no tendency to involute, they may represent a significant, lifelong cosmetic problem.

Figure 23-7

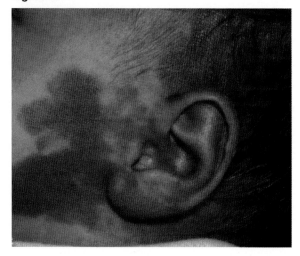

Port-wine stain The tunable pulsed dye laser is a successful modality in the treatment of disfiguring port-wine stains. Success is related to the fact that hemoglobin preferentially absorbs laser energy at the 595 to 600 nm wavelength.

Figure 23-8

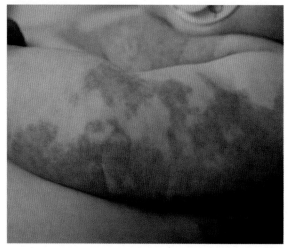

The very brief pulse duration prevents the heat from spreading from the blood vessels into the surrounding connective tissue, and the danger of scarring is thus minimized.

Figure 23-9

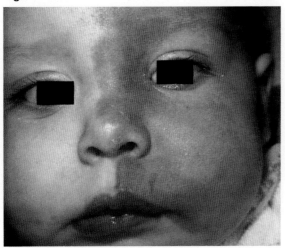

Sturge-Weber syndrome Certain port-wine stains, occurring on the face, may be associated with ocular and cerebral vascular malformations. It is now recognized that the danger of this occurrence correlates with the exact location of the skin lesions, and is related to the embryonic vasculature of the face.

Figure 23-10

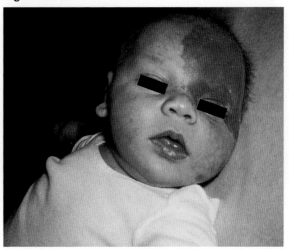

Children with port-wine stain involving the forehead are at risk for seizures, neurodevelopmental abnormalities, and glaucoma. Port wine stains occurring on other parts of the face appear to carry little or no risk.

Figure 23-11

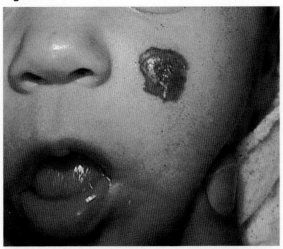

Hemangioma Infantile hemangioma is the most common benign vascular tumor that may occur during infancy. The vast majority of hemangiomas do not require treatment, and resolve spontaneously over time. Hemangiomas may be present at birth, or more commonly, develop during the first few months of life. The most rapid growth occurs during those months, and, for most, continues until 6 months of age. Some hemangiomas continue to increase in size until 1 year of age. Resolution of the hemangioma takes several years, and in some cases, may not be complete.

Figure 23-12

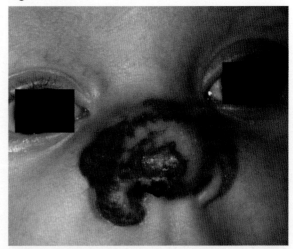

An additional important risk related to hemangioma is disfigurement and scarring. This is most significant for lesions involving the central face and, especially, the nose. In some cases, depending on the morphology, location, and growth stage of the hemangioma, early intervention is critical. The treatment of choice is oral propranolol, but topical timolol can be used to treat very superficial lesions.

Figure 23-13

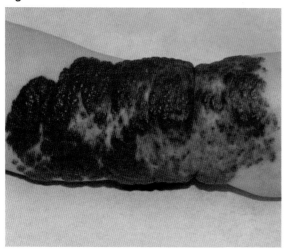

Hemangioma Illustrated in Fig. 23-13 is an example of segmental hemangioma. In contrast the localized nodular lesions seen in previous figures, this lesion is a plaque from which areas of vascular proliferation arise.

Figure 23-14

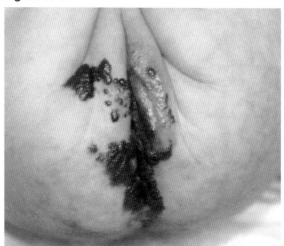

Segmental hemangiomas in the diaper area may be associated with a variety of underlying anatomic abnormalities. The acronym LUMBAR syndrome denotes *L*ower body hemangioma and other cutaneous defects, *U*rogenital anomalies, ulceration, *M*yelopathy, *B*ony deformities, *A*norectal malformations, arterial anomalies, and *R*enal anomalies.

Figure 23-15

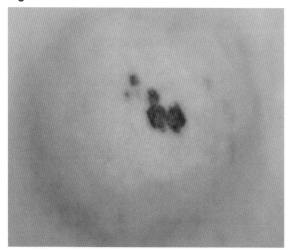

Hemangioma The hemangiomas in Figs. 23-15 and 23-16 have a large deep component and a superficial overlying area of vascular discoloration. The lesion in Fig. 23-16 is beginning to show spontaneous involution of the superficial component. Note that the central part of the superficial component is lightening and becoming blue-gray.

Figure 23-16

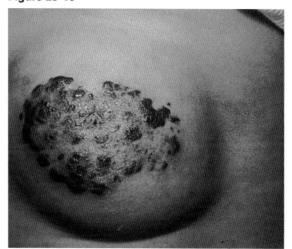

When deep hemangiomas involute, redundancy of overlying skin may remain. Frequently no treatment is needed, but if necessary, and depending on the location, plastic surgery may be required to improve appearance. Pulsed dye laser is of value in treating the residual superficial component of such a lesion.

Figure 23-17

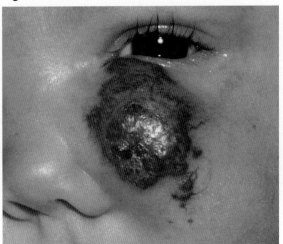

Hemangioma Hemangiomas that are close to the eye may result in astigmatism, strabismus, amblyopia, and even permanent vision loss. These changes result from the mass effect of the growing vascular lesion on the cornea, and from obstruction of the visual axis.

Figure 23-18

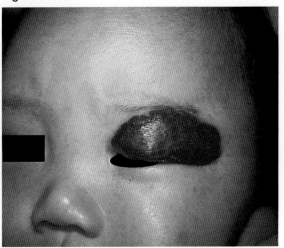

Infants with significant periorbital involvement should be managed in conjunction with an ophthalmologist.

Figure 23-19

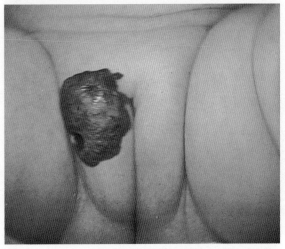

Hemangioma Figures 23-19 and 23-20 illustrate the spontaneous regression of a hemangioma. Although the resolution of the vascular portion is complete, there remains a fibrofatty mass with abnormal skin surface at the location of the original lesion.

Figure 23-20

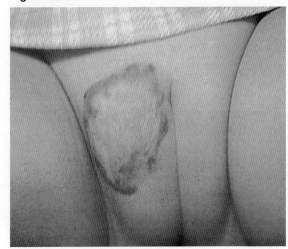

In general, depending on the size and location of the lesion, plastic surgery may be possible. In other cases, the patient and family may decide that surgical treatment is unnecessary.

Figure 23-21

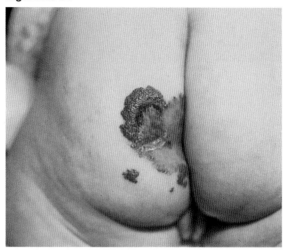

Figure 23-22

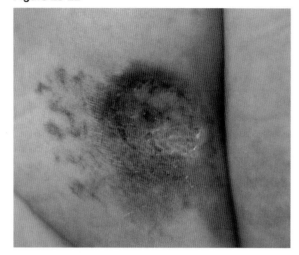

Hemangioma (ulcerated) During the growth phase of hemangiomas, especially in the groin area and buttocks (Figs. 23-21 and 23-22), ulceration may develop. The initial sign of ulceration, which is the most common complication of hemangioma, may be an area of crusting which may then enlarge and bleed. Ulcerated lesions on the scalp (Fig. 23-23) are more prone to bleeding given the increased vascularity of that area, and life-threatening bleeding has been reported in a number of hemangiomas.

Ulcerated hemangiomas, especially in the diaper area, are often extremely painful. Proper wound care, appropriate medications for pain control, along with the use of topical antibiotics such as mupirocin or metronidazole, will facilitate healing and decrease pain in the area of involvement.

Figure 23-23

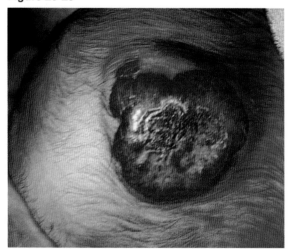

Figure 23-24

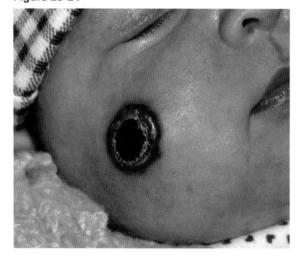

Hemangioma (ulcerated) The presence of odor or purulent drainage in an ulcerated hemangioma should prompt concern for the presence of infection, which should be treated with systemic antibiotics based on the results of bacterial culture. Becaplermin gel (topical platelet-derived growth factor) has been shown to speed the healing of ulcerated hemangiomas. Pulsed dye laser can also be helpful, and excision may be considered in lesions that will eventually require surgical removal because of scarring.

Illustrated in Fig. 23-34 is a facial hemangioma with significant ulceration. Ulcerated hemangiomas almost always heal with scarring, and so rapid and effective treatment in lesions occurring on the face is most important. Oral propranolol, now the first line systemic treatment for hemangioma, is also of value in hemangiomas that have ulcerated or are about to ulcerate.

Figure 23-25

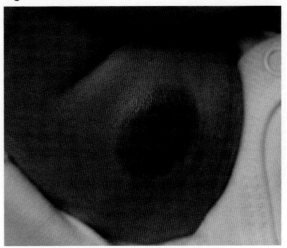

Rapidly involuting congenital hemangioma (RICH) This fairly unusual vascular lesion is present at birth, and occurs most often on the extremities, head, or neck. RICH often appears as a round or oval soft tissue mass covered with telangiectasias, and surrounded by a ring of pallor. Rarely, RICH has been associated with decreased platelets or heart failure due to increased output.

Figure 23-26

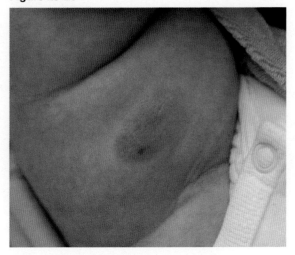

Pictured in Fig. 23-26 is the same lesion, in the process of spontaneous involution. Usually, RICH involutes by one year of age, but it often resolves with an area of redundant or atrophic skin.

Figure 23-27

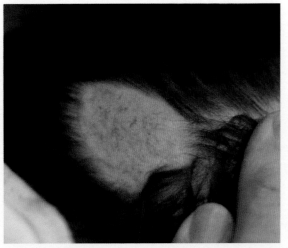

Noninvoluting congenital hemangiomas (NICH) This form of congenital hemangioma usually presents as a round to oval plaque with colors that range from blue to purple to red. Telangiectasias are often seen in the surface of the lesion, and, as in NICH, there is often a rim of pallor. Enlarged veins sometimes occur in the surrounding skin. These lesions do not resolve, and, in fact, tend to grow with the child.

Figure 23-28

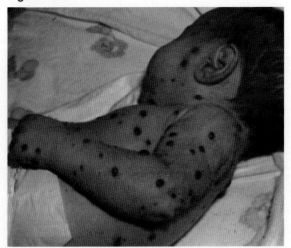

Disseminated hemangiomatosis Pictured in Fig. 23-28 is a neonate with multiple small hemangiomas. Children with this degree of cutaneous involvement may suffer from visceral hemangiomatosis. Liver, spleen, lungs, and the gastrointestinal and central nervous systems may be involved. Risks include high-output congestive heart failure, thrombocytopenia, and neurologic complications. If a complete workup establishes the presence of extensive visceral disease, early systemic therapy with propranolol is advisable.

Figure 23-29

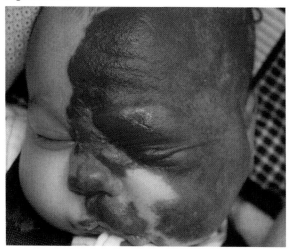

PHACE syndrome Patients with a segmental facial hemangioma may have PHACE syndrome, consisting of a *p*osterior fossae malformation in the brain, large facial *h*emangioma, *a*rterial anomalies of the head and neck, *c*oarctation of the aorta and other cardiac defects, and *e*ye abnormalities. Sternal clefts have been reported in some patients with PHACE syndrome. When patients present early, many are mistaken to have port-wine stains, but these lesions grow and are truly hemangiomas.

Figure 23-30

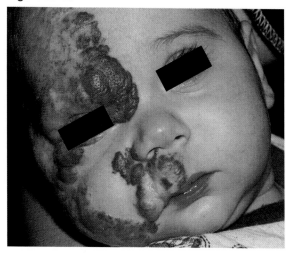

When presented with a patient with a large facial hemangioma, imaging studies of the brain must be done. Patients should also be evaluated by a pediatric ophthalmologist and pediatric cardiologist. Some patients also have hypothyroidism.

Figure 23-31

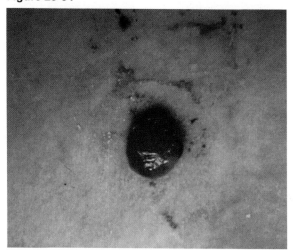

Pyogenic granuloma This is a commonly acquired lesion that may develop at the site of an obvious or unnoticed trauma. It is the result of a local vascular proliferation. Typically, a pyogenic granuloma grows rapidly, and there is often a history of spontaneous bleeding.

Figure 23-32

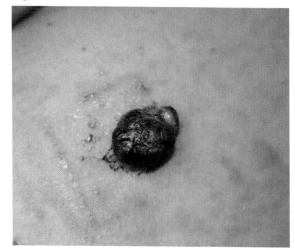

The lesion is usually a red papule or nodule, and it can be located anywhere on the body. The surface is usually friable, with a collarette of epidermis at the base. Treatment consists of thorough electrodessication and curettage.

Figure 23-33

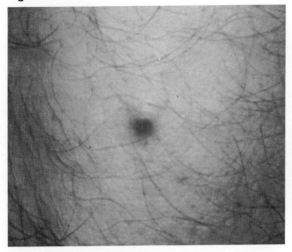

Figure 23-34

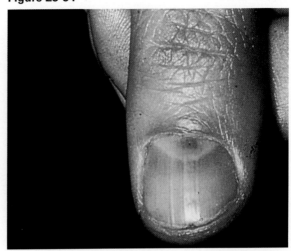

Glomovenous malformation (glomus tumor) Vascular shunts are special structures abundant in acral parts of the body that have a large area and a relatively small volume, such as the fingertips, the nose, and the pinnae of the ears. They are much sparser elsewhere. Their function is to alter circulation under the stimulus of cold in such a manner as to conserve heat by turning off much of the arterial circulation. Their structure is of a myoepithelium, that is, a conglomeration of epithelial cells that have contractile ability. Such tissue sometimes becomes benignly hyperplastic and somewhat bulky.

The purplish nodule in Fig. 23-33 is typical of the glomus tumor. Solitary glomus tumors are often located in the nail bed, as in Fig. 23-34, and may give rise to severe episodes of paroxysmal pain. The subungual lesions seem to be more common in females. Excision of painful lesions is the treatment of choice. In addition, a rare syndrome of multiple glomus tumors exists. These lesions tend to be asymptomatic. The condition is inherited in autosomal dominant fashion and is associated with defects in the glomulin gene.

Figure 23-35

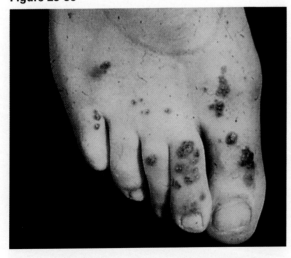

Figure 23-36

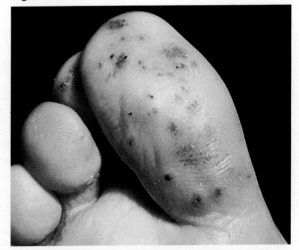

Angiokeratoma (angiokeratoma of Mibelli) Angiokeratoma of Mibelli is distinguished by the development of hyperkeratosis on small papular angiomas. The feet and lower extremities are common sites for this condition.

These lesions arise during adolescence. Papular lesions of the same sort are common on the scrotum where hyperkeratosis does not develop. These are sometimes labeled *angiokeratoma of Fordyce*. At first glance, one might think the condition, as illustrated in Figs. 23-35 and 23-36, might be verruca vulgaris. Biopsy distinguishes with certainty.

Figure 23-37

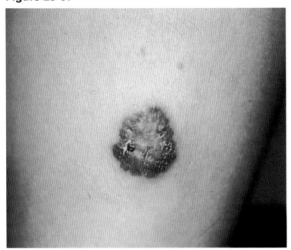

Solitary angiokeratoma This lesion usually develops on the lower extremities, sometimes in response to trauma. The lesion pictured in Fig. 23-37 could easily be mistaken for a melanoma or a pigmented basal cell carcinoma. Biopsy is indicated, and the combination of dilated blood vessels, hyperkeratosis, and acanthosis enables the dermatopathologist to make the correct diagnosis.

Figure 23-38

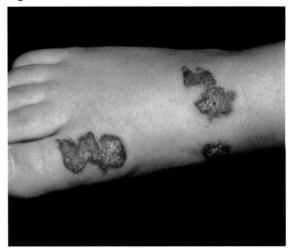

Angiokeratoma circumscriptum This vascular ectasia may be present at birth but has been reported to develop in childhood and even adulthood. There is a higher incidence in females. Lesions are most commonly found on the lower extremities but may be found elsewhere. Lesions consist of small nodules or larger plaques characterized by a dark red to purple color and a warty, hyperkeratotic scale sometimes in a linear distribution. These lesions may bleed when traumatized.

Figure 23-39

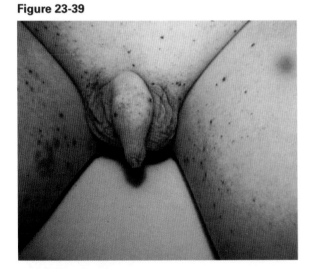

Fabry disease (angiokeratoma corporis diffusum) This serious condition is a sphingolipidosis associated with an enzyme anomaly that leads to the deposition of a ceramide trihexoside in the smooth muscle of blood vessels. The cutaneous lesions are tiny papules that are angiomatous. When this happens in the blood vessels of the heart, kidneys, eyes, and nervous system, symptoms of functional disturbance and failure appear. Fucosidosis and sialidosis may cause a similar clinical appearance.

Figure 23-40

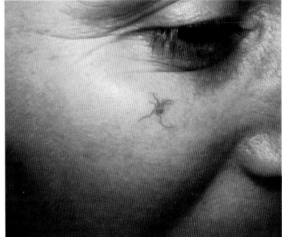

Spider angioma (nevus araneus) This is a trivial and common childhood angioma, highly characteristic in its central vascular punctum, from which radiates fine vessels that give the entire lesion the fanciful appearance of a spider in its web. Such lesions are usually solitary, and the face is a common site for them. The dorsa of the hands are another common site. Compression of the central vessel on diascopy will blanch the lesion, which will then refill from the central portion. Persistent lesions are easily treated by laser.

Figure 23-41

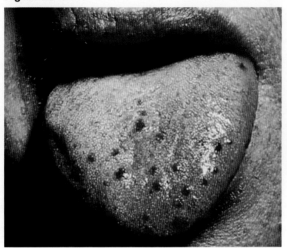

Figure 23-42

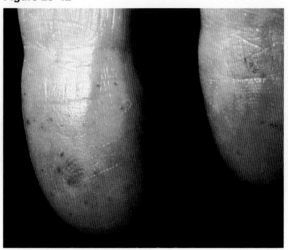

Hereditary hemorrhagic telangiectasia (Osler-Rendu-Weber syndrome) This is an autosomal dominant syndrome with both cutaneous and visceral involvement. It is due to genetic mutations that involve signaling of TGF-β. In most children with the disease, the presenting symptom is recurrent epistaxis. Patients go on to develop vascular papules that stud the lips, tongue, palate, and nasal mucosa. The ears, palms, soles, digital tips, and nail beds are other common sites for lesions.

As the disease progresses, melena and hematemesis may develop as a result of gastrointestinal involvement. A significant number of patients with this syndrome have hepatic and pulmonary arteriovenous fistulas. The latter may lead to cyanosis, shortness of breath, polycythemia, and digital clubbing. Patients must be monitored carefully for hemorrhage in the liver, brain, urinary bladder, and retina and for the development of a secondary anemia.

Figure 23-43

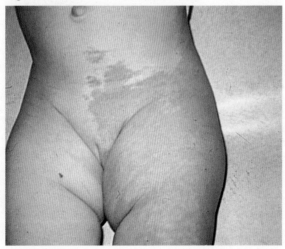

Figure 23-44

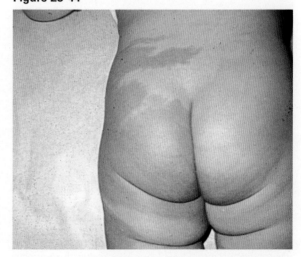

Klippel-Trénaunay-Weber syndrome This is a condition in which capillary, venous and/or lymphatic, malformations are associated with overgrowth of the involved extremity. The involved limb may have increased length or circumference, and may be warmer to the touch.

A combination of port-wine stain and vascular malformations may be present from birth. The osteohypertrophy usually develops during the first several years of life. Figures 23-43 and 23-44 are the front and back views of an infant who has a large, lightly colored port-wine stain. Over time, increased vascularization and enlargement of the limb may develop. MRI is needed to determine the extent of bone and soft tissue involvement.

Figure 23-45

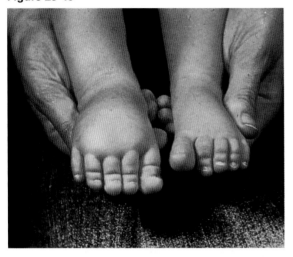

Milroy disease This term refers to a form of primary lymphedema that is inherited in autosomal dominant fashion. The swelling of the feet and legs is either unilateral or bilateral. The edema is pitting at first, but fibrosis of the lower extremities gradually leads to a firmer and more persistent enlargement. Over time, the overlying epidermis may become verrucous and hyperkeratotic.

Figure 23-46

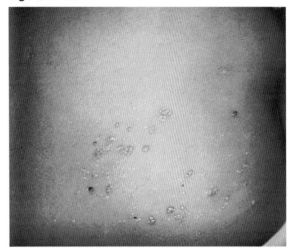

Lymphangioma The proliferation of lymphatic channels in the skin or subcutaneous tissue may give rise to lesions with a variety of clinical appearance. Most lymphangiomas develop during the first 2 years of life and some are present at birth. The cluster of clear vesicles pictured here is termed *lymphangioma circumscriptum*. The lesions are benign but may be distressing because of their tendency to increase in size and number over time and occasionally to become irritated or superinfected.

Figure 23-47

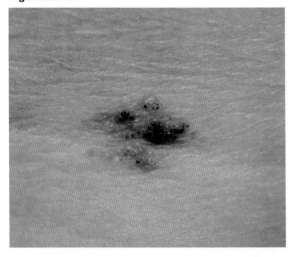

Lymphangioma Illustrated in, Figs. 23-47 and 23-48 are additional examples of lymphangioma circumscriptum. This figure shows why the appearance of these glistening papules is sometimes compared to frogspawn and also demonstrates a mixed hamartoma composed of both lymphatic channels and blood vessels. The surgical treatment of lymphangioma circumscriptum is complicated by the fact that the associated lymphatic channels may be deeper than can be clinically appreciated. The result is a high rate of recurrence. Laser surgery may be a reasonable approach for some of these lesions.

Figure 23-48

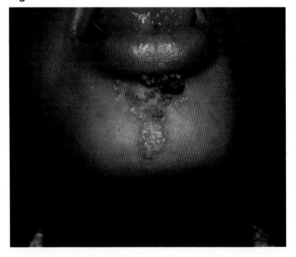

Lymphangioma circumscriptum is usually localized to the neck, proximal extremities, abdomen, tongue, and mucous membranes. The lesion pictured here is in an unusual location. The surface is hyperkeratotic, and one can imagine confusing this lymphangioma with a large verruca or epidermal nevus.

Figure 23-49

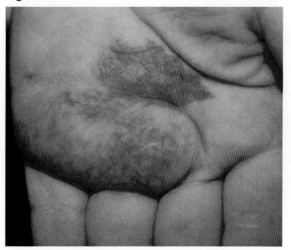

Figure 23-50

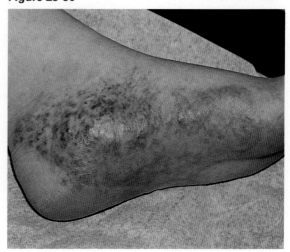

Vascular malformations These are congenital malformations that consist of capillary, venous, arterial, or lymphatic abnormalities. There are often combined malformations that comprise different types of vessels. Vascular msalformations are divided into slow-flow (port-wine stains, venous malformations, and lymphatic malformations) and fast-flow (arterial abnormalities with A-V shunting).

Vascular malformations are present at birth and grow proportionately with the child. Some vascular malformations may not manifest themselves until adolescence or adulthood. Figures 23-49 and 23-50 represent venous malformations on the hand and foot. Some vascular malformations require only reassurance, while others are disfiguring and affect function in various ways. These lesions worsen over time in some patients, and longitudinal multidisciplinary care through childhood and adolescence may be required.

Figure 23-51

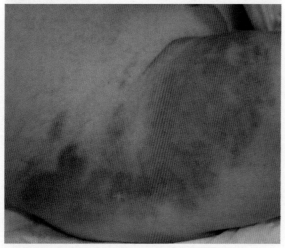

Figure 23-52

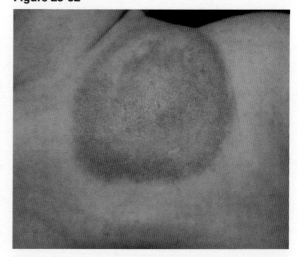

Tufted angioma This is a benign vascular tumor which may be congenital, or develop during childhood. Sites of predilection are the trunk and proximal extremities, and lesions range up to 20 cm in diameter. The most common presentation is an area of vascular erythema with underlying induration and nodularity. Blue or violaceous discoloration, and hyperhidrosis and/or hypertrichosis may be presenting features.

Infants with tufted angiomas are at risk for Kasabach-Merritt phenomenon, a consumption coagulopathy associated with hemolytic anemia and thrombocytopenia. A variety of surgical and nonsurgical approaches have been recommended for treatment of children who develop these serious hematologic complications of tufted angioma.

Figure 23-53

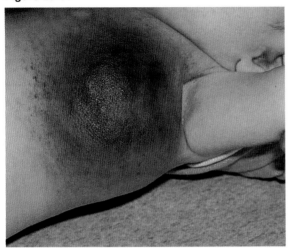

Figure 23-54

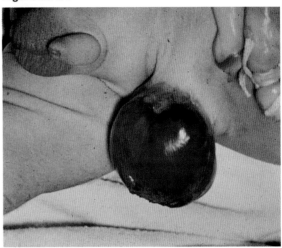

Kaposiform hemangioendothelioma This benign vascular neoplasm, like as tufted angioma, may be associated with Kasabach-Merritt phenomenon, a potentially life-threatening consumptive coagulopathy. The lesions are usually located on the trunk and extremities and very rarely involve the face or scalp. The most common presentation is a warm, tender, indurated plaque with erythematous or bluish discoloration. Lesions may also present as bulging masses, as seen in Fig. 23-54.

Diagnosis is based on a biopsy showing spindle cells in nodules and slit-like blood vessels. The treatment of this disorder depends on whether Kasabach-Merritt phenomenon is present, and how severe it is. Options for treatment include vincristine and sirolimus.

Figure 23-55

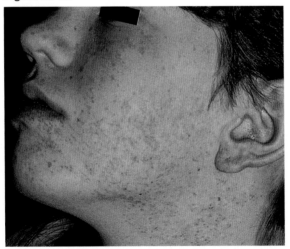

Unilateral nevoid telangiectasia This benign dermatologic condition appears to be more common in females, and is more common in the teenage years than during childhood. Vascular skin lesions, consisting of erythematous lines and punctuate red macules, develop on a single extremity, the side of the back and chest, or on one side of the neck and face, as pictured in Fig. 23-55. In some case, the whitish halo that surrounds each vascular lesion is the most prominent feature. When this disorder poses a significant cosmetic problem, it can be treated with pulsed dye laser.

Neoplastic Disorders

Figure 24-1

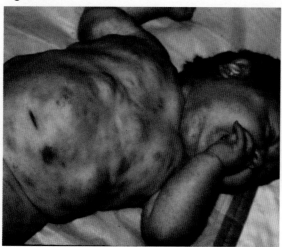

Leukemia cutis A dermal infiltrate of leukemic cells results in the papulonodular lesions, or plaques, that are illustrated here in Fig. 24-1. Such primary involvement of the skin is relatively rare in childhood leukemia. The wide variety of secondary manifestations of leukemia includes petechiae and ecchymoses and pyoderma gangrenosum.

Figure 24-2

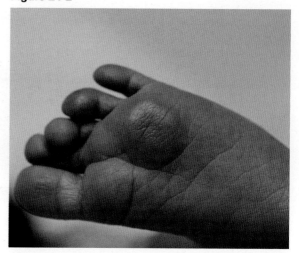

In this example of congenital leukemia cutis, the violaceous nodule could easily be confused with a hemangioma or vascular malformation. In addition, Sweet's syndrome (Fig. 16-24), an eruption of erythematous plaques, with a polymorphonuclear dermal infiltrate may be associated with leukemia. Also, children receiving chemotherapy are prone to bacterial and fungal infections of the skin, severe varicella, and ulcerative or chronic herpes simplex.

Figure 24-3

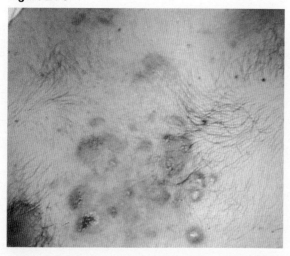

Hodgkin disease Like other lymphoproliferative disorders, Hodgkin disease may have both specific and nonspecific cutaneous manifestations. Figure 24-3 illustrates a relatively rare event in children with Hodgkin disease: the direct infiltration of malignant cells into the skin. A biopsy analysis of these brownish papules, nodules, and plaques reveals a histology similar to that of affected lymph nodes. These lesions may occasionally ulcerate, and pruritus is a distressing symptom.

Figure 24-4

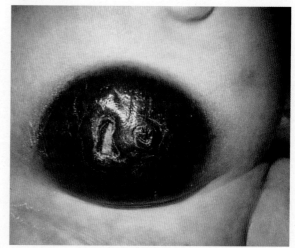

Chloroma Also known as granulocytic sarcoma, this lesion may be seen in acute and chronic myelocytic leukemias. The lesions, which are infiltrates of masses of leukemic cells, occasionally present with a green color due to myeloperoxidase activity.

Figure 24-5

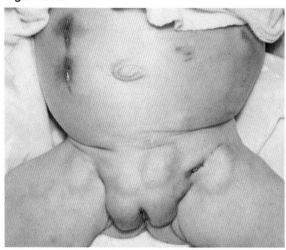

Neuroblastoma, metastatic This malignant tumor of the autonomic nervous system occurs most frequently in young children. Metastatic disease is often present at the time of diagnosis. Cutaneous metastases appear as bluish papules or nodules involving the trunk or extremities.

Figure 24-6

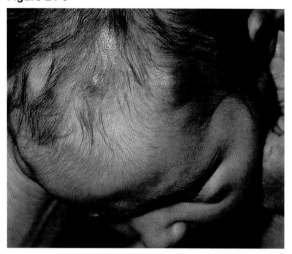

The lesions are sometimes noted to blanch upon stroking and may sometimes exhibit increased sweating. Children who are under 1 year of age at the time of diagnosis, as was the case in the patient in Fig. 24-6, may experience spontaneous regression of their illness. The prognosis in older children and in those with very widespread disease tends to be poor.

Figure 24-7

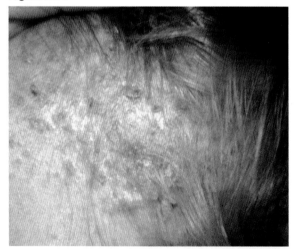

Langerhans cell disease This disorder is the result of a clonal proliferation of Langerhans cells and can involve a variety of organ systems. This is a spectrum of disease that encompasses acute disseminated LCD (formerly Letterer-Siwe disease), chronic multifocal LCD (formerly Hand-Schüller-Christian disease), and chronic focal LCD (eosinophilic granuloma). Figure 24-7 shows the characteristic skin involvement of Langerhans cell disease, which can present with a seborrheic-like, scaly, erythematous eruption on the scalp, face, and ears.

Figure 24-8

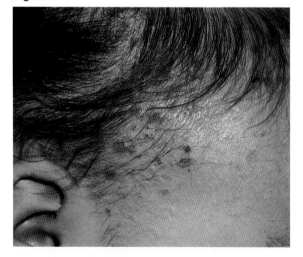

Figure 24-8 shows a more papular presentation, also in the scalp. Diagnosis is made with skin biopsy, which demonstrates the presence of large oval cells with S100 and CD1a positivity. In some cases, the presence of Birbeck granules on electron microscopy is used to confirm the diagnosis. Langerhans cell histiocytosis may be accompanied by hepatosplenomegaly, lymphadenopathy, anemia, and thrombocytopenia.

Figure 24-9

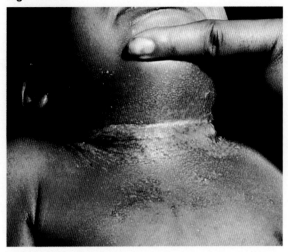

Langerhans cell disease (cont'd.) An eruption accompanied by erosive and granulomatous changes may be seen in the neck folds, as in Fig. 24-9, or in the axillae (Fig. 24-10).

Figure 24-10

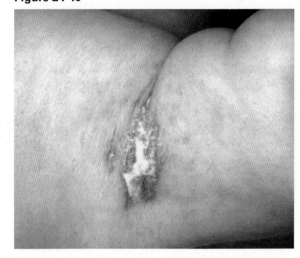

In both of these cases, the differential diagnosis would include streptococcal intertrigo (Figs. 3-19 to 3-22), *Candida* (Figs. 6-49 and 6-50), and psoriasis (Figs. 12-26 and 12-27).

Figure 24-11

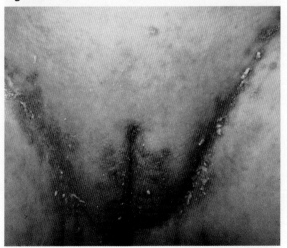

Langerhans cell disease In general, an unusual or recalcitrant diaper rash of this general appearance should alert the physician to consider the diagnosis. The diaper area may occasionally be the first area of involvement for infants.

Figure 24-12

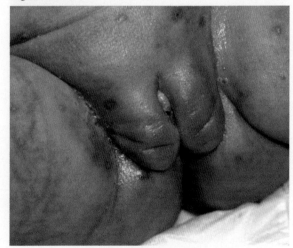

The inguinal creases appear erythematous, with scaling, fissuring, and a white mucoid material that may be the result of a secondary candidal infection. The presence of individual erythematous papular and petechial lesions will aid in the diagnosis.

Figure 24-13

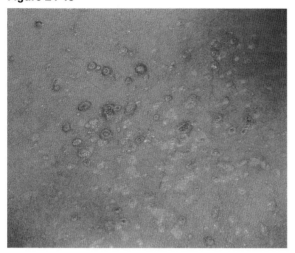

Figure 24-14

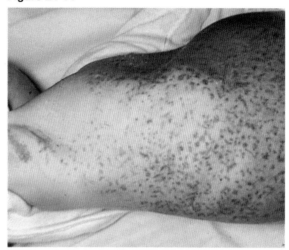

Langerhans cell disease (cont'd.) Figures 24-13 and 24-14 illustrate the papular lesions that may be seen. The child shown in Fig. 24-14 is covered with numerous reddish-brown crusted papules that may become hemorrhagic. Rarely, this clinical picture is present at birth.

The prognosis of children with Langerhans cell histiocytosis is extremely variable but is certainly worse in patients who develop organ dysfunction from their disease. The decision to initiate chemotherapy should be based on the extent of organ involvement and clinical course of the individual patient.

Figure 24-15

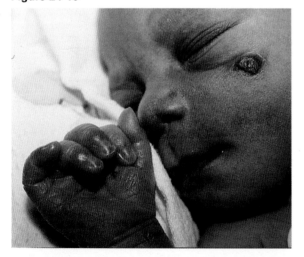

Figure 24-16

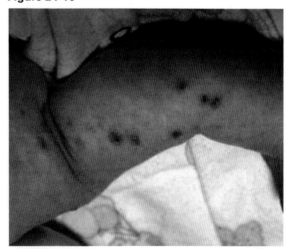

Congenital self-healing reticulohistiocytosis (Hashimoto-Pritzker disease) This rare condition may present with solitary or multiple nodules (Fig. 24-15) or in a generalized form with vesicles, papules, pustules, and crusts (Fig. 24-16). Mucous membranes are spared. Lesions are almost always present at birth, but new lesions may erupt in the early neonatal period.

Most cases have only cutaneous involvement, but all patients should be evaluated for other organ involvement. The lesions typically resolve without any treatment within a few months. Ongoing monitoring is essential even after apparent clinical resolution since other manifestations of Langerhans cell disease may occur at a later date.

Figure 24-17

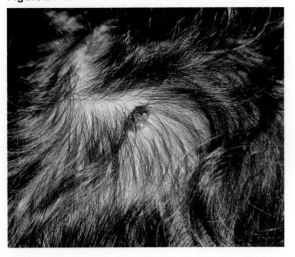

Basal cell carcinoma It is well known that children with the basal cell nevus syndrome, and children who have received radiation therapy for other malignancies are at risk for basal cell carcinoma. The patient in Fig. 24-17 developed a basal cell carcinoma after receiving radiation for a brain tumor.

Figure 24-18

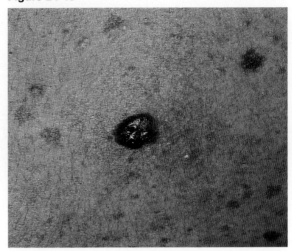

In addition, we now recognize that basal cell carcinoma may occur in healthy children (Fig. 24-18) who have had excessive sun exposure and may carry a genetic predilection for this form of skin cancer. The lesions are pearly and telangiectatic papules or nodules, and treatment is surgical excision.

Figure 24-19

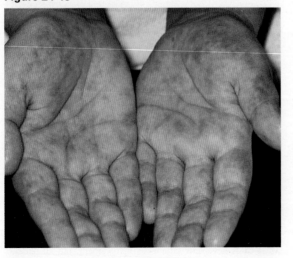

Graft-versus-host disease (GVHD) This disorder is most frequently seen in children who have received a bone marrow transplant. The acute phase, pictured in Fig. 24-19, is characterized by a macular, papular, or morbiliform eruption favoring the face, palms, and soles. Diarrhea and elevation of liver

Figure 24-20

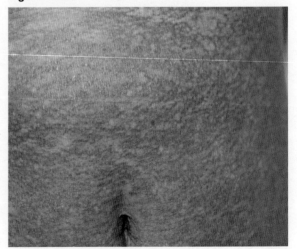

function enzymes often accompany this clinical finding. Some children with acute GVHD go on to develop a more chronic form. Manifestations of this include a lichenoid skin eruption (Fig. 24-20), hyperpigmentation, and a form of generalized scleroderma.

Figure 24-21

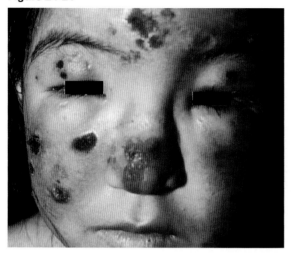

Hydroa vacciniforme-like cutaneous T-cell lymphoma (CTCL)
The benign form of hydroa vacciniforme (figs. 11-13 and 11-14) is characterized by photo-related vesicles that evolve into crusting and varicelliform scars, with no related systemic symptoms. However, a severe form of hydroa vacciniforme, which also includes facial edema and larger areas of ulceration, has also been described.

Figure 24-22

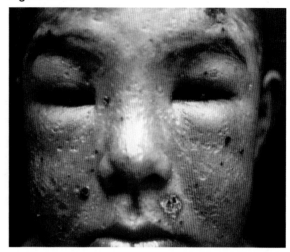

This disorder appears to be most common in indigenous populations of Mexico and Central America. Children with the severe form of hydroa vacciniforme develop wasting, fever, and hepatosplenomegaly. Lobular or septal panniculitis may also develop along with vasculitis. In a number of children, progression to non-Hodgkin lymphoma has been reported to occur.

Figure 24-23

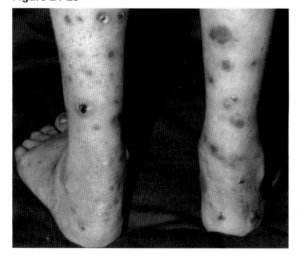

Hydroa vacciniforme-like cutaneous T-cell lymphoma (CTCL)
These patients often have severe insect bite hypersensitivity. The lesions pictured in Fig. 24-23 may be a manifestation of this, or of cutaneous vasculitis.

Figure 24-24

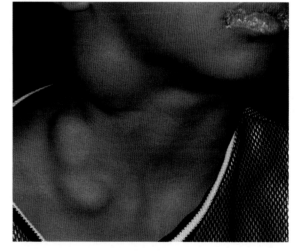

Rosai-Dorfman disease (sinus histiocytosis with massive lymphadenopathy) The signs of this disorder are significant cervical lymphadenopathy, sometimes associated with malaise, weight loss, and low-grade fever. Skin lesions are yellow to brown papules, nodules or plaques, but these occur in a minority of patients. Although various viral etiologies have been proposed, the cause of this disorder is unknown. In most cases, it resolves without treatment over a period of several months.

Figure 24-25

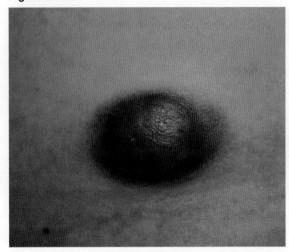

Dermatofibrosarcoma protuberans This is a fibrohistiocytic tumor of low malignant potential that rarely occurs in children. The tumor may be present at birth. Delays in diagnosis may occur because the tumor may mimic other entities such as vascular lesions, atrophic plaques and fibromas. Treatment is wide local excision or MOHS micrographic surgery.

Adnexal Dysplasias

Figure 25-1

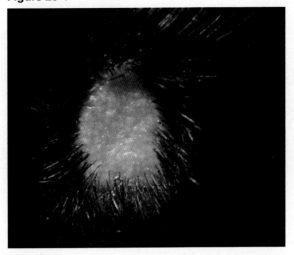

Nevus sebaceous This congenital lesion is composed of hamartomatous sebaceous glands and abortive hair follicles. It usually presents at birth as a yellow nodule or pebbled, hairless plaque on the scalp, forehead, or neck. Figure 25-1 shows the color and shape of the congenital lesion. With the loss of the effect of maternal hormones during the first few months of life, the lesion may quickly flatten and lose its distinctive color.

Figure 25-2

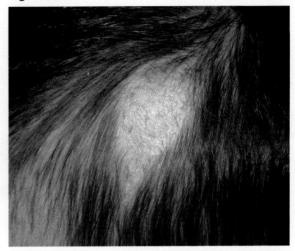

During puberty, the nevus sebaceous again becomes raised, yellow, and verrucous. After this change, and usually during adulthood, nevus sebaceous may give rise to a wide variety of benign and malignant neoplasms. These include basal cell hamartomas, keratoacanthomas, syringocystadenoma papilliferum, basal cell epitheliomas, and, rarely, squamous cell carcinomas.

Figure 25-3

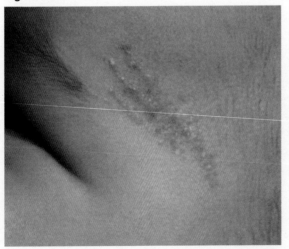

Nevus sebaceous Figures 25-3 and 25-4 illustrate examples of nevus sebaceous occurring on the face, In infancy, facial lesions have a characteristic yellow color and pebbly surface. In both infants, the lesions are linear. Nevus sebaceous, especially when occurring on the face, follows the lines of Blaschko. These lines of normal cell development indicate a form of genetic mosaicism, and are seen in a wide variety of cutaneous disorders.

Figure 25-4

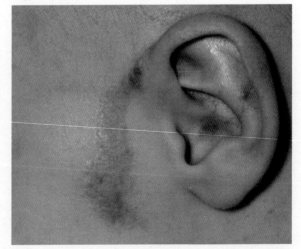

Widespread nevus sebaceous occasionally indicates a complex syndrome—linear nevus sebaceous syndrome: Patients may develop skeletal, ocular, and neurological abnormalities, Nevus sebaceous syndrome shares features with epidermal nevus syndrome (Figs. 15-53 and 15-54).

Figure 25-5

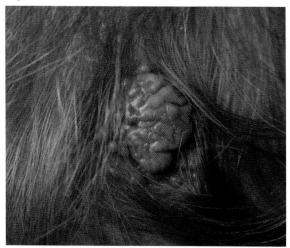

Nevus sebaceous Figure 25-5 illustrates an unusual variant-cerebriform nevus sebaceous. The term refers to the "brain-like" convolutions on the surface. The salmon red color is typical for this form of nevus sebaceous.

Figure 25-6

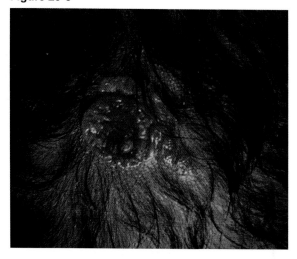

Figure 25-6 illustrates a syringocystadenoma papilliferum arising within a nevus sebaceous. This is a benign neoplasm.

Figure 25-7

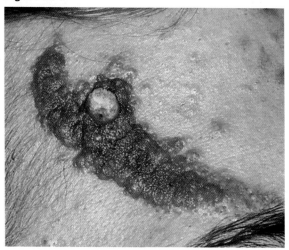

Nevus sebaceous Figure 25-7 shows another nevus sebaceous on which basal cell carcinoma has developed. In this case, the color appears more brown and blackish in the main lesion, but the yellow color can still be appreciated in the small outlying papules. The nodule near the center represents the malignant change.

Figure 25-8

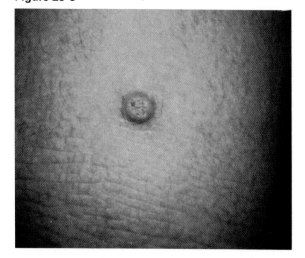

Clear cell hidradenoma This benign eccrine sweat gland tumor occurs as a solitary lesion in most cases. Most commonly, the growth appears as a small intraepidermal nodule. Ulceration or discharge of serous material rarely occurs. The lesion is harmless and may easily be excised.

Figure 25-9

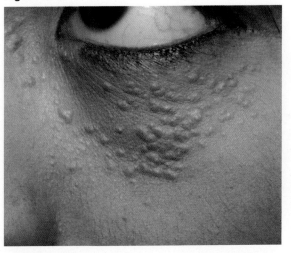

Syringoma These very small papules are adenomas of intraepidermal eccrine ducts. Most commonly, syringomas develop on the eyelids of girls during adolescence. They have no malignant potential, but the lesions are usually multiple and therefore the cause of cosmetic concern.

Figure 25-10

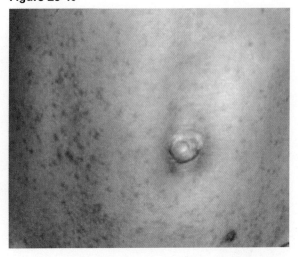

Figure 25-10 illustrates multiple lesions on the abdomen. Rarely, a child or adolescent will develop successive crops of syringomas on the skin of the anterior neck, antecubital fossa, trunk, axilla, and groin. This condition, termed *eruptive syringoma*, is sometimes inherited in autosomal dominant fashion. Syringomas may also be seen with increased frequency in patients with Down syndrome.

Figure 25-11

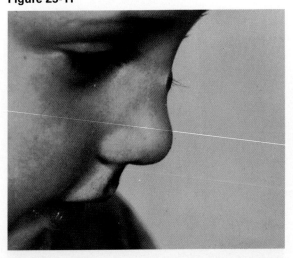

Dermoid cyst These lesions present in the newborn as soft, round, subcutaneous tumors that may be freely movable or bound down beneath the overlying epidermis. They represent ectodermal hamartomas and occur at the site of closure of embryonic clefts. The vast majority of dermoid cysts are found near the lateral eyebrow or on the forehead. The neck is the next most common location. The lesion pictured in Fig. 25-11 has protruding hair and was present at birth.

Figure 25-12

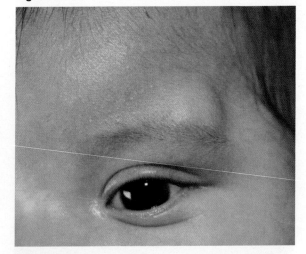

In Fig. 25-12 there is a typical mass just lateral to the eyebrow. Histologic examination of these lesions reveals combinations of epidermis, dermis, sweat glands, sebaceous glands, and hair. Surgical excision is generally the treatment of choice. Imaging may be required in advance of surgery to determine the underlying anatomy.

Figure 25-13

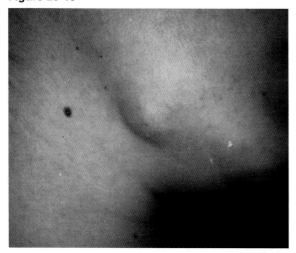

Figure 25-14

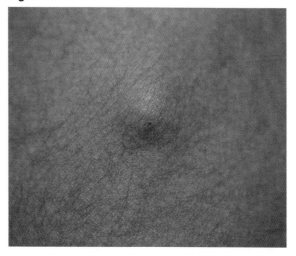

Epidermal cyst The lesions that were long termed *sebaceous cysts* are now renamed *epidermal cysts*, because their points of origin are not the sebaceous glands, and their content is not purely sebum. Epidermal cysts are exceedingly common lesions on the face and trunk. They consist of an epithelium-lined cavity that is filled with a caseous mixture of lipid and proteinaceous matter.

They may have no apparent opening onto the surface of the skin, as in Fig. 25-13, or they may have a small aperture, as shown in Fig. 25-14. They have no malignant potential, but may sooner or later require surgical removal because of the size, location, or secondary infection. Uncomplicated epidermal cysts may be excised by clean dissection.

Figure 25-15

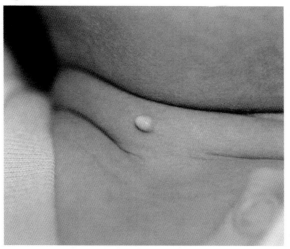

Congenital giant milium of the anterior neck Figure 25-15 illustrates a very superficial milia or epidermal inclusion cyst seen on the anterior neck in a newborn. These are not associated with any underlying abnormalities. Deeper cysts must be imaged up to rule out underlying malformations.

Figure 25-16

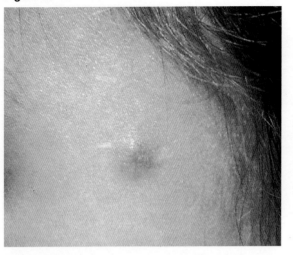

Pilomatricoma (benign calcifying epithelioma of Malherbe)
This solitary benign tumor arises most commonly during childhood, usually on the face or upper extremities. Pilomatricomas
range in size from 0.5 to 3.0 cm, although they are occasionally
even larger.

Figure 25-17

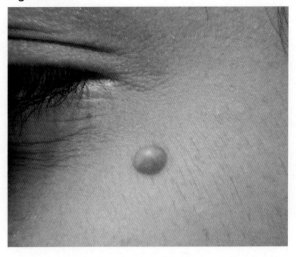

They appear as hard, freely movable dermal nodules. The skin
overlying the lesion is usually normal but is sometimes erythematous or bluish (as in Fig. 25-17). The overlying surface may
feel irregular and exhibit a "tent sign."

Figure 25-18

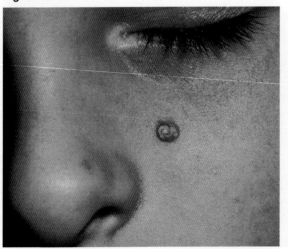

Pilomatricoma Over time, many pilomatricomas become calcified developing a yellow-white color. Sometimes the calcification
may extrude, as seen in this figure, having a firm consistency.
Pilomatricomas may clinically resemble epidermal cysts. Surgical excision is the treatment of choice.

Figure 25-19

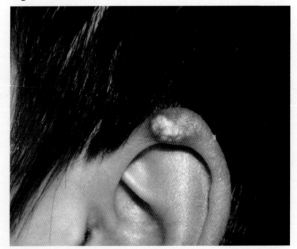

Extensive calcification is seen in this pilomatricoma of the pinna
of the ear. Multiple pilomatricomas are rare and are occasionally
associated with myotonic muscular dystrophy.

Figure 25-20

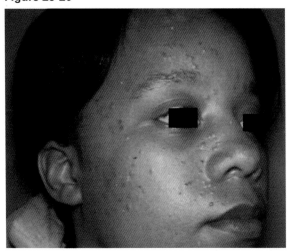

Trichoepithelioma Trichoepithelioma is a benign neoplasm that differentiates toward hair structures. Lesions of this type may be multiple or solitary. Figures 25-20 and 25-21 illustrate patients with multiple trichoepitheliomas. Individuals with this condition have numerous firm, rounded, skin-colored papules that are located mainly near the nasolabial folds.

Figure 25-21

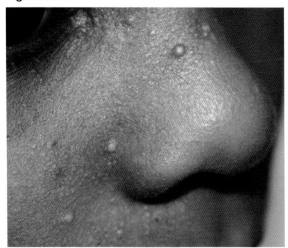

In more extensive cases, the rest of the face may become involved. The lesions usually begin to emerge during puberty, and the tendency for them to develop is inherited in autosomal dominant fashion.

Figure 25-22

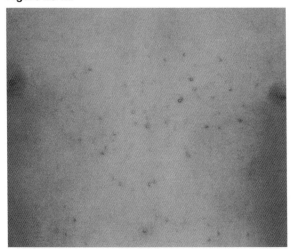

Eruptive vellus hair cysts This condition is characterized by the rapid appearance of numerous small pigmented and flesh-colored papules. The tiny, dome-shaped lesions are usually clustered on the chest but may also involve the proximal extremities, buttocks, and back. The onset of this asymptomatic condition usually occurs during mid-childhood.

Figure 25-23

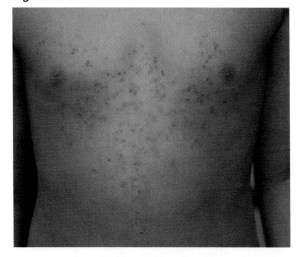

Biopsy analysis of a lesion reveals a mid-dermal cyst containing laminated keratinous material. Autosomal dominant inheritance of this condition is sometimes observed, sometimes in conjunction with steatocystoma multiplex (Fig. 25-24). Spontaneous resolution occurs frequently.

Figure 25-24

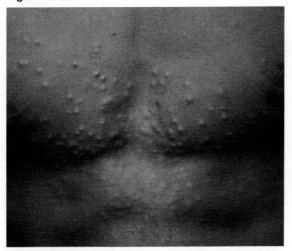

Steatocystoma multiplex This condition is characterized by multiple sebaceous gland cysts, occurring most frequently on the chest and back. It is associated with defects in Keratin 17 and is inherited in an autosomal dominant fashion. There is an association with eruptive vellus hair cysts (Figs. 25-22 and 25-23). The disorder usually presents at puberty.

Figure 25-25

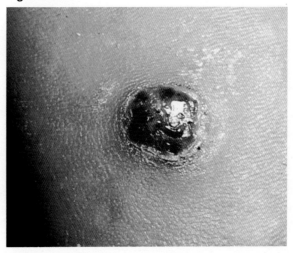

Eccrine poroma This is a solitary benign tumor that is more common in adults but is occasionally seen in adolescents. Eccrine poromas are usually located on the sole of the foot, although they may rarely occur in a variety of other areas. The vascular appearance of the lesion, as shown in Fig. 25-25, could lead to confusion with pyogenic granuloma. Treatment consists of complete surgical excision.

Figure 25-26

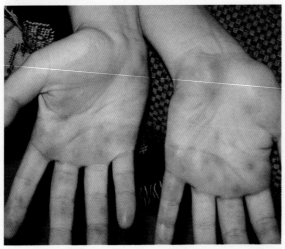

Palmoplantar eccrine hidradenitis This entity is characterized by the acute onset of painful erythematous papules and nodules located on the palms and/or soles in otherwise healthy children. Histopathology is remarkable for a neutrophilic infiltrate involving eccrine structures.

Figure 25-27

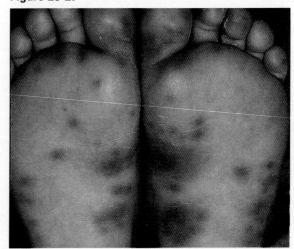

The cause is not always certain although there are numerous reports of cases associated with hot tub use and cutaneous pseudomonas infection, in which case it may be referred to as *hot hand-foot syndrome*. The condition is self-limited.

Figure 25-28

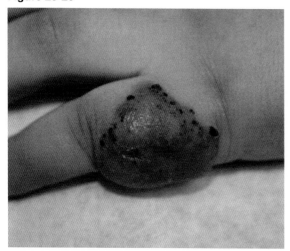

Figure 25-29

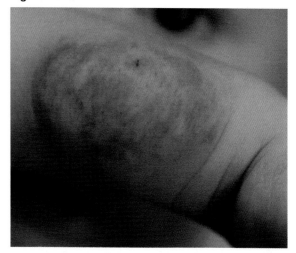

Eccrine angiomatous hamartoma This is a benign combined vascular and eccrine hamartoma. It may be present at birth or arise during early childhood, and the most common location is on the distal extremities.

The lesions, which can be single or multiple, are violaceous, brown or skin-colored, and generally present as either a nodule or a plaque. Other variable features are hyperhidrosis, hypertrichosis, and pain. This benign tumor tends to grow with the child, and, in some cases, surgical excision may be performed to alleviate pain or to improve appearance.

Benign and Malignant Pigmented Lesions

Figure 26-1

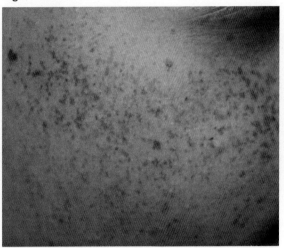

Ephelis This is the learned word for a freckle. The plural is ephelides (pronounced ĕf-ĕl-ī-dēz). These brown macules are exceedingly common on the face in some children. They appear after exposure to sunlight and are more common in children with very fair skin or red hair. They tend to disappear in adult life. Histologically, these lesions show increased amounts of epidermal melanin but no abundance of melanocytes.

Figure 26-2

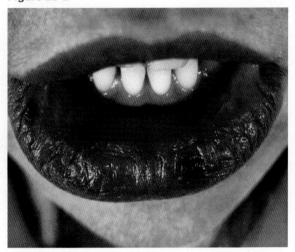

Lentigo This tan-to-brown to almost brown-black macular lesion may be found on any area of the body surface, which includes mucous membranes. There is no relation to ultraviolet light exposure. The illustration here is of lentigines on the lip. Lentigines may be present at birth and tend to increase in number during childhood and adult life. Histologically, there is a proliferation of melanocytes and elongation of the rete ridges. Lesions of this sort show no tendency to resolve spontaneously.

Figure 26-3

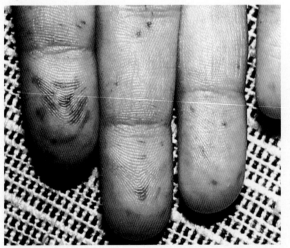

Peutz-Jeghers syndrome This autosomal dominant syndrome is notable for highly characteristic lentigines seen on the vermilion of the lips and adjacent skin, on the buccal mucosa, and on the palmar aspect of the fingertips. Figures 26-3 and 26-4 are good representations of the lentigines in a typical case.

Figure 26-4

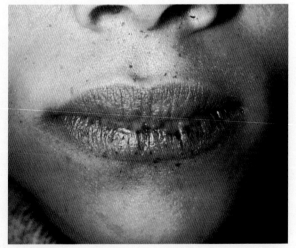

Patients with this syndrome may also have gastrointestinal polyps throughout the GI tract but most frequently in the jejunum. These benign hamartomas have very little malignant potential but may be the cause of obstruction, diarrhea, bleeding, or intussusception. Unlike common lentigines, the cutaneous lesions in these patients tend to fade during adult life. Mucous membrane lesions persist.

Figure 26-5

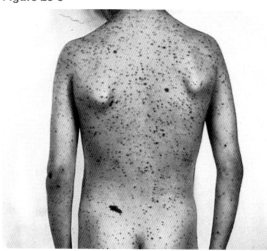

Figure 26-6

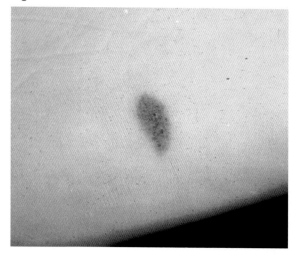

Multiple lentigines syndrome This autosomal dominant syndrome features numerous small lentigines, which are present at or soon after birth and cover the entire cutaneous surface. Previously known as the mnemonic LEOPARD syndrome, the common findings are summed up as follows in which *l* stands for lentigines, *e* for electrocardiographic conduction defects, *o* for ocular hypertelorism, *p* for pulmonary stenosis, *a* for abnormalities of genitalia, *r* for retardation of growth, and *d* for deafness. Mutations in the *PTPN11, RAF1,* or *BRAF* genes cause multiple lentigines syndrome.

Junctional nevus The macule of hyperpigmentation pictured in Fig. 26-6 is the most common form of nevocytic nevus in childhood. The so-called junctional nevus is a benign lesion that is composed of melanocytic nevus cells along the dermoepidermal junction. Lesions of this sort may arise in crops after the first year of life. As nevus cells migrate into the dermis, the typical junction nevus becomes a compound nevus. This process usually occurs during adolescence and early adulthood.

Figure 26-7

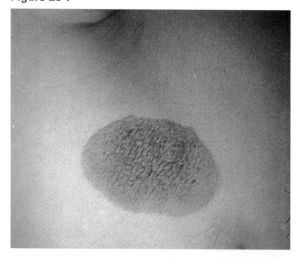

Figure 26-8

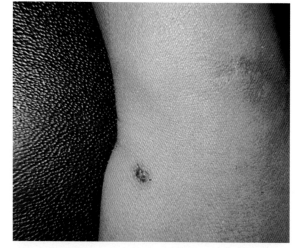

Compound nevus The ordinary mole has great variety in intensity of brown color, size, shape, and location. Those termed *compound nevi* are composed of melanocytes that are gathered into thèques or nests at the dermoepidermal junction and in larger, less compact collections deeper in the dermis. Shown in Fig. 26-7 is a plaque that is light brown and of fairly large size as compound nevi go. Figure 26-8 shows a papule that is reddish-brown and of a more usual size. Such lesions are thought to start out

as junctional nevi, which then go on to more melanocytic proliferation; melanocytes continue to drop off and down, becoming collections in the dermis. At any time in the development of compound nevi, melanocytes are found both at the dermoepidermal junction and in the dermis. Generally speaking, these lesions are benign and remain so. If cosmetically objectionable, they may be excised or shaved off. Histologic examination of all surgically removed pigmented lesions is advisable.

Figure 26-9

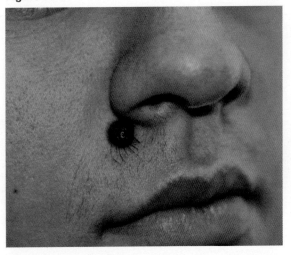

Figure 26-10

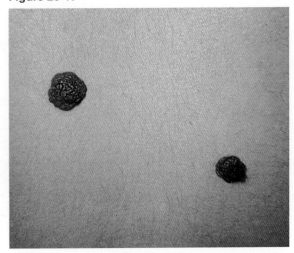

Intradermal nevus Figures 26-9 and 26-10 illustrate common moles in which the collections of melanocytes are entirely intradermal. Such lesions do not show any thèques or nests of melanocytes at the dermoepidermal junction. They too come in a great variety of colors, shapes, sizes, and sites. Intradermal nevi

are the end stage of development of junction and compound nevi. As with junction and compound nevi, they are extremely common and benign. Like compound nevi, they may be ablated by shaving or elliptical excision. Treatment by these methods does not increase the possibility of malignant transformation.

Figure 26-11

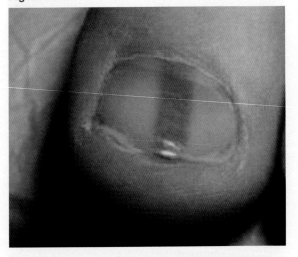

Figure 26-12

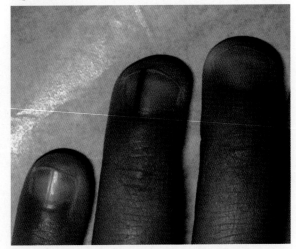

Melanonychia This lesion presents as a brown or black longitudinal streak along the nail. The pigmentation is most commonly caused by increased melanin by melanocytes in the nail unit. Melanonychia may be caused by physiologic factors such as racial pigmentation, trauma, dermatologic conditions, infection, medication, or systemic disease. In children, melanonychia is often caused by nevi.

The biggest concern in the evaluation of a pigmented lesion of the nail is the development of malignant melanoma. Although rare, it is reported in children. These nail lesions should be followed closely and biopsy, when necessary, can aid in management.

Figure 26-13

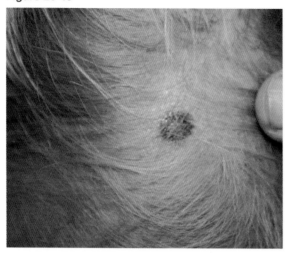

Eclipse scalp nevus Some children will develop nevi in the scalp that are larger than average, and not homogeneous in color. The lesion pictured in Fig. 26-13 is known as an eclipse nevus and is one of the most common scalp nevi found in children. It has a lighter, reddish brown or tan center that may be elevated, a brown rim, and at times a stellate border. Dermoscopy is a useful tool to aid in diagnosing these benign nevi.

Figure 26-14

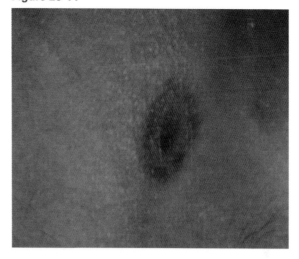

Cockarde nevus This clinical variant of benign acquired melanocytic nevus has a distinct targetoid appearance. There is a central papule, an intermediate zone of lighter pigment, and a surrounding pigmented ring. Histologic examination reveals a central compound nevus with junctional activity extending toward the outer edge. There is no evidence that lesions of this type have a particular potential for malignant degeneration.

Figure 26-15

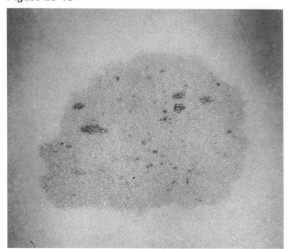

Speckled lentiginous nevus (Nevus spilus) This is a solitary flat area of light-brown pigmentation that may vary in size. Illustrated in Figs. 26-15 and 26-16 is the tendency for numerous

Figure 26-16

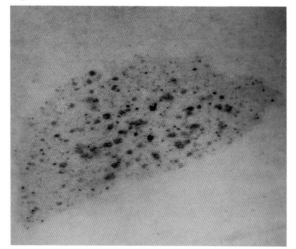

brown or black freckles of pigmentation to develop on top of the larger and lighter-colored macule. There is a low risk of malignant change in these lesions. Careful follow-up is advised.

Figure 26-17

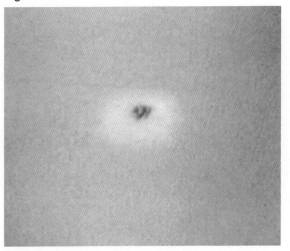

Figure 26-18

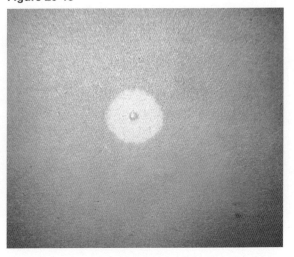

Halo nevus This is a relatively common condition in which an area of depigmentation develops around an existing melanocytic nevus. Lesions of this type are not unusual during childhood. They may be single or multiple. Figure 26-17 shows a small halo around a typical compound nevus. Over time, the nevus itself may depigment (Fig. 26-18) and disappear, and the skin color of the entire area may return to normal. The development of a

halo around a nevus is probably due to an immune response to the melanocytes of the original lesion. Halo nevi are more common in children with vitiligo and have been very rarely seen in association with malignant melanoma at another site. For most halo nevi no treatment is required. When biopsy analysis is performed, there is a dense lymphohistiocytic infiltrate around the central pigmented lesion.

Figure 26-19

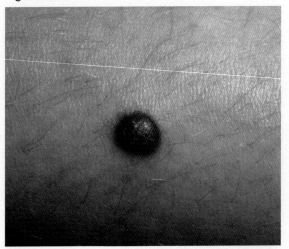

Figure 26-20

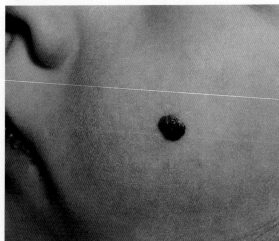

Spitz nevus This melanocytic lesion most often occurs during childhood. Spitz nevi are usually solitary, dome-shaped papules or nodules. They frequently arise on the face and extremities. The red to red-brown color of the papular lesions in Figs. 26-19 and 26-20 is fairly typical. At times, the lesion may appear as a

red papule mimicking a vascular lesion or a wart. Occasionally, they may be flesh-colored or brown-black. There is often a history of rapid growth. There are little data on the natural history of these lesions, but the customary treatment consists of a conservative complete excision.

Figure 26-21

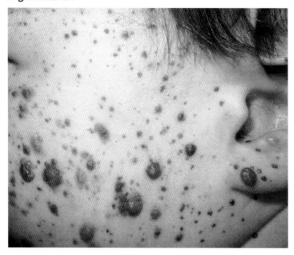

Multiple and agminated Spitz nevi Rarely, a patient may present with multiple Spitz nevi on an underlying light tan macular base. These patients must be closely observed for the possible development of malignant melanoma.

Figure 26-22

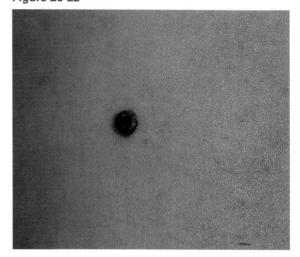

Pigmented spindle cell nevus This lesion shown in Fig. 26-22, first described by Reed, is a variant of a Spitz nevus that is heavily pigmented. Although this lesion is benign, clinically it may mimic a malignant melanoma. Biopsy of such a lesion is advised.

Figure 26-23

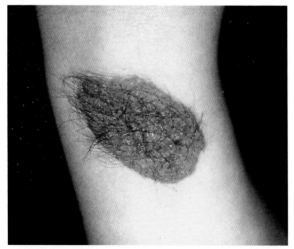

Congenital melanocytic nevus This pigmented lesion is present at birth in about 1 percent of all infants. The typical appearance is a flat, tan, or brown macule of irregular shape. The lesion may be studded with fine papules or may even be nodular. As illustrated in Fig. 26-23, a congenital melanocytic nevus may develop numerous coarse hair. Biopsy of a lesion reveals nevus cells in the deep dermis between collagen bundles and adjacent to adnexa. Because the true incidence of malignant melanoma arising in small congenital melanocytic nevi is uncertain, management remains controversial.

Figure 26-24

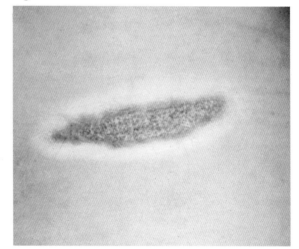

The lesion shown in Fig. 26-24 is surrounded by a border of depigmentation. The occurrence of a halo congenital melanocytic nevus is fairly unusual. The spontaneous regression of a portion of a pigmented lesion is probably due to a host antibody response to a subset of melanocytes. This phenomenon is sometimes associated with the development of melanoma. However, in most cases, the formation of such a halo is a benign event. Complete and spontaneous resolution of even very large congenital melanocytic nevi may occur.

Figure 26-25

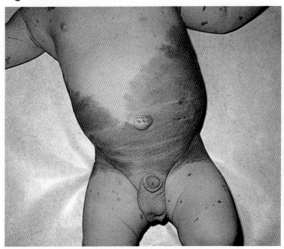

Figure 26-26

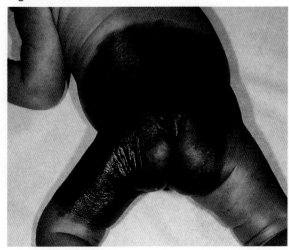

Congenital melanocytic nevus A congenital melanocytic nevus may cover large parts of the cutaneous surface. A lesion in the distribution illustrated here in Fig. 26-25 is sometimes referred to as a bathing trunk nevus. The possibility of malignant melanoma developing within such a large congenital melanocytic nevus represents a significant problem. Because of the increased potential for malignant change, the excision of giant congenital melanocytic nevi has been recommended whenever feasible. The use of inflatable tissue expanders enables the surgeon to remove large portions of lesions like the one shown in Fig. 26-26 without skin grafting. Patients with congenital melanocytic nevi on the scalp or midback, or with multiple satellite lesions, may be at risk for leptomeningeal melanocytosis or other neurologic defects.

Figure 26-27

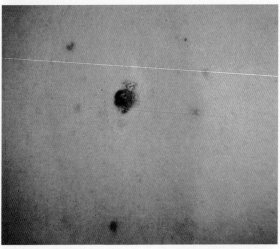

Figure 26-28

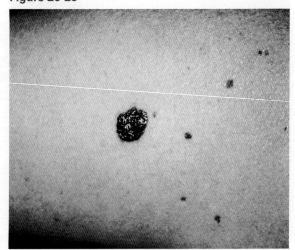

Malignant melanoma Less than 2 percent of all melanomas occur during childhood. Nonetheless, attention must be paid to signs and symptoms suggestive of this potentially fatal disease. Variegations of color are of particular concern. Irregular or notched borders, bleeding, and ulceration are other signs of malignant change. The patient may give a history of itching, and the parents may have noted rapid growth of the lesion. Because the prognosis of a melanoma is most closely related to the thickness of the lesion at the time of treatment, emphasis should be on early diagnosis.

Figure 26-29

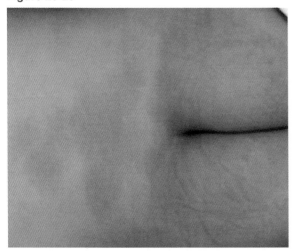

Dermal melanocytosis (mongolian spot) This very common cutaneous lesion is caused by a collection of melanocytes scattered through the deep dermis. The sacral location shown in Fig. 26-29 is by far the most frequent, but dermal melanosis may be present in other areas as well (Fig. 26-30).

Figure 26-30

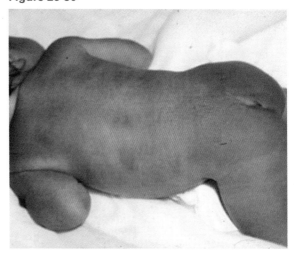

Dermal melanocytosis is found in many African-American and Asian newborns and are significantly less common among white infants. The areas of blue-gray pigmentation are usually present at birth and almost always fade during the first years of life.

Figure 26-31

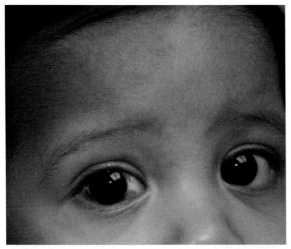

Nevus of Ota This rare dyschromia is characterized by a persistent bluish-gray discoloration of the skin around the eye. The proliferation of melanocytes in the upper dermis may extend to the forehead, malar area, and nose. Ocular involvement always includes the sclera, as in this patient, and sometimes the iris, conjunctiva, and optic disc. Nevus of Ota is considered a benign dermatosis, but melanoma on the ipsilateral side has been known to occur.

Figure 26-32

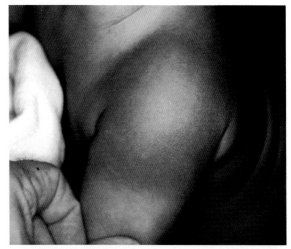

Nevus of Ito The occurrence of a pathological process identical to nevus of Ota but occurring on the skin of the deltoid, scapular, and clavicular regions is termed *nevus of Ito*. The color tends to be somewhat browner than the Mongolian spot because of the distribution of melanocytes higher in the dermis. In contrast to the Mongolian spot, these lesions tend to persist through adult life.

Figure 26-33

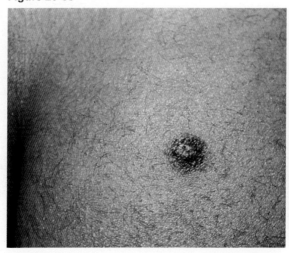

Blue nevus Collections of melanocytes deep in the dermis produce a blue macule or papule such as one illustrated in Fig. 26-33. The physics of color in the skin is such that melanin high in the dermis makes for black coloration, and melanin low in the dermis makes for blue coloration. Blue nevi are small, dome-shaped nodules that are often located on the dorsa of the hands or feet. They frequently arise during childhood. The common blue nevus has little or no potential for malignancy. Malignant degeneration of a cellular blue nevus occurs rarely.

Figure 26-34

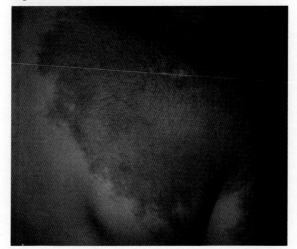

Figure 26-35

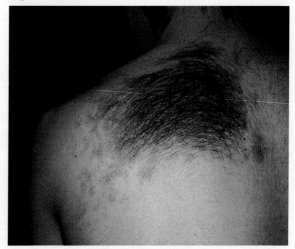

Becker nevus This lesion is an irregular, pigmented macule that most commonly arises in males at puberty, although it may be seen in females. The light-brown area of pigmentation, which may be quite large, eventually develops thick hairs. The most typical location for Becker nevus is on the shoulder or upper back. Less commonly, lesions arise on the forearm, upper chest, abdomen, and rarely, the lower extremity. Becker nevus has no malignant potential, and therefore surgical removal is not necessary. The pigmentation and hypertrichosis both tend to persist into adult life.

Miscellaneous Pigmentary Disorders

Figure 27-1

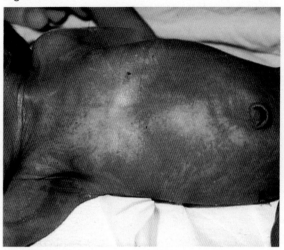

Pigmentary mosaicism This condition is characterized by areas of hypopigmentation following the lines of Blaschko. These are present from birth or evolve during early childhood. The lesions may be generalized, with individual areas of hypopigmentation assuming blotchy, whorled, or streaked patterns.

Figure 27-2

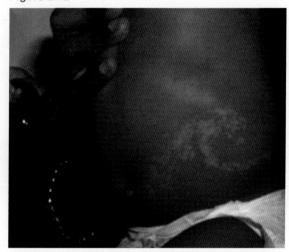

A very small number of patients with this pigmentary disorder have central nervous system disease, usually manifest as seizures or mental retardation. Other reported abnormalities include skeletal and ocular defects. This condition was formerly called hypomelanosis of Ito or incontinentia pigmenti achromians.

Figure 27-3

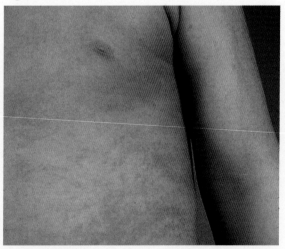

Pigmentary mosaicism In this form of mosaicism, there are lines of hyperpigmentation that follows lines of Blaschko. In this patient, there is a linear pattern on the extremities and a whorled pattern on the trunk. This condition was formerly referred to as "linear and whorled nevoid hypermelanosis." The hyperpigmentation may be present at birth or develops shortly thereafter, spreading during the first 2 years of life, at which time it stabilizes.

Figure 27-4

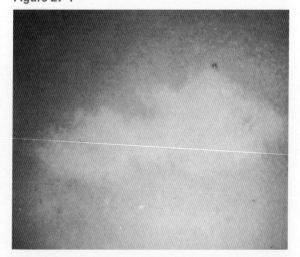

Nevus depigmentosus (achromicus) These are localized areas of hypopigmentation that are usually present at birth. The lesions may be irregular in size and shape and occasionally follow a linear or segmental pattern. Electron microscopic study of these areas suggests that melanosomes are not being transferred from melanocytes into surrounding keratinocytes. There are no associated abnormalities. It is best considered as a more subtle form of pigmentary mosaicism, also resulting from a somatic mutation during embryogenesis.

Figure 27-5

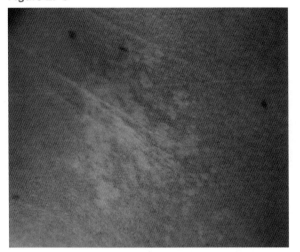

Figure 27-6

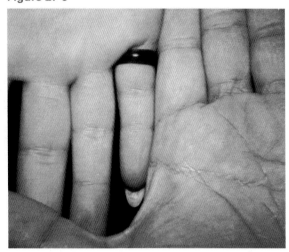

Nevus anemicus This benign lesion develops at birth or in early childhood. Rubbing the area causes the surrounding skin to turn red, while the area itself maintains its white color. Nevus anemicus does not represent a loss of pigment, but rather a constriction of blood vessels, due to a local increased sensitivity to catecholamines.

Carotenemia The vegetable pigment carotene is widely distributed in carrots, lettuce, squash, and many other vegetables and fruits. A diet that is very rich in these foods results in a yellowish-orange discoloration of the skin. This appearance is usually localized to the palms and soles (note the hand on the left in Fig. 27-6) but may also involve the skin of the face. The presence of normal sclera distinguishes the clinical appearance of this condition from that of jaundice. Return to normal skin color follows a reduction in dietary intake of carotene.

Figure 27-7

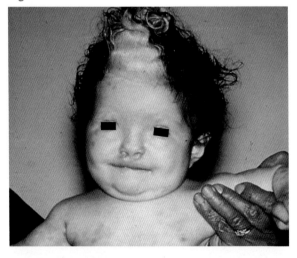

Figure 27-8

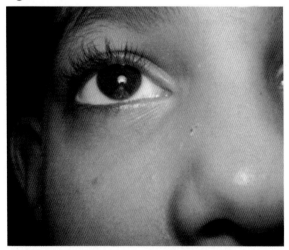

Waardenburg syndrome This genetic disorder is transmitted as an autosomal dominant, with variable penetrance. It is characterized grossly by partial albinism in the form of a white forelock (Fig. 27-7), broad nasal root (Figs. 27-7 and 27-8), hypertrichosis of the inner portions of the eyebrows, lateral displacement of the medial canthi (Figs. 27-7 and 27-8), partial or complete heterochromia of the irides (Fig. 27-8), and complete or unilateral deafness. In children with skin of color, blue irides, vitiligo, and pigmentary changes in the fundi may be seen. There are no other constitutional symptoms, but the hearing loss and unusual appearance may pose handicaps.

Figure 27-9

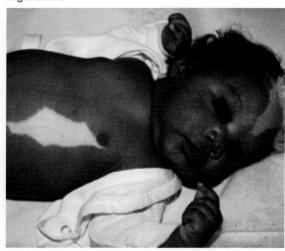

Piebaldism Patients with this autosomal dominant condition have congenital patches of depigmentation. Most have a white forelock, with involvement of adjoining scalp and forehead in a triangular pattern. There may be other areas of involvement on the trunk and extremities. Electron microscopic examination of affected areas reveals a complete absence of melanocytes.

Figure 27-10

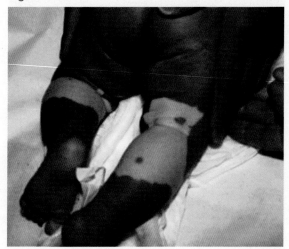

Piebaldism The presence of islands of normal pigmentation within the areas of involvement is a common finding in piebaldsim. Piebaldism is caused by mutations of the c-kit proto-oncogene, which is related to melanoblast migration, proliferation, differentiation, and survival.

Figure 27-11

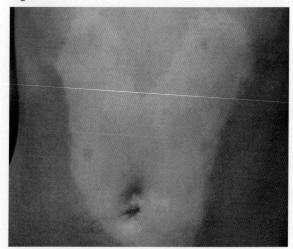

Piebaldism Figure 27-11 shows a geographic area of depigmentation on the abdomen and chest, again with islands of normal pigmentation. Management must include the appropriate use of sunscreen lotions on depigmented skin.

Figure 27-12

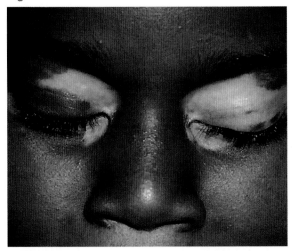

Vitiligo About one-half of patients with vitiligo have onset of their disease during childhood or adolescence. Patients may present with hypopigmented and depigmented macules of various sizes and shapes. The area of involvement surrounding the eye in Fig. 27-12 represents one fairly typical distribution.

Figure 27-13

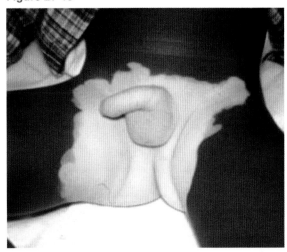

Vitiligo may involve the skin around the mouth, rectum, and genitalia. The frequent presence of antibodies to melanocytes in individuals with vitiligo suggests an autoimmune etiology. A number of other autoimmune disorders, including Addison disease and Hashimoto thyroiditis, are more common among patients with vitiligo and their relatives.

Figure 27-14

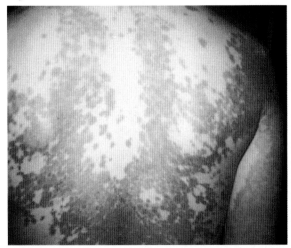

Vitiligo Figure 27-14 illustrates a fairly extensive case of vitiligo. The condition tends to progress and may even become universal. A variety of treatment modalities are commonly employed, with varying degrees of success. In many patients, the application of topical corticosteroids or topical immunomodulators, along with natural sunlight exposure or narrow band UVB phototherapy, may induce repigmentation.

Figure 27-15

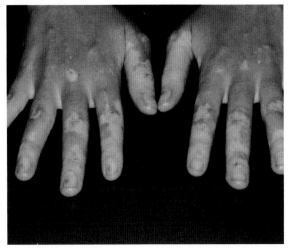

Varying combinations of topical or oral psoralens and ultraviolet A light (PUVA) are also used in the treatment of vitiligo. The pattern shown in Fig. 27-15, with involvement of the distal fingers (and often toes) is particularly difficult to treat.

Figure 27-16

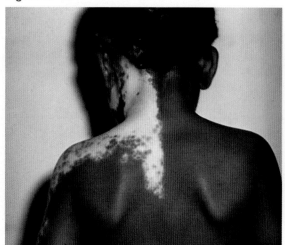

Vitiligo (cont'd.) Segmental vitiligo is characterized by smaller patches of depigmented skin that are generally unilateral and in a limited area; approximately 20 percent of patients with vitiligo in childhood have this form of the disease.

Figure 27-17

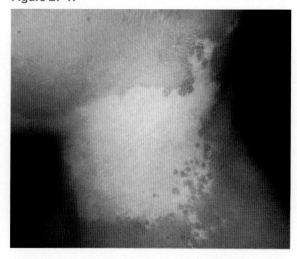

Figure 27-17 is another example of segmental vitiligo. Very rarely, patients with the segmental form of the disease go on to develop the generalized and symmetrical form. The treatment, consisting of topical corticosteroids and light, or psoralens, is essentially the same as that previously discussed.

Figure 27-18

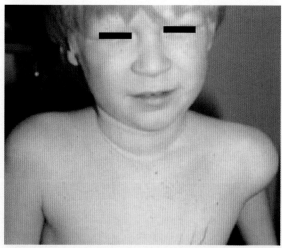

Albinism This condition is characterized by congenital hypopigmentation of the skin, hair, and eyes. Almost all of the many varieties are inherited in autosomal recessive fashion. Photophobia is a significant problem for most patients. The lack of protective melanin leads to extreme sun sensitivity and results in a high incidence of actinic keratoses, basal cell carcinomas, and squamous cell carcinomas. The avoidance of sun exposure by using protective clothing and sunscreen preparations is critical.

Figure 27-19

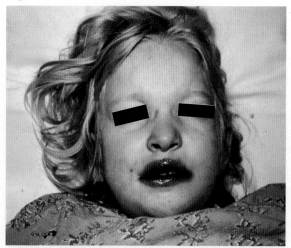

Chédiak-Higashi syndrome This genetic disorder, recessive in mechanism of transmission, is extremely rare. It is characterized by albinism, photophobia, lymphadenopathy, hepatosplenomegaly, and susceptibility to pyogenic infection. The peripheral blood smear reveals giant granules within lymphocytes. The high incidences of serious infection and lymphoreticular malignancy contribute to a poor prognosis.

Figure 27-20

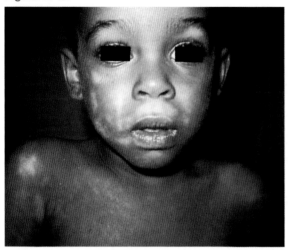

Figure 27-21

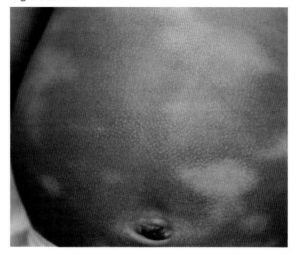

Postinflammatory hypopigmentation A wide variety of dermatologic diseases may leave either temporary or permanent hypopigmentation. The pigmentary change in these two figures is the result of atopic dermatitis. Postinflammatory hypopigmentation can usually be easily differentiated from vitiligo.

The lesions that follow inflammatory skin disease are less well defined and are more off-white than stark white. For most children, postinflammatory hypopigmentation is temporary. Parents should be reassured that even the most disfiguring patterns of pigmentary alteration will resolve with proper therapy and time.

Figure 27-22

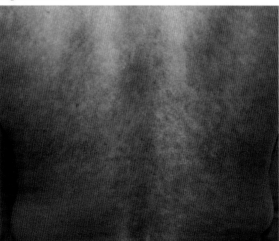

Progressive macular hypomelanosis This condition appears to be most prevalent among teenagers and young adults and more common in females. It is characterized by the unexplained development of pale, round coalescing hypopigmented macules on the back, chest, and abdomen. This disorder may be mistaken for tinea versicolor or pityriasis alba. Proposed treatments include topical benzoyl peroxide and clindamycin and narrow band ultraviolet B.

Figure 27-23

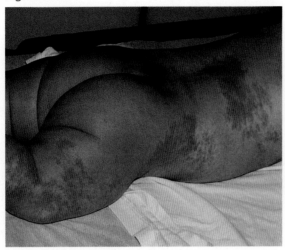

Figure 27-24

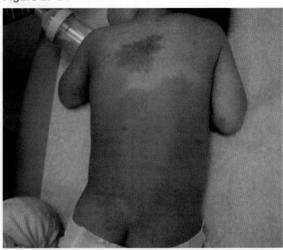

Phakomatosis pigmentovascularis This is a group of conditions characterized by nevus flammeus in combination with other birthmarks. The other lesions may be blue spots (dermal melanocytosis), nevus spilus, or nevus anemicus.

This patient shown in Fig. 27-24 has a large area of vascular discoloration accompanied by an area of dermal melanocytosis. According to one of several classification systems, this would be termed *type IIA*.

SECTION

28

Dermatitis Artefacta

Figure 28-1

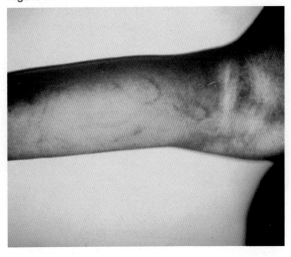

Child abuse The physical abuse of children accounts for many deaths each year in the United States. Physicians who care for children must acquaint themselves with the signs of battering, sexual abuse, and nutritional deprivation. For the protection of children, the laws in all states require the reporting of all cases of suspected child abuse. Illustrated in Fig 28-1 are typical loop marks in a child who was struck with a doubled-over rope or electrical cord.

Figure 28-2

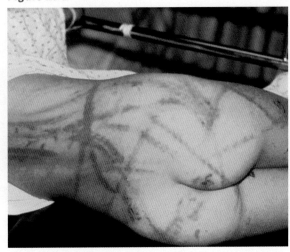

The presence of ecchymoses or scars on the lower back or buttocks is almost always the result of physical abuse. Slap marks, human bites, and lash marks each leave bruises of a distinctive shape and distribution. The presence of bruises of this sort is the evidence of force used without restraint and is a definite sign of child abuse.

Figure 28-3

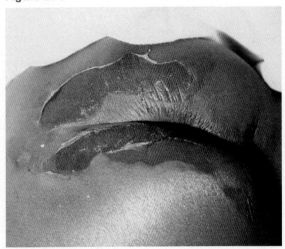

Child abuse Ten percent of the cases of physical abuse in children involve the deliberate infliction of burns as a form of punishment. Cigarette burns, which appear as uniform round erosions, are often located on the palms and soles. Second-degree burns may also occur when a child is held against a radiator or hot plate. Illustrated here are two burns that resulted from forcible immersion in hot water.

Figure 28-4

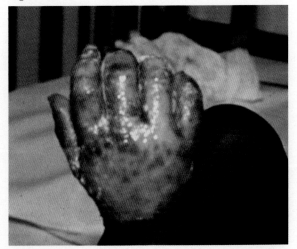

Symmetrical blistering of the perineum (Fig. 28-3) is the evidence of a child being lowered into a hot bath. Figure 28-4 is illustrative of forcible immersion of a hand. In general, the presence of an injury for which the history seems implausible should alert the physician to the possibility of child abuse. A delay in seeking medical assistance for the care of an injury should also cause concern.

Figure 28-5

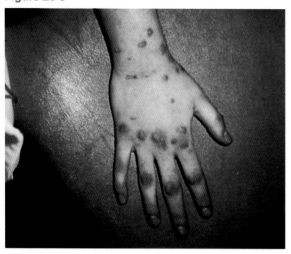

Figure 28-6

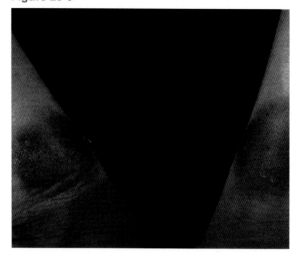

Factitial dermatitis Injuries to the skin that are induced by the patient or another individual are termed *factitial dermatitis*. This entity, when it occurs in childhood, may be related to a variety of emotional disturbances in either parent or child. The lesions in Fig. 28-5 are self-inflicted wounds caused by bites. Some are scars and others are inflammatory lesions.

The distribution and morphology of lesions of this type are not consistent with any known cutaneous disease, and there is usually no credible history for their development. Other methods of inducing self-injury include scratching, picking, and gouging. The hypertrichosis in Fig. 28-6 resulted from repeated biting on the skin in a child with severe mental retardation. Self-mutilation of this type is also seen in Lesch-Nyhan syndrome.

Figure 28-7

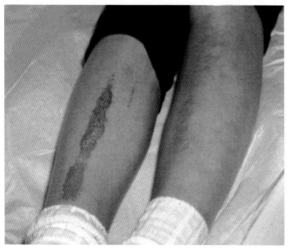

Figure 28-8

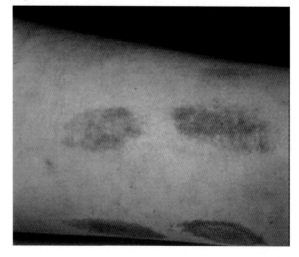

Factitial dermatitis Figures 28-7 and 28-8 show erosions that are suspiciously sharply demarcated from the surrounding skin, and peculiarly shaped. Self-induced injury of this sort is associated with a wide range of emotional disturbances or psychiatric disease.

Healing of lesions can sometimes be facilitated by occlusion of the area of skin that is being repeatedly injured. Psychiatric referral is often of value.

Figure 28-9

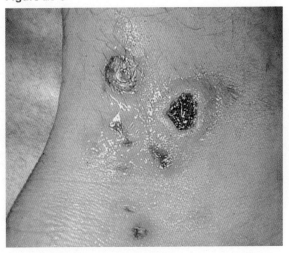

Figure 28-10

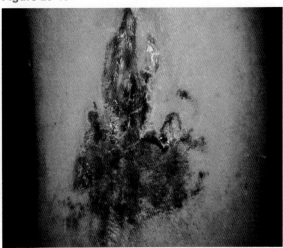

Factitial dermatitis (cont'd.) Figure 28-9 shows lesions that might have been produced by fingernails. The first step in evaluating a child with possible facititial dermatitis is to rule out other causes of the skin lesions. Diseases that have been mistaken for signs of child abuse include bullous impetigo (Figs. 3-3 and 3-4) (which can resemble cigarette burns), and urticaria multiforme (Figs. 16-21 to 16-23) which can resolve with ecchymoses.

Figure 28-10 shows factitial lesions that were caused by caustic chemicals. A particular cause of factitial dermatitis in children is termed *Munchausen syndrome by proxy.* In this condition, a disturbed parent attempts to create the appearance of illness in a child. The presence of this syndrome signals a high level of physical danger for the child, and cases of this sort must be promptly reported to social service agencies as a form of child abuse.

Figure 28-11

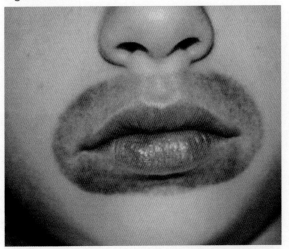

Figure 28-12

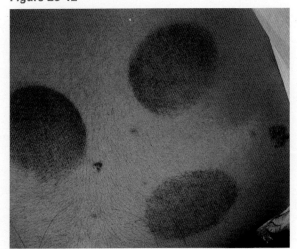

Factitial dermatitis The presence of a localized purpuric eruption in the circumoral area may not indicate a serious disease. This condition is caused by sucking on a glass or cup, creating a negative pressure around the mouth, resulting in the presence of purpura.

Cupping This method has been used in traditional Chinese medicine and a wide variety of other medical traditions since 3000 BC. A vacuum is created in a glass cup by placing a small amount of alcohol at the bottom of the cup, then lighting it and immediately placing it on to the skin. The suction created results in a circular area of purpura that is sharply demarcated.

Figure 28-13

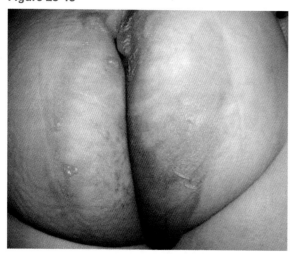

Senna laxative-induced blistering dermatitis Infants and toddlers ingesting senna-based laxatives may rarely develop a burnlike eruption on the buttocks. The eruption tends to occur after the buttock has been exposed to a loose stool for a few hours in a patient given this medication. It is important to differentiate this from a scald from hot water immersion as seen in Fig. 28-3.

Figure 28-14

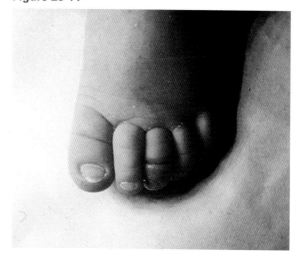

Pseudoainhum The word ainhum means "to saw." True ainhum is limited geographically to Africa and usually presents as a groove encircling the small toe. Pseudoainhum refers to a condition that is clinically similar but caused by a wide variety of disease processes. In children, congenital constricting bands may be a cause. More commonly, pseudoainhum occurs as an artifact from the wind of a cord or a long hair buried around a digit. In Fig. 28-14, the third toe is affected by a groove whose cause was indeed a buried hair.

Figure 28-15

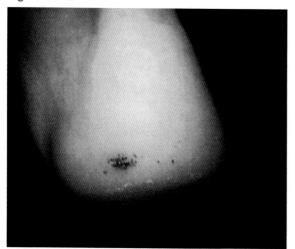

Talon noir (black heel) Stigmata caused by certain operations in occupations and avocations are characteristic. The bump on the radial aspect of the middle finger of a scribe and the callused fingertips of a violinist are examples. The illustration here is of punctate and ecchymotic hemorrhages in a heel of a basketball player. There is something about basketball playing in its jumps, twists, and turns that promotes this type of lesion. Its only significance is that it should not be mistaken for malignant melanoma.

Figure 28-16

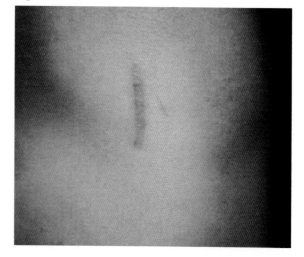

Tattoos The deposition into skin of inert materials that produce colored effects may be accidental or premeditated. The usual material that enters the skin accidentally is carbon from mischance, such as fire blast, abrasion on dirty surfaces, and stabs of sharp pencils. Figure 28-16 shows a stripe of blue color resulting from an incised wound incurred in a fall on a tarred pavement.

Disorders of Nails
and Hair

Figure 29-1

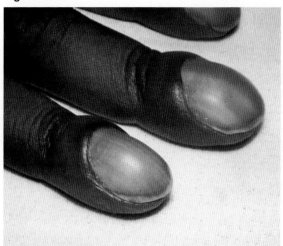

Clubbed nails Increased curvature of the nail plate may be due to a wide variety of causes. In this patient, the large, convex nails are a hereditary anomaly and were found to be present in both father and brother. Other causes of clubbing of the nails in children include cyanotic congenital heart disease, cystic fibrosis, and chronic inflammatory bowel disease.

Figure 29-2

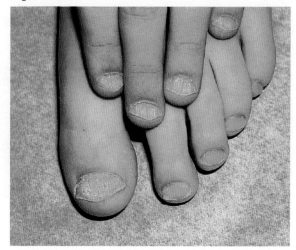

Trachyonychia Any skin disease that affects the nail matrix may result in an abnormal nail plate. There are children, though, who only manifest dystrophy of the nail without any other cutaneous lesions. The nails have a rough, sandpaper-like quality as well as longitudinal ridging and occasional splitting at the distal nail edge. When all nails are involved, the condition that has been termed *twenty nail dystrophy of childhood*. Similar nail changes can be seen in lichen planus and alopecia areata. In many patients the condition spontaneously regresses.

Figure 29-3

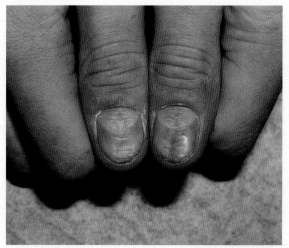

Traumatic onychodystrophy (Habit tic deformity) Trauma to the nail plate or nail folds can produce a wide variety of nail deformities. The one pictured in Fig. 29-3 is the result of a habit tic. This common nail dystrophy is characterized by a longitudinal canal that runs down the center of the entire nail plate. It is caused by manipulation of the proximal nail fold by the index finger of the same hand.

Figure 29-4

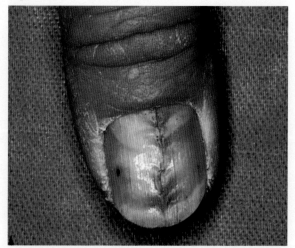

Dystrophia unguis mediana canaliformis This is a rare condition of unknown etiology that usually involves the thumb. It consists of a canal that runs near the center of the length of the nail plate. Small cracks that extend laterally from the linear canal give the appearance of an inverted fir tree. This deformity tends to resolve spontaneously over a period of months but often recurs.

Figure 29-5

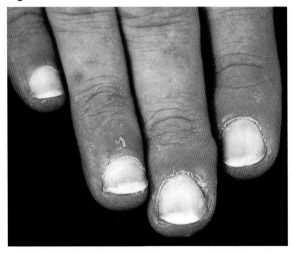

Figure 29-6

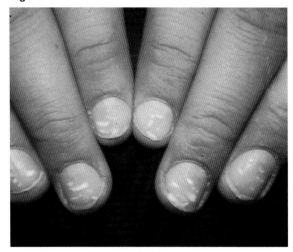

Leukonychia totalis This is a rare nail disorder that is inherited in autosomal dominant fashion. The color of normal nail plates beyond the lunulae is normally pink from the blood in the blood vessels of the nail bed. The whiteness shown in Fig. 29-5 is due to an abnormality in the nail plate. The nails may also be brittle.

Leukonychia striata The horizontal white streaks pictured in Fig. 29-6 are the result of abnormal keratinization of the nail plate. The tendency toward leukonychia striata is sometimes inherited in an autosomal dominant fashion. In other cases, it can be attributed to vigorous manicuring, to trauma, or to a wide variety of systemic illnesses. In many patients, there is no obvious cause, and the streaks resolve spontaneously.

Figure 29-7

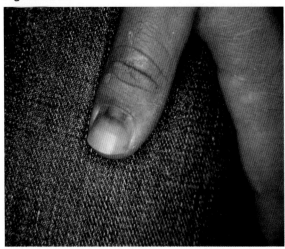

Figure 29-8

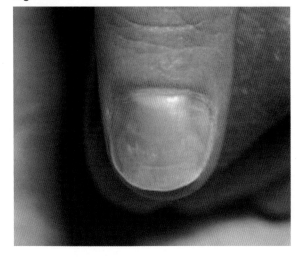

Onycholysis This word means separation (*-lysis*) of nails (*onycho-*) from nail beds. There are many causes for such a development. The commonest are mechanical. Nails worn long are frequently lifted by being snagged. Excessive soaping and soaking in heavy housework promote separation.

Figures 29-7 and 29-8 illustrate onycholysis associated with drug-induced photosensitivity. Figure 29-7 illustrates a reaction to tetracycline, and Fig. 29-8 to doxycycline. Doxycycline, frequently used in the treatment of acne, is a particularly common cause of photosensitivity.

Figure 29-9

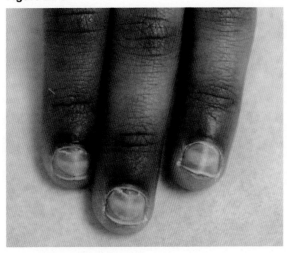

Onychomadesis Figure 29-9 illustrates separation of the nail plate from the matrix with continued attachment to the nail. The process may eventuate in shedding of the nail. Onychomadesis has been associated with infection, and is particularly common after atypical hand-foot-mouth disease (Figs. 5-59 to 5-62). Other causes include pemphigus vulgaris (Figs. 17-1 to 17-4). Oncyhomadesis may occur after chemotherapy or as a side effect of antiepileptic medications.

Figure 29-10

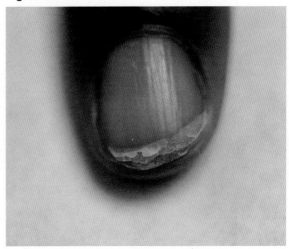

Onychoschizia This disorder is characterized by lamellar splitting of the nails. It is a form of nail brittleness and is usually the result of practices, such as dish washing, that require repeated wetting and drying of the nails. The problem can sometimes be prevented by the use of plastic or rubber gloves with cotton liners.

Figure 29-11

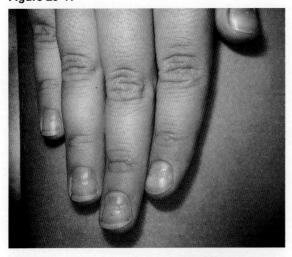

Beau lines These transverse lines or furrows begin at the proximal nail fold and grow out with the nail. They represent a brief interference of nail growth secondary to physical stress such as an illness or nutritional deficiency. The lines are not noticed until several weeks after the precipitating event.

Figure 29-12

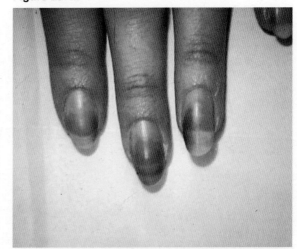

Discoloration of nail plates Many chemicals can discolor nail plates. Solutions of potassium permanganate and silver nitrate stain nail plates brown-purple and jet black, respectively. In the case illustrated in Fig. 29-12, the stain is derived from resorcinol. Such stains are harmless and can be easily removed by superficial scaling with the edge of a glass slide.

Figure 29-13

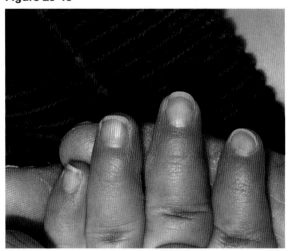

Nail-patella syndrome This entity, also known as hereditary osteo-onychodysplasia, is a genetic disease linked to a mutation in the gene encoding transcription factor LMX1B, mapped on the long arm of chromosome 9 (9q34).

Figure 29-14

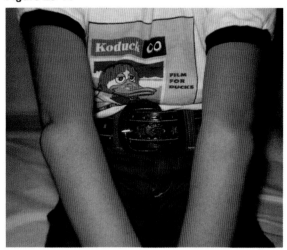

The manifestations include fingernail dysplasia, absent or hypoplastic patellae, the presence of posterior conical iliac horns, and abnormalities of the radial heads. Patients are also at risk for kidney disease and glaucoma.

Figure 29-15

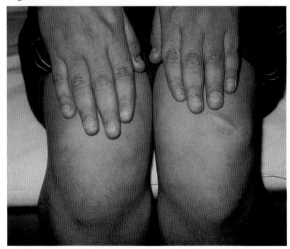

Nail-patella syndrome The nail change of triangular lunulae is considered pathognomonic (Fig. 29-13). Various other dysplastic nail changes may also be seen. Toenails are rarely affected. Elbow abnormalities include limitation of motion or subluxation of the radius (Fig. 29-14).

Figure 29-16

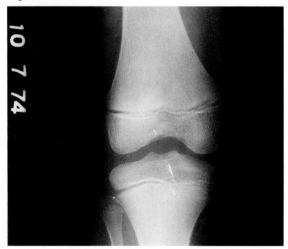

Absent or hypoplastic patellae may lead to knee pain and instability (Figs. 29-15 and 29-16). Patients should be monitored closely for evidence of kidney involvement.

Figure 29-17

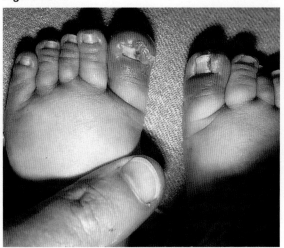

Congenital ingrown toenail Shortly after birth deformity of the great toe, unilaterally or bilaterally, may occur. Thickening of the lateral nail folds and hyponychium with erythema, edema, and sometimes secondary infection may occur. The growth of the nail may protrude through this thickening at its distal end. This condition is sometimes due to congenital malalignment of the nail plates. Surgical treatment is rarely necessary, as the condition is self-limited with good resolution. Secondary infection should be treated if present.

Figure 29-18

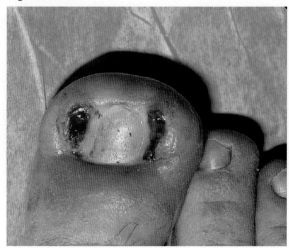

Ingrown toenail Improper trimming of nails may lead to the formation of an ingrown toenail. The lateral or medial nail fold becomes erythematous, edematous, and painful with the nail growing into the fleshy portion of the folds. Secondary infection and the formation of granulation tissue typically ensue. Surgical treatment is often necessary when local wound care measures fail to alleviate this condition.

Figure 29-19

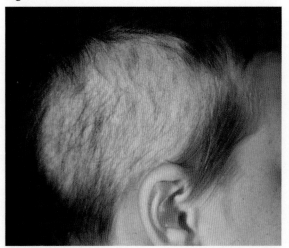

Trichotillomania This is a form of alopecia that is caused by the child's twisting or pulling of his or her own hair. This cause of hair loss is usually easy to recognize. There is often, but not always, a parental awareness of hair-pulling behavior—sometimes while the child is studying or watching television or at bedtime. The area of hair loss is usually asymmetric and follows an irregular pattern. Examination of the involved area reveals hair that are broken off at different lengths. There is never the total hair loss of alopecia areata or the scaling and erythema of tinea capitis.

Figure 29-20

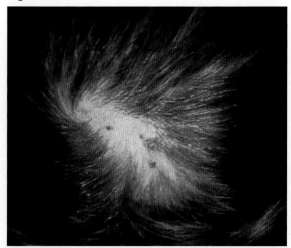

In most cases, trichotillomania is evidence of an innocent and benign habit that is best compared to nail biting. However, trichotillomania may sometimes be evidence of more severe emotional distress or a manifestation of obsessive-compulsive disorder. In addition, children who swallow their plucked hair may develop a gastric trichobezoar.

Figure 29-21

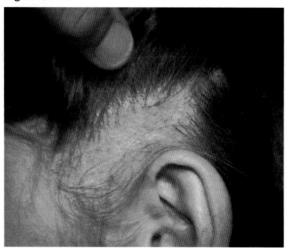

Traumatic alopecia Another traumatic form of alopecia is due to hairstyles that feature braiding with excessive tension. The alopecia in this condition is limited to the line of the hair part or to the margins of the scalp. Careful examination reveals broken hair of varying lengths and sometimes a localized folliculitis. The application of heat or of chemicals to straighten hair will also damage the hair shafts and cause traumatic alopecia. An example of this phenomenon is illustrated in Fig. 29-21. For most cases of traumatic alopecia, a change in hairstyle is the only treatment that is required.

Figure 29-22

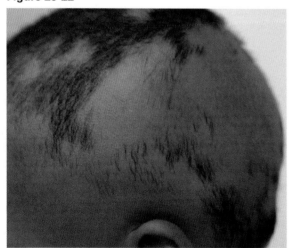

Alopecia areata The children pictured in these two figures are typical of the most common presentation of alopecia areata. There is usually a history of the abrupt onset of hair loss in one or several circumscribed round or oval patches. There is no history of pruritus or scaling. The occasional association of alopecia areata with diseases such as lymphocytic thyroiditis and vitiligo suggests a possible autoimmune etiology.

Figure 29-23

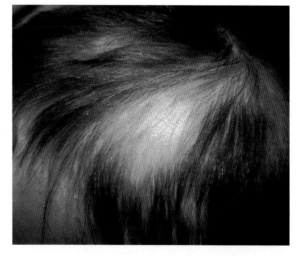

Fortunately, spontaneous regrowth occurs in most patients over a period of 6 months to 1 year. Prognosis is less favorable in patients with more widespread disease and earlier onset.

Figure 29-24

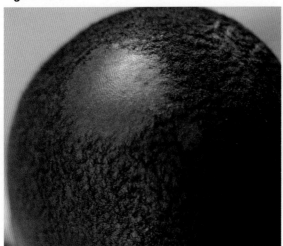

Alopecia areata (cont'd.) During the initial onset, parents and children should be counseled with cautious optimism, but forewarned that progression of the disorder may occur or that it may recur after a period of complete recovery. Treatments include topical and intralesional corticosteroids, topical anthralin, and a variety of topical allergens, such as squaric acid.

Figure 29-25

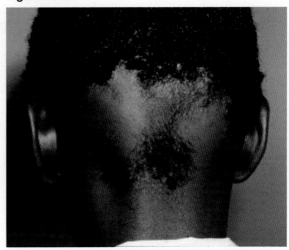

Illustrated in Fig. 29-25 is ophiasis, a form of alopecia in which hair loss progresses along the margin of the scalp. Both ophiasis and extensive alopecia areata carry a poorer prognosis for regrowth.

Figure 29-26

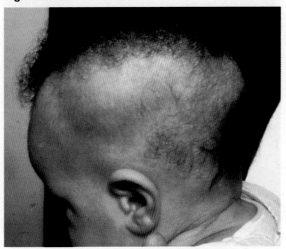

Alopecia areata Figures 29-26 and 29-27 show examples of alopecia areata that are progressing toward alopecia totalis. Topical agents that cause either an irritant or contact dermatitis of the scalp may sometimes stimulate hair growth. However, they may not affect the tendency toward progression and repeated recurrences in patients with severe involvement.

Figure 29-27

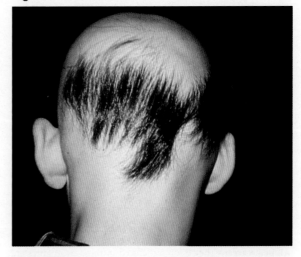

The use of intralesional steroids in patients with such extensive disease would be extremely painful. Certainly, alopecia areata has enormous implications for the self-image of the affected child or adolescent. Wigs are sometimes helpful. Patients and families should be advised of the availability of support groups related to this disease.

Figure 29-28

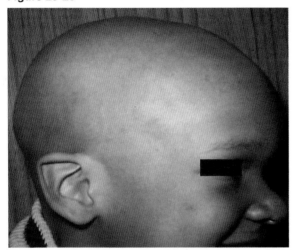

Alopecia universalis This is the severest expression of the alopecia areata disease process. Complete loss of scalp hair is termed *alopecia totalis*. The patient pictured in Fig. 29-28 has also lost all of his eyebrows, eyelashes, and axillary, body, and pubic hair. Hence, alopecia universalis. The prognosis in this situation is particularly poor, with little chance of responding to therapy or of experiencing spontaneous recovery.

Figure 29-29

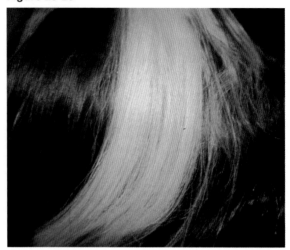

Alopecia areata (recovered) Figure 29-29 shows regrowth of hair in a patch of alopecia areata. The oddity is that the regrowth was with white hair. The phenomenon is not unusual and is temporary. Eventually the regrowth will be in a color that is normal for the patient. It also frequently happens that regrown hair is temporarily of different texture. In time, assuming no relapse, completely normal color and texture supervene.

Figure 29-30

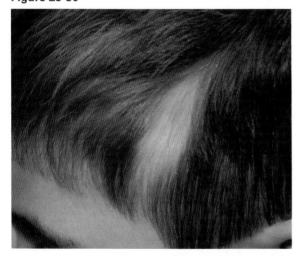

Temporal triangular alopecia This condition may be present at birth but more frequently develops during early childhood. There is absence of hair in the temporal region of the scalp, either on one side or bilaterally. The area of involvement may be either triangular or lancet-shaped. There is no clinical evidence of inflammation or scarring, and there is no known treatment.

Figure 29-31

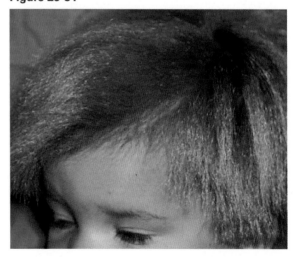

Uncombable hair syndrome This syndrome presents during infancy or childhood with "spun glass" hair. The hair is blond, grows slowly, and is extremely difficult to comb or manage. Subtle longitudinal grooves may be noted on light microscopy and are clearly seen with a scanning electron microscope. Autosomal dominant inheritance is seen in some cases, and the condition may improve as the patient grows older.

Figure 29-32

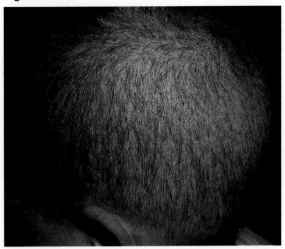

Monilethrix This word means "beaded hair" and designates a condition in which the hair varies in thickness along its length. Inheritance is autosomal dominant. The result is that the hair remains dry and brittle and fractures easily.

Figure 29-33

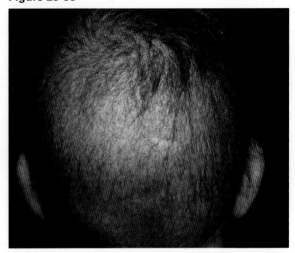

Children with this condition may have normal neonatal hair, but the hair that begins to grow in the second or third month of life will fracture before reaching a normal length. The condition may resolve spontaneously over time or persist into adult life. Keratosis pilaris (Figs. 15-63 to 15-65) is almost always associated.

Figure 29-34

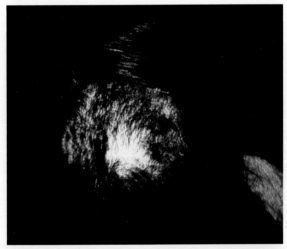

Trichorrhexis nodosa This is another anomaly of hair growth. It is characterized by dry, fragile hair and results in patches of partial alopecia. The second word in the condition's name derives from the presence of whitish nodes along the hair shaft. These nodes are the site of breakage. This disorder is sometimes, though very rarely, associated with argininosuccinic aciduria and mental retardation. The acquired forms are far more common and seem to be the combined result of trauma to the hair and a genetic predisposition.

Figure 29-35

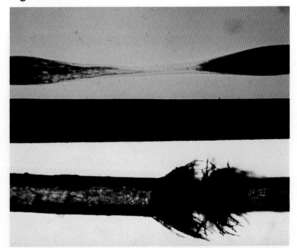

Monilethrix and trichorrhexis nodosa (magnified appearance of hair shafts) Use of a hand lens or low-power magnification by microscope reveals the anomalies in the hair shafts. The upper part of the Fig. 29-35 shows the hair in monilethrix. The nodes are strung on a thin, internodal shaft. The lower part of the picture shows the distinctive appearance of the hair in trichorrhexis nodosa. The nodes look like brushes or brooms. Breakage of hair occurs at the weak internodes of monilethrix and at the brush-like nodes of trichorrhexis nodosa.

Figure 29-36

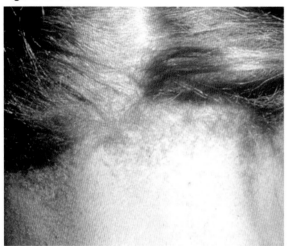

Pili torti The title means twisted *(torti)* hair *(pili)*. The gross clinical appearance is of diffuse alopecia and dry, fragile hair. Pili torti is seen in association with a number of enzyme deficiencies and hereditary syndromes, including citrullinemia and Bazex syndrome. It may also be associated with sensorineural hearing loss. No effective treatment is available.

Figure 29-37

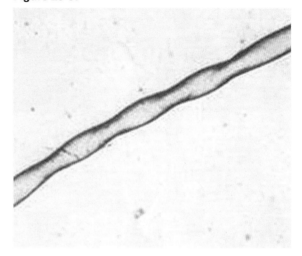

Magnification of hair in this condition reveals spiral twists at irregular intervals along the long axes of the shafts.

Figure 29-38

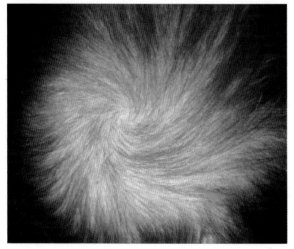

Loose anagen syndrome Dramatic thinning of the hair is usually noted during early childhood. Some cases are familial, and affected siblings appear to have blonder and thinner hair than family members who are unaffected by the disorder.

Figure 29-39

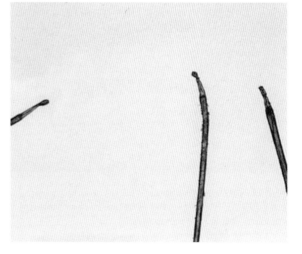

A hair pull examination reveals easily plucked hairs that are in the anagen phase. Microscopic examination of pulled hair reveals the "rumpled sock" appearance of an abnormal hair bulb (Fig. 29-39). In many patients, the hair thinning improves with age.

Figure 29-40

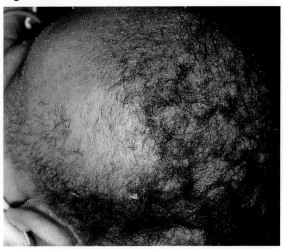

Trichothiodystrophy The term *trichothiodystrophy* describes brittle hair with abnormally low sulfur content. Trichothiodystrophy is sometimes associated with intellectual impairment, decreased fertility, short stature, ichthyosis, and photosensitivity. The hair is short, sparse, and brittle, as illustrated in Fig. 29-40.

Figure 29-41

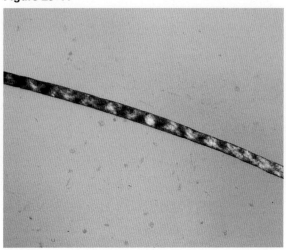

Examination of the hair shaft under polarizing light microscopy reveals alternating light and dark bands giving the hair a "tiger-tail" appearance. The disorder is transmitted in an autosomal recessive fashion. It is unknown whether the different syndromes that include trichothiodystrophy are distinct entities or represent a single variable syndrome.

Figure 29-42

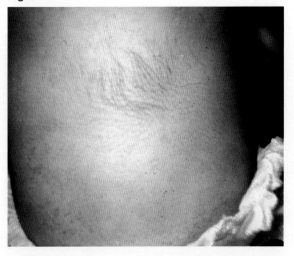

Nevoid hypertrichosis Illustrated in Fig. 29-42 is a hamartoma consisting entirely of hair follicles. A small lesion of this type is completely benign and unimportant.

Figure 29-43

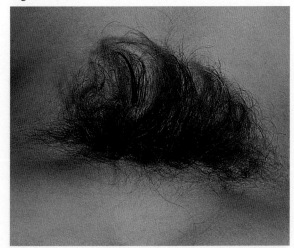

The presence of a patch of hypertrichosis overlying the mid-lower back ("faun tail nevus") may signal the presence of spina bifida occulta, diastematomyelia, or duplication or tethering of the spinal cord. A thorough neurologic investigation is warranted in such cases. CNS lesions of this type may eventually lead to a neurologic defect and require neurosurgical correction. The simultaneous presence of other skin lesions, such as lipoma, hemangioma or port-wine stain, increases the possibility of a spinal cord abnormality.

Figure 29-44

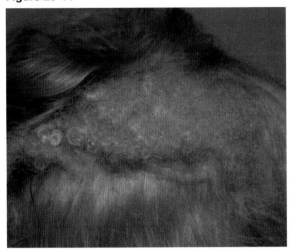

Wooly hair nevus This term is used to describe a patch of tightly coiled or unruly hair. The area of involvement may be normal at birth, with slow evolution during early childhood. Although generalized wooly hair is associated with several genetic syndromes, wooly hair nevus is a benign condition, and is not hereditary.

Figure 29-45

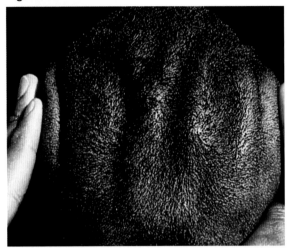

Cutis verticis gyrata Scalp skin sometimes develops redundantly as a congenital anomaly or in association with a disease such as acromegaly or Noonan syndrome. The consequence is furrowed wrinkling of hyperplastic skin in a pattern that suggests the pate of a bulldog, in whom the condition is natural. There are cases that are so extreme that hygiene of the scalp is difficult and the cosmetic appearance disturbing. Plastic surgery is a reasonable treatment.

Miscellaneous Anomalies

Figure 30-1

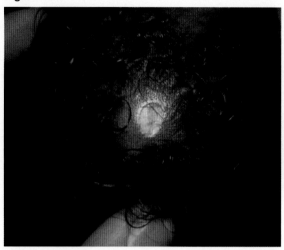

Aplasia cutis congenita This not uncommon disorder is characterized by congenital localized areas of missing skin. These may present as ulcers, or may have already healed by the time of birth. The most common location is the vertex of the scalp. Figure 30-1 depicts a child born with superficial erosion.

Figure 30-2

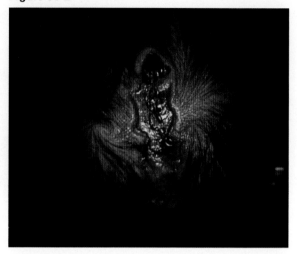

Shown in Fig. 30-2 is a child with a significant ulcer as a presentation of aplasia cutis congenita. Lesions of this type inevitably heal with scarring, and with an area of alopecia. Most infants have a single lesion, although multiple lesions may occur.

Figure 30-3

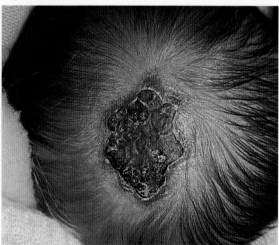

Aplasia cutis congenita Although the occurrence of this condition is usually an isolated event, it may be seen in a number of syndromes. In Adams-Oliver syndrome, distal limb reduction abnormalities are found in association with solitary midline scalp defects. SCALP syndrome is the constellation of nevus *S*ebaceus, *C*entral nervous system malformations, *A*plasia cutis congenita, *L*imbal dermoid, and *P*igmented nevus.

Figure 30-4

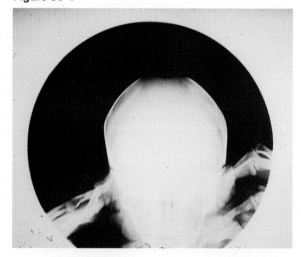

This radiograph represents a case of aplasia cutis congenita associated with a significant underlying skull defect. When this occurs, there is a higher risk of infection and bleeding. These smaller bony defects usually heal in a few months. The larger lesions may require neurosurgical repair.

Figure 30-5

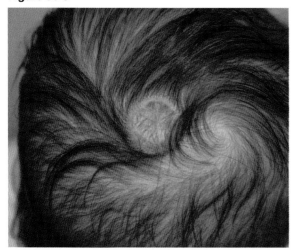

Aplasia cutis congenita Sometimes a thicker, darker growth of hair may be seen around the lesion of aplasia cutis congenita on the scalp. The "hair collar sign" may be a marker for cranial dysraphism such as encephalocele, agenesis of the corpus callosum, and heterotopic brain tissue. This may be a forme fruste of a neural tube defect.

Figure 30-6

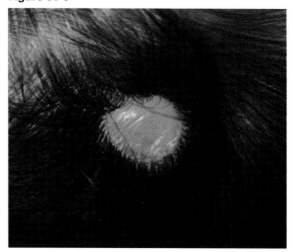

Figures 30-5 and 30-6 show a membranous variety of aplasia cutis congenita. Although lesions of this type may be mistaken for bullae, the location and hair collar signify that this is a defect of skin closure covered by a thin membrane.

Figure 30-7

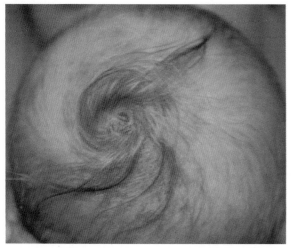

Aplasia cutis congenita Seen in Fig. 30-7 is another infant with a "hair collar" sign. In this patient, there is aplasia cutis congenita with both a vascular stain and a whorl of hair. This combination of cutaneous findings might raise particular concern about an underlying abnormality and should prompt appropriate imaging of the brain.

Figure 30-8

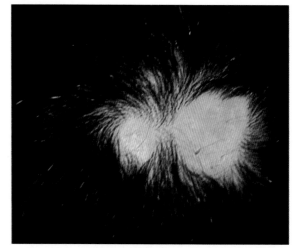

This is an example of a lesion of aplasia cutis congenita that has healed into a scar. This process may occur in utero or shortly after birth. Figure 30-8 pictures a lesion that healed postpartum. Note that the defect involved the full thickness of skin and resulted in destruction of the hair bulbs. In consequence, the scar, healed by secondary intention, is bald and may require plastic surgery in the future.

Figure 30-9

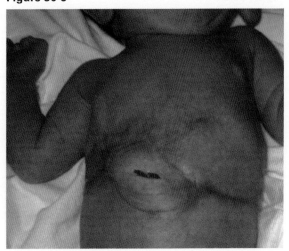

Fetus papyraceus A particular variant of aplasia cutis congenita results from the in utero demise of a twin. Affected infants have symmetric "butterfly-shaped" involvement of the trunk and sometimes fibrous bands encircling the extremities. The remains of the twin fetus ("fetus papyraceus") may be embedded in the placenta.

Figure 30-10

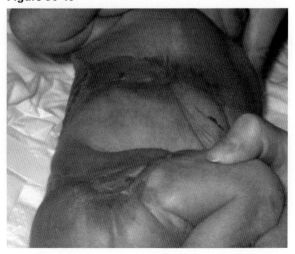

The skin abnormalities that occur in the surviving infant may be result of disseminated intravascular coagulation. Additional findings in such patients include clubbing of the hands and feet, nail dystrophy, and developmental delay, sometimes accompanied by spastic paraparesis.

Figure 30-11

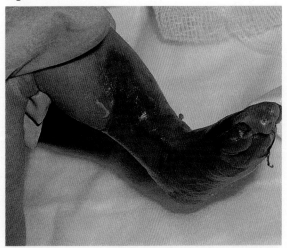

Aplasia cutis congenita limited to legs and feet In some infants, the occurrence of aplasia cutis congenita which is limited to the distal lower extremities is a presenting sign of epidermolysis bullosa. In other patients, it is benign and not associated with a genetic blistering disorder.

Figure 30-12

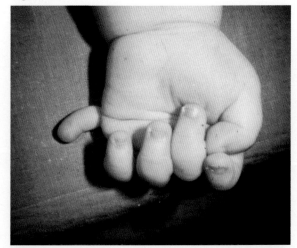

Supernumerary digits Supernumerary digits, such as other supernumerary structures, come in all degrees of development, from merest suggestion to nearly full reduplication. Figure 30-12 shows a fairly well-developed extra digit containing bones, musculature, and nerves and situated in a common site just beyond the last natural finger. More commonly, the vestige consists of a small nubbin of soft tissue in the same location. Treatment is by surgical excision.

Figure 30-13

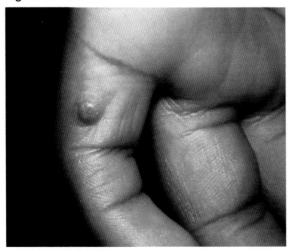

Amputation neuroma Although surgical removal of a supernumerary digit is a technically simple operation, a rare complication is illustrated in Fig. 30-13. It is an amputation neuroma, a knot of neural tissue formed at the site of the wound of an operation for removal of a structure that had nerves within it. Such a lesion can be tender to touch, spontaneously painful, and possibly productive of phantom symptoms. Reexcision is necessary.

Figure 30-14

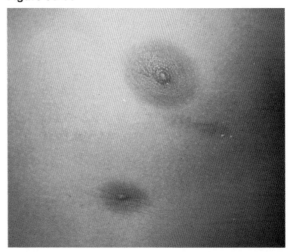

Supernumerary nipple Supernumerary nipples are exceedingly common in both sexes. In women, more than mere nipples, considerable mammary glands may develop along the "milk lines" from axillae to pubes. In males, one or a pair of supernumerary nipples is common enough; two, even three, complete pairs are still not rare. The degree of development may be from vestiges that could be taken for common pigmented moles to well-developed ones like those pictured in Fig. 30-14.

Figure 30-15

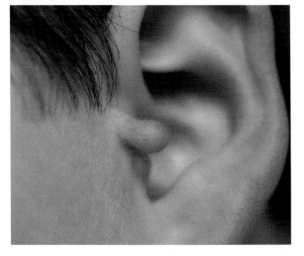

Auricular tags Supernumerary vestiges of the external structures of ears are common. Accessory tragi and auricular tags with or without communication to deeper structures may be deceptively simple.

Figure 30-16

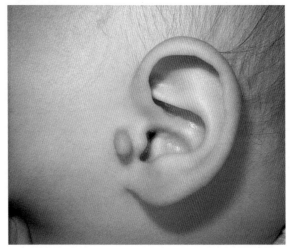

Sometimes, however, such structures bear cartilage within them and communicate with the more important structures in the external canal or middle ear.

Figure 30-17

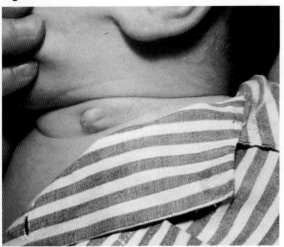

Auricular tag In Fig. 30-17 there is a bit of reduplicated auricular tissue that had been displaced onto the neck. Again, the anomalous tissue could be easily excised if it had no communication deeper and upward. In the latter event, more thorough dissection of the entire structure would be required.

Figure 30-18

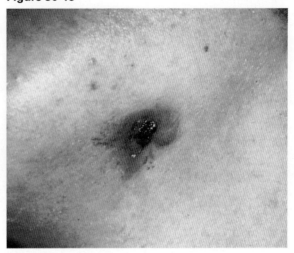

Dental sinus Infection at or around the apex of a tooth may become an abscess that drains in the overlying skin. There may be a channel from a tooth in the lower jaw onto the skin over the mandible, on the underside of the chin or jaw, or on the neck. The presenting lesion may appear, like the one pictured in Fig. 30-18, as a superficial pyoderma, or an infected cyst. Excision of the entire lesion is required.

Figure 30-19

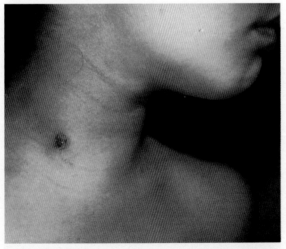

Branchial-cleft cysts The embryogenesis of the head and neck requires that many structures have to come together perfectly from both sides. An occasional failure of perfect coaptation is to be expected. Cleft palate and cleft lips are well known and easily recognizable. More subtle is failure of perfect development of the branchial arches.

Figure 30-20

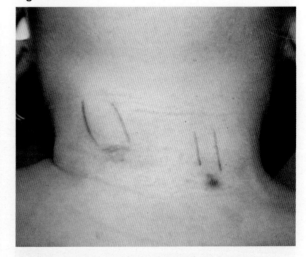

The usual clinical lesion is an insignificant-looking papule or small cystic mass on one side of the neck, anteriorly off center. Figure 30-19 shows such a lesion. Figure 30-20 shows a much rarer bilateral anomaly of this nature. Surgical ablation of such embryonic errors can be complicated, and requires tracing the unexpected twists and turns of such cysts and sinuses from important structures of the region.

Figure 30-21

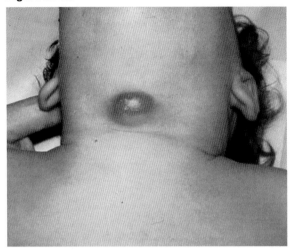

Figure 30-22

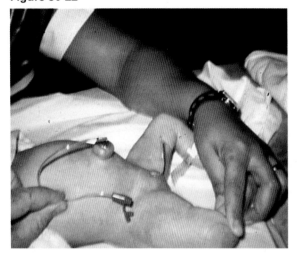

Thyroglossal cyst Figure 30-21 shows another example of a dysraphism of midline structures. Thyroglossal cysts and fistulas are similar in appearance to branchial cleft malformations but are usually midline and located near the hyoid bone. These lesions may become complicated because of enlargement or secondary infection. Careful excision is recommended.

Anomalies of umbilical maldevelopment A number of developmental abnormalities may accompany an umbilicus with abnormal appearance. Figure 30-22 shows an umbilicus that gives exit to a patent urachus. The persistent urachus is due to failure of closure of the allantoic duct. This diagnosis is usually suggested by the presence of a clear liquid discharge from the umbilicus.

Figure 30-23

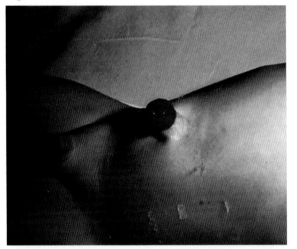

Figure 30-24

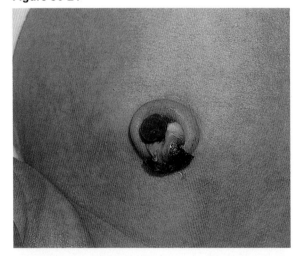

Omphalomesenteric remnants An umbilical polyp noted at birth may represent the presence of omphalomesenteric remnants. The bright red polyp shown in Fig. 30-23 is a remnant of the distal portion of the omphalomesenteric duct. Any portion of the duct may persist and lead to the formation of sinus tracts, congenital bands, cysts, and fistulas. The mucosal lining of this lesion may represent small intestine, stomach, or colon.

Fistulas of the duct, Meckel diverticulum, and ileal prolapse may accompany this malformation. The presence of an omphalomesenteric band or Meckel diverticulum may lead to intestinal obstruction during the neonatal period or later in childhood. Treatment in all cases is surgical. Note in Fig. 30-24 the presence of the prominent red remnant with the umbilical cord still attached. This lesion is not to be confused with an umbilical granuloma (Fig. 30-25).

Figure 30-25

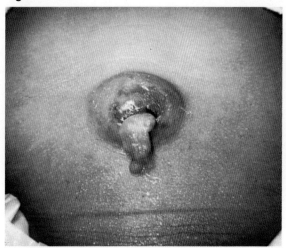

Umbilical granuloma It is normal for the umbilical cord to separate about 6 to 8 days after birth and for the resulting wound to heal within 2 weeks. Pictured in Fig. 30-25 is the formation of heaped-up granulation tissue at and in the umbilicus—the so-called umbilical granuloma. Treatment by repeated cauterization with silver nitrate is usually successful.

Figure 30-26

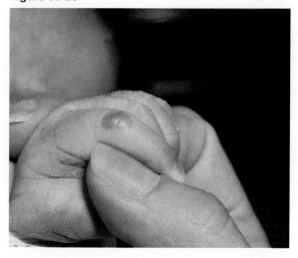

Sucking blister The oval blister pictured in Fig. 30-26 was present at birth and is a result of normal sucking behavior in utero. Sucking blisters are fairly common and are usually located on the forearm, wrist, or hand. They are most often solitary and involve only one upper extremity. However, lesions involving both hands, or even involving a foot, are sometimes seen. The sucking blister resolves spontaneously as soon as bottle or breast is offered as a dietary substitute.

Figure 30-27

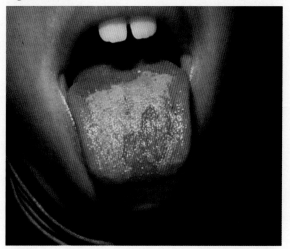

Geographic tongue This benign condition is characterized by denudations of the lingual surface in patches of redness that shift in position from time to time over hours and days.

Figure 30-28

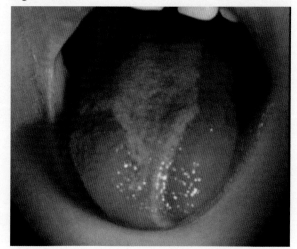

The cause of the condition is the loss of filiform papillae of the tongue epithelium. No treatment is effective. The condition is largely asymptomatic except for slight tingling associated with foods with a strong taste. Geographic tongue is more common in patients with psoriasis.

Figure 30-29

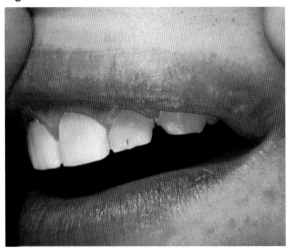

Fordyce condition The face abounds in sebaceous glands. Normally their distribution stops sharply at the junction of the skin and vermilion of the lips. Commonly, however, ectopic sebaceous glands are found within the lips under the vermilion and sometimes within the oral mucosa of the lips and even in the buccal mucosa. The condition is harmless and may have been present long before the patient or parents became aware of it. No treatment is required or available.

Figure 30-30

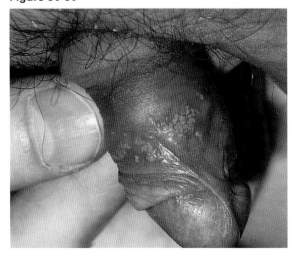

Tyson glands The prepuce of the penis has sebaceous glands, known as Tyson glands, that open directly to the surface of the skin. These glands appear as very small yellow papules and may be prominent in some males, as is seen in Fig. 30-30.

Figure 30-31

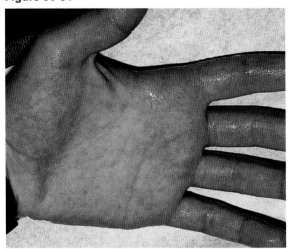

Hyperhidrosis This disorder entails excessive sweating that may be localized to specific body regions. Figure 30-31 represents palmar hyperhidrosis. The most common locations are palms, soles, axilla, and groin. There is usually no association with underlying disease, but the sweating itself can be a significant cause of emotional distress. Treatments include topical aluminum chloride, oral anticholinergics, iontophoresis, and the injection of botulinum toxin.

Figure 30-32

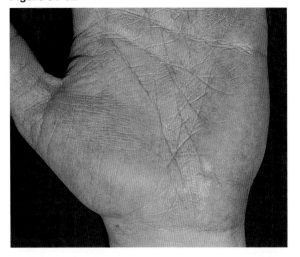

Aquagenic wrinkling of the palms This rare entity is characterized by prominent wrinkling of the skin on the palms after brief immersion in water. It is seen as white or translucent papules, which may coalesce into larger plaques. Patients may experience stinging or burning. The lesions usually persist for several hours. This condition may occur in patients with cystic fibrosis.

Figure 30-33

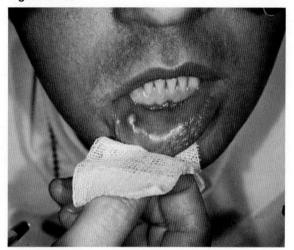

Mucocele The lower lip is studded with cells that produce mucus. Mucoceles are cysts deriving from such cells. They appear as papules that are visibly and palpably filled with highly viscous fluid. They are harmless and asymptomatic but require extirpation because they make themselves felt when within the mouth and are cosmetically objectionable when on the lips. When reasonably small, like the one pictured in Fig. 30-33, electrodessication and curettage are sufficient; larger lesions may require scalpel surgery.

Figure 30-34

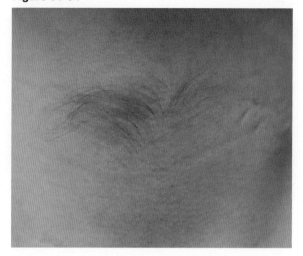

Anterior Cervical Hypertrichosis This disorder is a rare form of localized hair growth, and is characterized by a tuft of terminal hair on the anterior neck, just above the laryngeal prominence. The disorder may be congenital or acquired. Neurologic disorders, especially peripheral sensory and motor neuropathy, have been observed in a very small subset of these patients.

Figure 30-35

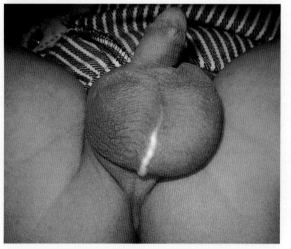

Median raphe cyst of the scrotum This is an embryologic developmental abnormality. The typical lesion is a mobile translucent cyst and these cysts may be single or multiple. In some cases, this malformation presents as a canal-like lesions in the ventral midline part of the penis and perineum.

Figure 30-36

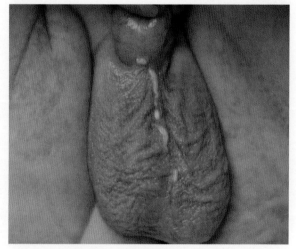

Median raphe cysts tend to persist, and may eventually be complicated by infection. Treatment consists of surgical excision.

Figure 30-37

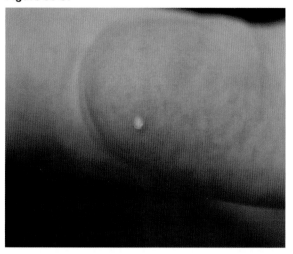

Calcified heel stick nodule Following heel sticks to draw blood in the neonatal period, some infants may develop small areas of calcification. Although more commonly reported in high-risk neonates receiving multiple heel sticks, this may also be seen in infants who receive just one.

Figure 30-38

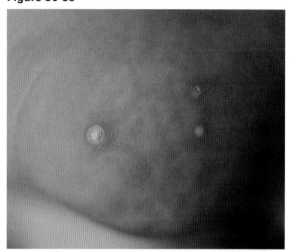

Lesions may be single or multiple and are typically white or yellow firm papulonodules that may be tender. The lesions usually appear 4 to 12 months after birth and are sometimes confused with warts. Spontaneous resolution is common but may take as long as 2 years.

Figure 30-39

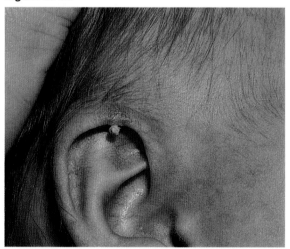

Calcified ear nodule Calcifications of this type may be present at birth or develop during early childhood. The lesions are solitary, firm, white nodules, usually measuring less than 1 cm in diameter.

Figure 30-40

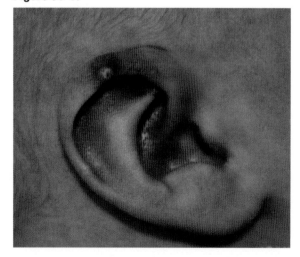

The ears are a particularly common location, as pictured in Figs. 30-39 and 30-40. Ulceration and extrusion of calcified material may occur. The treatment of choice is surgical excision.

Figure 30-41

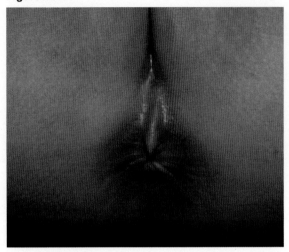

Infantile pyramidal perianal protrusion This fairly common lesion is a small fleshy protrusion from the median raphe, usually anterior to the anus. It is most common in girls and usually develops during infancy. There are no associated symptoms. Pyramidal protrusions are sometimes confused with genital warts. No treatment is required.

Figure 30-42

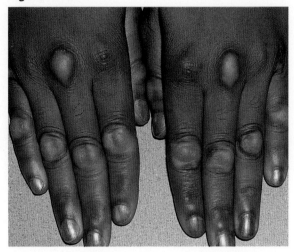

Knuckle pads These are benign, asymptomatic, smooth, well circumscribed skin-colored papules, nodules, or plaques occurring on the dorsal aspect of the metacarpophalangeal and interphalangeal joints. There may be a history of repeated trauma although many cases are idiopathic and some are familial. There are no effective treatments for knuckle pads, but it is important to remove the source of repeated trauma. Sometimes keratolytic agents are used to soften the lesions.

Figure 30-43

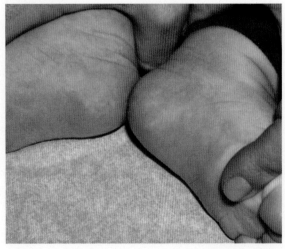

Precalcaneal fibrolipomatous hamartoma These are soft, subcutaneous nodules occurring on the plantar region of the heel. There are no overlying epidermal changes. They are usually symmetrical, and are painless.

Figure 30-44

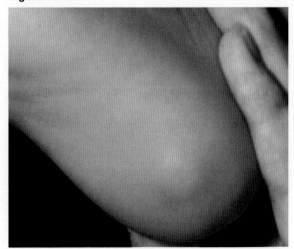

Lesions of precalcaneal fibrolipomatous hamartoma may be present at birth or develop soon thereafter. In some patients, they persist at least until adolescence, but they do not create difficulty walking.

Figure 30-45

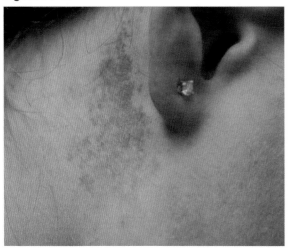

Terra firma-form dermatosis This cutaneous condition of unknown etiology presents with a dirty brown appearance in the affected areas. Parents feel that their children are not bathing correctly, but when washed with soap and water the discoloration persists. The neck is a common area of involvement, although the condition can affect the trunk, extremities, and the scalp. Treatment involves rubbing the affected area with isopropyl alcohol.

Figure 30-46

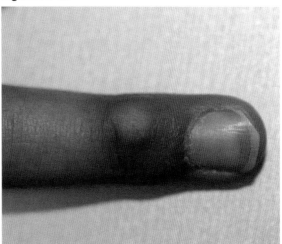

Writing callus Also called writer's bump, this is a thickening of the skin produced by localized pressure and friction on the skin by a pen or pencil.

Figure 30-47

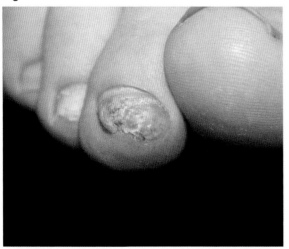

Subungual exostosis This is a benign tumor that occurs on the distal phalanges of the toe. Children and young adults are mainly affected. The lesion is a small, pink or flesh-colored, hard nodule that projects beyond the inner free edge of the nail, and it is often painful.

Figure 30-48

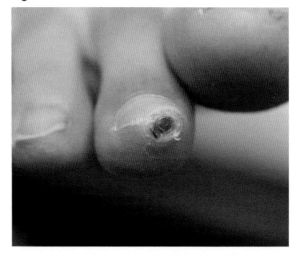

The lesion may become hyperkeratotic, and may lift the overlying nail. Lesions may mimic a wart or a pyogenic granuloma. Diagnosis is made by X-ray of the digit, and complete excision or curettage by a qualified surgeon is the treatment.

Figure 30-49

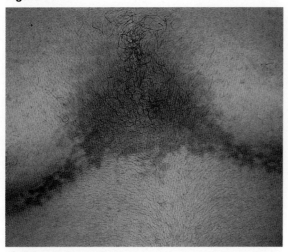

Confluent and reticulated papillomatosis This disorder is characterized by the presence of reticulated areas of scale and hyperpigmentation, usually favoring the upper back and upper chest. It is more common in teenagers and may also be more frequent in patients with obesity and acanthosis nigricans.

Figure 30-50

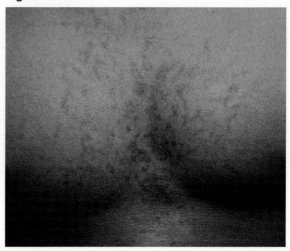

Clinically, confluent and reticulated papillomatosis may resemble tinea versicolor and must be differentiated from this more common disorder. For reasons unknown, treatment with doxycycline, minocycline, and a variety of other antibiotics has been shown to be effective.

Figure 30-51

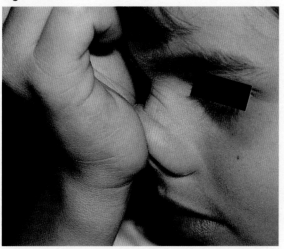

Nasal crease papules Some children will develop milia or comedonal-like lesions on the transverse nasal crease which has been caused by the repetitive upward movement of the tip of the nose from manipulation as demonstrated in Fig. 30-51. Many of these patients have nasal allergies.

Figure 30-52

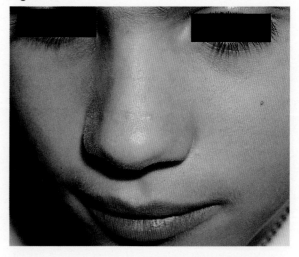

The resultant lesions occur in a linear fashion in the transverse nasal crease. Occasionally lesions may become inflamed. Topical retinoids may be helpful in removing these lesions. However, the lesions will continue to occur with continued manipulation.

Note: Reference numbers in this index are the figure numbers.